Handbook of Clinical Pharmacology

Handbook of Clinical Pharmacology

Editor: Herbert Walker

AMERICAN
MEDICAL PUBLISHERS
www.americanmedicalpublishers.com

AMERICAN
MEDICAL PUBLISHERS
www.americanmedicalpublishers.com

Cataloging-in-Publication Data

Handbook of clinical pharmacology / edited by Herbert Walker.
p. cm.
Includes bibliographical references and index.
ISBN 979-8-88740-142-3
1. Clinical pharmacology. 2. Drugs. 3. Pharmacology. I. Walker, Herbert.
RM301.28 .H36 2023
615.1--dc23

American Medical Publishers,
41 Flatbush Avenue,
1st Floor, New York,
NY 11217, USA

ISBN 979-8-88740-142-3 (Hardback)

Contents

Preface

Every book is initially just a concept; it takes months of research and hard work to give it the final shape in which the readers receive it. In its early stages, this book also went through rigorous reviewing. The notable contributions made by experts from across the globe were first molded into patterned chapters and then arranged in a sensibly sequential manner to bring out the best results.

Clinical pharmacology is a medical discipline concerned with the study of drugs and their effect on humans. It is involved in the understanding of drug interaction, therapeutic efficacy and safety in humans. It is a translational discipline underpinned by science of pharmacology, which is involved in the observational and experimental assessment of effects and disposition of drugs in humans. The fundamental goal of clinical pharmacology is to produce data for optimum utilization of drugs. There are various branches that fall under the domain of clinical pharmacology. These include pharmacodynamics, pharmacokinetics, rational prescribing, toxicology, drug interactions, drug development, molecular pharmacology and pharmacogenomics. This book unfolds the innovative aspects of clinical pharmacology which will be crucial for the progress of this field in the future. Also included herein is a detailed explanation of the various concepts and applications of this field of study. This book will serve as a valuable source of reference for graduate and post graduate students.

It has been my immense pleasure to be a part of this project and to contribute my years of learning in such a meaningful form. I would like to take this opportunity to thank all the people who have been associated with the completion of this book at any step.

Editor

1

Development of Lipid–Polymer Hybrid Nanoparticles for Improving Oral Absorption of Enoxaparin

Bo Tang [1,2,3], Yu Qian [1] and Guihua Fang [1,*]

1 School of Pharmacy, Nantong University, 19 Qixiu Road, Nantong 226001, China; tangbo@ntu.edu.cn (B.T.); syfsxyhh18@163.com (Y.Q.)
2 School of Pharmacy, Shenyang Pharmaceutical University, 103 Wenhua Road, Shenyang 110016, China
3 Yabang Medical Research Institute, 66 Changhong Road, Changzhou 213145, China
* Correspondence: fangguihua@ntu.edu.cn

Abstract: Enoxaparin, an anticoagulant that helps prevent the formation of blood clots, is administered parenterally. Here, we report the development and evaluation of lipid–polymer hybrid nanoparticles (LPHNs) for the oral delivery of enoxaparin. The polymer poloxamer 407 (P407) was incorporated into lipid nanoparticles to form gel cores and ensure high encapsulation efficiency and the controlled release of enoxaparin. In vitro results indicated that 30% of P407 incorporation offered higher encapsulation efficiency and sustained the release of enoxaparin. Laser confocal scanning microscopy (LCSM) images showed that LPHNs could not only significantly improve the accumulation of enoxaparin in intestinal villi but also facilitate enoxaparin transport into the underlayer of intestinal epithelial cells. In vivo pharmacokinetic study results indicated that the oral bioavailability of enoxaparin was markedly increased about 6.8-fold by LPHNs. In addition, its therapeutic efficacy against pulmonary thromboembolism was improved 2.99-fold by LPHNs. Moreover, LPHNs exhibited excellent biocompatibility in the intestine. Overall, the LPHN is a promising delivery carrier to boost the oral absorption of enoxaparin.

Keywords: enoxaparin; lipid–polymer hybrid nanoparticles; oral; intestinal absorption

---

1. Introduction

Heparin is an anticoagulant that prevents the formation of blood blots, and it has shown great prevention and therapeutic efficacy in terms of deep-vein thrombosis (DVT), pulmonary embolism (PE), and venous thrombosis [1] clinically. Low molecular weight heparin (LMWH) is obtained from unfractionated heparin (UFH) by chemical and enzymatic depolymerization [2]. Enoxaparin, one of the most commonly used LMWH, holds a longer half-life in vivo than UFH, which reduces the administration frequency [3]. However, its oral absorption is still low due to its large molecular weight, high anionic charges, and first-pass effect in the liver [4–6]. Therefore, it is administered via the parenteral route, which is less convenient and has lower compliance for patients. To translate the administration route from injection to oral delivery, it is quite crucial to increase the oral absorption of LMWH [7,8]. With the advances in nanotechnology, polymer- and lipid-based nanocarriers such as polymeric micelles [9], polymeric nanoparticles [10], lipid nanocapsules [11], microemulsions [12], and solid lipid nanoparticles [13] have been intensively used to facilitate the oral absorption of LMWH. Rationally designed nanocarriers are able to overcome the hurdles encountered during the absorption process through following ways, including (1) protecting drugs from acidic degradation in the stomach; (2) increasing the intestinal epithelial permeability; (3) facilitating intestinal lymphatic transport [13–18].

Solid lipid nanoparticles (SLNs) are colloidal drug delivery systems consisting of surfactant-stabilized lipids that are solid both at room and body temperature [13]. They integrate the advantages of liposomes, polymeric nanoparticles, and emulsions. In addition, SLNs possess a solid lipid core matrix, so they are used to encapsulate lipophilic drugs in most cases [19,20]. Because LMWH is hydrophilic, the encapsulation efficiency of LMWH in the SLNs is low, which leads to insufficient therapeutic concentration in vivo. This is due to hydrophilic drugs having limited loading quantity and homogeneity in the lipid cores. To improve the encapsulation efficiency of LMWH in the SLNs, conjugating lipidic molecules with LMWH via chemical synthesis was reported in a previous study [13]. Although the oral absorption of LMWH is significantly improved in this way, there may be some problems associated with the chemical modification of LMWH. Since LMWH exerts its therapeutic effects by binding to antithrombin III (AT III) via a unique pentasaccharide motif [21], chemical synthesis may increase the risk of reducing or losing the activity of LMWH. To avoid the possibility of reducing or losing drug activity, a common alternative strategy is to prepare LMWH-loaded SLNs by a double emulsion (water-in-oil-in-water, W/O/W) method. However, the encapsulation efficiency of LMWH in the SLNs is still unsatisfactory. Therefore, a new encapsulation strategy is needed to further improve the encapsulation efficiency of LMWH.

It has been reported that hydrophilic viscosity-enhancing agents such as propylene glycol (PG) and polyethylene glycol (PEG) 400 and PEG 600 are able to increase the encapsulation efficiency of insulin in the SLNs [22]. Inspired by this, hydrogels may be an alternative. Hydrogels, a network of polymer chains, are often used for the delivery of hydrophilic drugs with higher drug loading [23]. Poloxamer 407 (P407) is a triblock copolymer consisting of a central hydrophobic block and two hydrophilic blocks of polyethylene glycol at both ends. P407-based hydrogels exhibit interesting nature at certain concentration levels. That is, they are in a liquid state below gelation temperature and turn into a viscosity-enhancing gel above gelation temperature [24,25].

Encouraged by the advantage of SLNs and hydrogels, we attempted to fabricate lipid–polymer hybrid nanoparticles (LPHNs) for the oral delivery of enoxaparin. In this study, poloxamer 407 is used to improve the encapsulation efficiency and control the release of enoxaparin. The lipid–polymer hybrid nanoparticles were characterized in terms of size and zeta potential, encapsulation efficiency, and particle morphology. In vitro release behavior was also investigated. The intestinal absorption was evaluated by laser confocal scanning microscopy. In addition, in vivo absorption, in vivo efficacy, and safety tests were performed by rat experiments. In all, we attempt to investigate whether lipid–polymer hybrid nanoparticles can increase encapsulation efficiency and boost the oral absorption of enoxaparin.

2. Materials and Methods

2.1. Materials

Enoxaparin (mean MW 4251 Da, 101 IU/mg) was purchased from Hangzhou Jiuyuan Gene Engineering Co., Ltd. (Hangzhou, China). Precirol ATO 5 (glyceryl palmitostearate) was kindly donated by Gattefosse (Lyon, France). Egg yolk lecithin (E80) was obtained from Lipoid KG (Ludwigshafen, Germany), and Tween 80 was purchased from BASF (Ludwigshafen, Germany). Poloxamer 407 (BASF, Ludiwigshafen, Germany) was purchased from Xi'an Yuelai Medical Technology Co., Ltd. (Xi'an, China). Fluorescein isothiocyanate (FITC) was obtained from Shanghai Golden Wheat Biotechnology Co., Ltd. (Shanghai, China). Tissue-Tek O.C.T. compound (SAKURA, Torrance, CA, USA) was purchased from Nantong Qixiang Biotechnology Co., Ltd. (Nantong, China). Activated partial thromboplastin time (APTT) assay kits were obtained from Nanjing Caobenyuan Biotechnology Co., Ltd. (Nanjing, China). All other chemicals were of analytical grade.

2.2. Preparation of Lipid–Polymer Hybrid Nanoparticles (LPHNs)

Enoxaparin-loaded LPHNs were prepared as follows. In brief, 12.5 mg of enoxaparin was dissolved in 0.5 mL-differentiated ratios of poloxamer 407 (P407) aqueous solution at 4 °C. Then, 10 mg E 80 and 40 mg Precirol ATO 5 were dissolved in 2 mL dichloromethane (DCM). DCM was dropped into 0.2 mL of P407 aqueous solution containing enoxaparin. Then, this mixed solution was ultrasonicated using a probe sonicator (Ningbo Xinzhi Biological Technology Co. Ltd., Ningbo, China) for 2 min at 500 W to obtain primary W/O emulsion. Subsequently, 2% Tween 80 aqueous solution added to the obtained primary emulsion followed by ultrasonication for 1 min at 380 W. Finally, the obtained formulation was transferred into a flask to remove the DCM at 34 °C, using a rotary evaporator (Eyela, Tokyo, Japan). The preparation method for enoxaparin-loaded SLNs was the same as that for enoxaparin-loaded LPHNs, except that no P407 was in the aqueous solution.

2.3. *In Vitro Characteristics*

2.3.1. Size, Zeta Potential, and Encapsulation Efficiency

The particle size and size distribution of prepared nanoparticles were measured by 90 plus zeta (Brookhaven, MS, USA) at room temperature. The zeta potential of nanoparticles was tested using the 90 plus zeta by electrophoretic laser doppler anemometry at room temperature. All the samples were diluted with deionized water, and measurements were taken in triplicate.

The encapsulation efficiency of enoxaparin in nanoparticles was determined by an ultra-filtration method [26]. An appropriate amount of nanoparticle dispersion was added in a Millipore Amicon®Ultra filteration tube (MWCO: 100 kDa). Free enoxaparin was separated from the nanoparticle dispersion by centrifugation at 2000 rpm for 15 min. To determine the total amount of the drug, including the free drug in the dispersion and encapsulated drug in the nanoparticles, an appropriate amount of nanoparticle dispersion was destroyed by DCM, and the released enoxaparin was extracted by deionized water. The enoxaparin in the ultrafiltrate and nanoparticle dispersion was determined by the Azure II colorimetric method using a multimode microplate reader (Bio Tek, Winooski, VT, USA) at 606 nm [27]. The linearity range of this method was determined between 0 and 6 μg/mL, with a linear correlation coefficient of 0.9973. All samples were measured in triplicate. The encapsulation efficiency (EE) of enoxaparin was calculated using the following equation:

$$EE\% = \frac{W_{totaldrug} - W_{freedrug}}{W_{totaldrug}} \tag{1}$$

where $W_{\text{total drug}}$ is the total amount of drug in the nanoparticle dispersion, and $W_{\text{free drug}}$ is the total amount of drug in the ultrafiltrate.

In addition, the prepared nanoparticle suspension was placed at 4 °C in a refrigerator for 1 week to determine whether the encapsulation efficiency changes with time.

2.3.2. Particle Morphology

The morphology of nanoparticles was examined by transmission electron microscopy (TEM). Samples of nanoparticles were diluted with deionized water, dropped onto a copper grid, and then stained with phosphotungstic acid. The samples were subjected to TEM (JEOL, Tokyo, Japan) after drying.

2.3.3. In Vitro Drug Release

In vitro release of enoxaparin from the nanoparticles was studied using the dialysis method, and an enoxaparin solution was used as control. Briefly, 2 mL of nanoparticle suspension was transferred into dialysis bags (Biosharp Biotechnology Co. Ltd., Hefei, China, MWCO: 14 kDa) and dialysis bags were immersed into a beaker containing 25 mL pH 6.8 phosphate buffer. Then, the beaker was placed in a 37 °C water bath with a magnetic stirring speed of 150 rpm. At a predetermined time point, the medium in the beaker was withdrawn, followed by replacement with the same volume of fresh release medium. The released enoxaparin content was determined by the Azure II colorimetric method, as mentioned in the previous part.

2.4. Intestinal Absorption

To investigate the intestinal absorption of nanoparticles, in vivo experiments were conducted in rats. All animal studies were conducted according to the guidelines of the local Institute Animal Ethical Care Committee (IAEC, 20180512-003). To visualize the intestinal absorption, fluorescein isothiocyanate (FITC) was used to label enoxaparin. FITC was conjugated with enoxaparin according to the method previously described [28]. Briefly, 2 mg of FITC dissolved in dimethylsulfoxide was slowly added to 0.1 M sodium carbonate, and then added in 50 mg of enoxaparin. The reaction was performed in a ice-water bath, with a stirring speed of 150 rpm in the dark. After 8 h, the reaction was stopped by adding an ammonium chloride solution. Then, the resulting FITC-enoxaparin conjugate was introduced into a dialysis bag (MWCO: 1000 Da) to remove the byproduct. The dialyzed product was lyophilized at −50 °C to obtain FITC-labeled enoxaparin. Male SD rats (200 ± 20 g) were given FITC-enoxaparin solution and FITC-enoxaparin LPHN2 by gavage at a dosage of 505 IU/kg. After 30 min, the rats were sacrificed, and then the jejunum was removed, washed, and fixed with 4% paraformaldehyde for 4 h at room temperature, and dehydrated with 20% sucrose solution. The segments were frozen in cryo-embedding media, sectioned at 20 μm, and placed on polysine-coated slides. The sections were fixed with 4% paraformaldehyde for 30 min and rinsed three times with pH 7.4 phosphate buffer, and the intestine sections were then incubated with 20 μL of 4′,6-diamidino-2-phenylindole (DAPI) for 10 min in the dark to stain the nucleus, followed by mounting with antifluorescence quenching reagent. Finally, the sections were observed under a Leica SP8 laser confocal scanning microscope.

2.5. In Vivo Pharmacokinetic Study in Rats

In vivo absorption of nanoparticles was studied in rats. Male SD rats (200 ± 20 g) were divided randomly into three groups, with four rats per group. After fasting for 24 h, the rats were given enoxaparin solution and enoxaparin-loaded LPHN2 by gavage at a dose of 1010 IU/kg. At predetermined time intervals (0, 1, 3, 5, 8, 12 h), blood samples (about 0.5 mL) were drawn from the rats. Plasma was obtained by centrifugation (6000 rpm, 10 min) and analyzed by measuring the activated partial thromboplastin time (APTT) value according to a standard commercial kit The absolute bioavailability (F) of orally administered formulations was calculated by comparing their AUC with that intravenous injection of enoxaparin solution (101 IU/kg).

2.6. In Vivo Efficacy in Mice

The in vivo prevention of pulmonary thromboembolism of nanoparticles was studied in mice. Male Kunming mice (18~22 g) were divided randomly into four groups, with 12 mice per group. Two groups were treated with enoxaparin solution and enoxaparin-loaded LPHN3 via intragastric administration at a single dosage of 1010 IU/kg, respectively. Two groups were given 100 μL of enoxaparin solution (101 IU/kg) and saline as control. Two hours after administration, all groups were intravenously injected with 100 μL of 1250 IU/kg thrombin to induce hind limb paralysis or death. The number of dead or paralyzed mice was recorded within 20 min; the results are shown as a percentage of protection.

2.7. Safety Evaluation

To investigate whether nanoparticles cause intestinal membrane damage or not, a histopathological examination was conducted. In this experiment, enoxaparin-loaded nanoparticles were given orally to rats at 1010 IU/kg, and physiological saline was given orally as a control. Then, the rats were sacrificed after 2 and 8 h. The jejunum was removed from rats and placed in 5% formaldehyde solution and stained with hematoxylin-erosin for histological studies.

2.8. Statistical Analysis

Statistical analysis was performed using a Student's t-test. Data were expressed as mean ± SD. Statistical significance was represented by * $p < 0.05$ and ** $p < 0.01$.

3. Results and Discussion

3.1. Preparation and Characterization of Lipid–Polymer Hybrid Nanoparticles

Double W/O/W emulsification technology was used to prepare enoxaparin-loaded lipid–polymer hybrid nanoparticles. Poloxamer 407 acted as the polymer core to load the drug. The schematic diagram of enoxaparin-loaded lipid–polymer hybrid nanoparticles is presented in Figure 1A. To screen the optimal amount of poloxamer 407, a control group (SLNs) was created with the absence of P407, and three different ratios (20%, 30%, 40%, *w/v*) of poloxamer 407 were tested. Their size and encapsulation efficiency are summarized in Table 1. The tested amount of P407 had no significant influence on particle size, polydispersity index, or zeta potential, but it led to different encapsulation efficiencies for enoxaparin. When the amount of P407 was set as 30%, the enoxaparin-loaded LPHN possessed a higher encapsulation efficiency of 65.72%. The results suggest that the addition of an appropriate concentration of P407 into the double emulsion could improve the encapsulation efficiency of enoxaparin. The higher encapsulation efficiency of LPHN2 could possibly be attributed to its appropriate viscosity. P407 is a thermo-sensitive polymer, and it can form gels when the ambient temperature is above gelation temperature. According to previous research [3,24,29], the increase in P407 concentration in the gel increases its viscosity. When the amount of P407 is 20%, its viscosity is not enough to restrain the enoxaparin in the internal gel core. Theoretically, the addition of 40% P407 could offer the highest encapsulation efficiency. However, the gel formed by 40% of P407 is too viscous to be dispersed well by ultrasonication, leading to lower encapsulation efficiency. Hence, LPHN2 was selected as the formulation in the following experiments. To investigate if the encapsulation efficiency of LPHN2 was changed with time, we tested the encapsulation efficiency after storage at 4 °C for one week. The encapsulation efficiency of LPHN2 stored at 4 °C for one week was 64.01%, which indicated that the encapsulation efficiency of LPHN2 could be kept unchanged for at least one week.

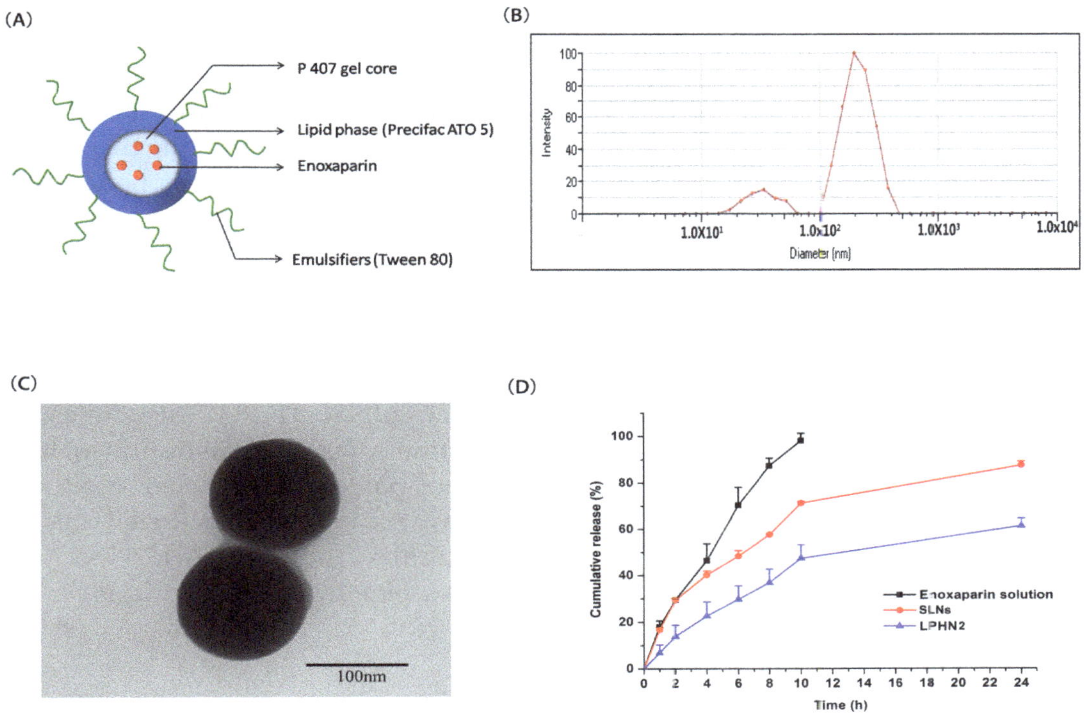

Figure 1. (**A**) Schematic representation of the structure of enoxaparin-loaded lipid hybrid nanoparticles. (**B**) The size distribution of lipid–polymer hybrid nanoparticle 2 (LPHN2). (**C**) The transmission electron microscopy (TEM) morphology of LPHN2. (**D**) In vitro release of profiles of enoxaparin from enoxaparin solution, enoxaparin-loaded solid lipid nanoparticles (SLNs), and enoxaparin-loaded LPHN2 ($n = 3$).

Table 1. Characterization of enoxaparin-loaded lipid-polymer hybrid nanoparticles at 3 different ratios of poloxamer 407 ($n = 3$).

Amount of P407	Size (nm)	PI	ζ Potential (mV)	EE (%)
0% (SLNs)	159.40 ± 1.59	0.293 ± 0.010	−21.83 ± 3.94	43.21 ± 3.79
20% (LPHN1)	149.70 ± 1.71	0.264 ± 0.030	−17.47 ± 1.20	43.14 ± 7.52
30% (LPHN2)	149.75 ± 2.45	0.293 ± 0.009	−14.71 ± 1.93	65.72 ± 14.33
40% (LPHN3)	153.19 ± 0.79	0.274 ± 0.002	−20.04 ± 1.59	59.47 ± 11.66

PI, polydispersity index; ζ potential, zeta potential; EE, encapsulation efficiency.

The average size of LPHN2 was about 150 nm, with a low PI (<0.30) (Figure 1B). In addition, there is a size distribution ranging from 10 to 100 nm in Figure 1B, which may be caused by the formation of Tween 80-based micelles in nanoparticle suspensions. The zeta potential of LPHN2 was slightly negative (−14.71 mV), which may be attributed to negatively charged egg lecithin in the surface of the LPHN.

Transmission electron microscopy (TEM) has been extensively used to observe the surface morphology of nanoparticles. The TEM image of LPHN2 is shown in Figure 1C, indicating that LPHN was spherical and about 150 nm in size, consistent with dynamic light scattering results.

The release of enoxaparin from LPHN2 was evaluated in pH 6.8 phosphate buffer and compared with the in vitro release of 0% P407-prepared SLNs and enoxaparin solution. The in vitro release profiles of enoxaparin solution, SLNs, and LPHN2 are shown in Figure 1D. Almost 98% of the drug released from the enoxaparin solution was within 10 h, which indicates that enoxaparin can diffuse freely through the dialysis bag. In contrast with the SLNs, there was a controlled and sustained release of enoxaparin from the LPHN2. Approximately 87% of the cumulative amount of enoxaparin was released from SLNs within 24 h. In the case of LPHN2, the percentage cumulative release of enoxaparin was about 61% within 24 h. The in vitro release result indicated that the incorporation of 30% P407 could control and sustain the enoxaparin release from LPHN compared with free P407 SLNs. There are two reasons to explain why LPH2 exhibited sustained release behavior in contrast with traditional lipid nanoparticles (SLNs). On the one hand, LPHN2 has higher encapsulation efficiency. For most of the drugs, they should diffuse from the nanoparticles first, and then release into the medium. Therefore, less amounts of free drugs could be released from the nanoparticles. On the other hand, the viscous gel core may delay drug diffusion from nanoparticles into the release medium.

3.2. Intestinal Absorption

The absorption of enoxaparin-loaded LPHN2 in the intestine of rats was visualized by LCSM after oral administration. Figure 2 shows the intestine fluorescence signals after the intragastric administration of FITC-labeled enoxaparin solution and LPHN2. The LCSM images suggest that a more intense fluorescence was observed in the intestine after administration of FITC-labeled enoxaparin-loaded LPHN2 in comparison with the administration of FITC-labeled enoxaparin solution. In addition, the fluorescence signal can be viewed under a layer of intestinal epithelial cells, as indicated by the red arrows. Therefore, the LCSM results indicate that the drug in LPHN2 was not only accumulated in the surface of intestinal villi but had also penetrated the underlayer of intestinal epithelial cells.

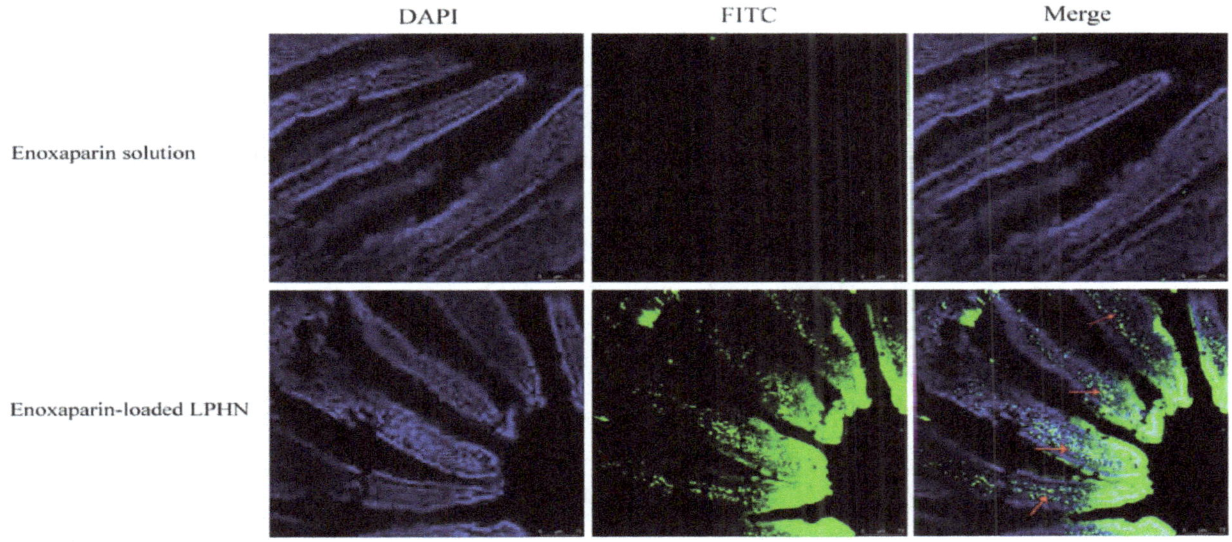

Figure 2. The LCSM images of the jejunum of rats at 0.5 h after administration of FITC-labeled (green) enoxaparin solution (the upper) and LPHN2 (the bottom). Cell nuclei of the jejunum sections were stained by DAPI (blue).

3.3. *In Vivo Pharmacokinetic Study in Rats*

In vivo pharmacokinetic behavior of enoxaparin-loaded LPHNs was investigated by measuring APTT in rats after intragastric administration, as shown in Figure 3. The main pharmacokinetic parameters are summarized in Table 2. The absolute bioavailability (F_{abs}) of enoxaparin-loaded LPHN2 was 14.2%, a 6.8-fold increase compared with enoxaparin solution. The results indicate that the oral bioavailability of enoxaparin could be improved by lipid–polymer hybrid nanoparticles. As we know, the basic mechanisms that nanoparticles could improve oral absorption of drugs are as follows [30,31]: (1) encapsulation of drug to avoid degradation in the gastrointestinal tract before reaching the absorption site; (2) improving intestinal epithelial cell uptake. For drugs that are unstable in the gastrointestinal tract, high encapsulation efficiency is the precondition of oral absorption enhancement by nanoparticles. There are several reasons that could explain why LPHNs enhance the oral absorption of enoxaparin. On the one hand, LPHNs have higher encapsulation efficiency to protect enoxaparin from degradation in the stomach. On the other hand, on the basis of the intestinal absorption of LPHNs, LPHNs could overcome the mucus layer to facilitate enoxaparin entry to under layer of intestinal epithelial cells, followed by absorption into the systemic circulation.

Table 2. Main pharmacokinetic parameters after peroral administration of enoxaparin formulations in rats at a dosage of 1010 IU/kg ($n = 4$). * $p < 0.05$ represents a significant improvement in absolute bioavailability in comparison with enoxaparin solution (p.o.).

Formulations	T_{max} (h)	$AUC_{0-12\,h}$ (s·h)	F_{abs} (%)
Enoxaparin solution (i.v.)	-	182.3 ± 44.2	100.0
Enoxaparin solution (p.o.)	0.5	37.6 ± 10.0	2.1
Enoxaparin-loaded LPHN2 (p.o.)	3	258.3 ± 93.1	14.2*

i.v. means intravenous injection; p.o. means peroral administration.

Despite the results that LPHNs can improve the oral bioavailability of enoxaparin, its absolute bioavailability is still not high enough. There are several reasons that may explain this: (1) The encapsulation efficiency of enoxaparin in the LPNH is about 65%, and almost 35% of enoxaparin is a free drug in LPHN dispersion, and free enoxaparin usually has low oral bioavailability; (2) the nanoparticles must overcome the mucus layer before they are transported across the epithelium.

Although one part of the nanoparticles can penetrate the mucus layer and be transported across the epithelium, other parts of the nanoparticle may be trapped in the mucus layer and eliminated from the gastrointestinal tract, owing to the mucus layer being renewed every 1~2 h [32]. Therefore more rationally designed nanocarriers with higher encapsulation efficiency and stronger mucus layer permeability are needed to further improve the absolute oral bioavailability of enoxaparin.

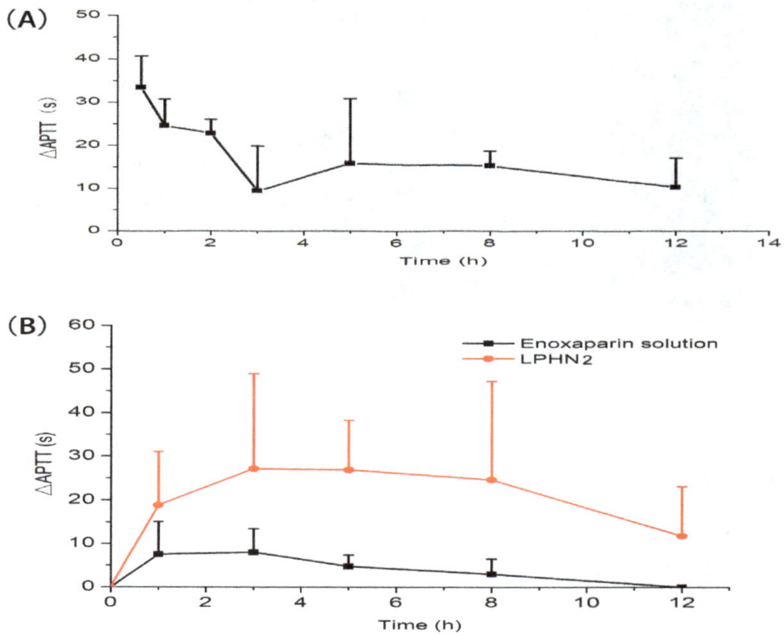

Figure 3. Mean Δ activated partial thromboplastin time (APTT) over time after a single intravenous injection of enoxaparin solution at a dosage of 101 IU/kg (**A**), and oral administration of enoxaparin solution and enoxaparin-loaded LPHN2 at a dosage of 1010 IU/kg (**B**) (n = 4).

3.4. In Vivo Efficacy

In vivo prevention of pulmonary thromboembolism of nanoparticles was studied in mice As shown in Table 3, the inhibition effect was 58.3% when enoxaparin solution was intravenously administered. The inhibition effect of enoxaparin-loaded LPHN2 was 50.0%, 2.99-fold higher than that of enoxaparin solution after oral administration, which further indicated that lipid–polymer hybrid nanoparticles are effective in improving oral absorption and the inhibition effect of enoxaparin against thrombin-induced thrombosis.

Table 3. Inhibition effect of pulmonary thromboembolism by orally administered various enoxaparin formulations (n = 12).

Formulations	Inhibition Effect (% protection)
Saline (i.v.)	8.3
Enoxaparin solution (i.v.)	58.3
Enoxaparin solution (p.o.)	16.7
Enoxaparin-loaded LPHN2 (p.o.)	50.0

i.v. means intravenous injection; p.o. means peroral administration.

3.5. Safety Evaluation

To investigate whether nanoparticles cause intestinal membrane damage or not, a histopathological examination was conducted. The results of pathological sections are shown in Figure 4. The histological studies indicated that there were no significant changes in the morphology and structure of the intestine exposed to enoxaparin-loaded LPHN2. The mucosal erosions and disruption of the enterocytes did not appear. Hence, LPHN is biocompatible in vivo as well as safe for the oral delivery of enoxaparin.

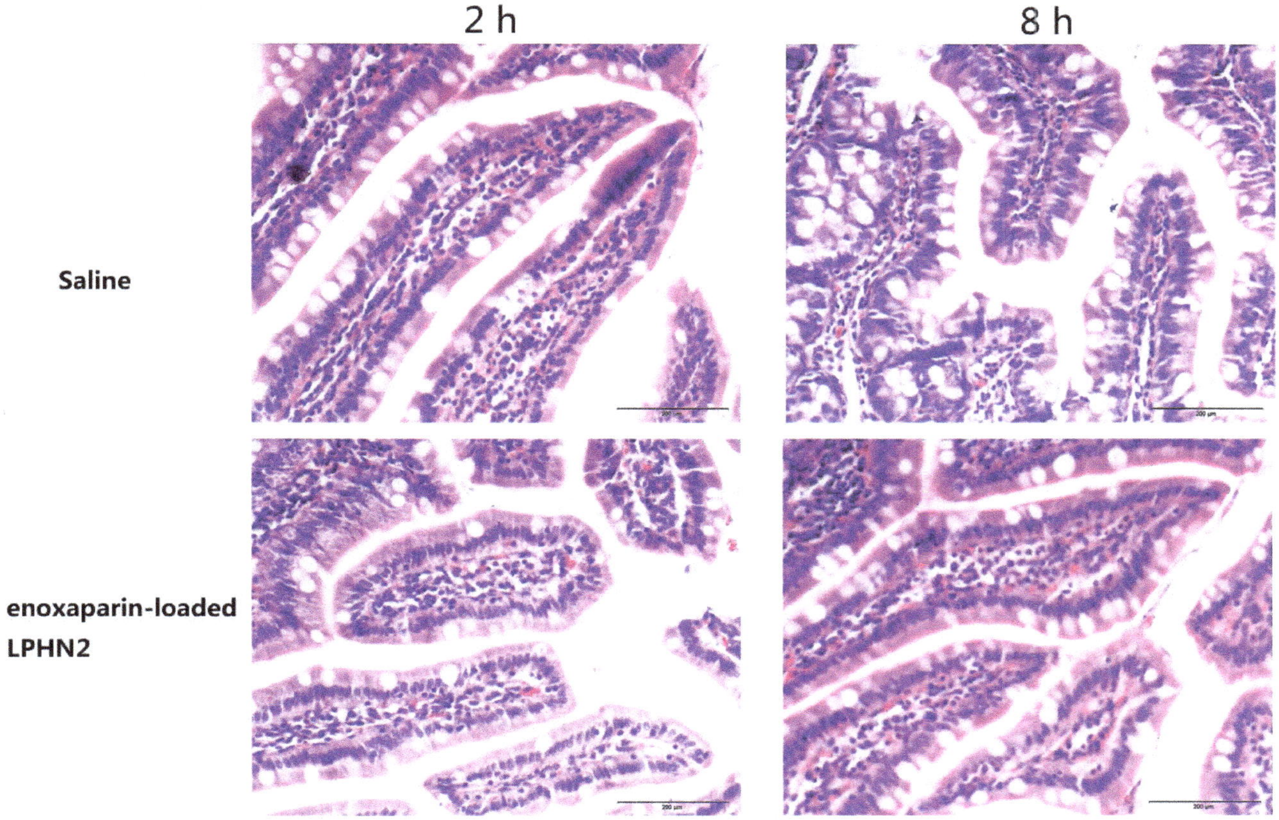

Figure 4. Morphology of intestinal mucosa of rats after oral administration of physiological saline- and enoxaparin-loaded LPHN2 after 2 and 8 h. Scale bar: 200 μm.

4. Conclusions

In summary, lipid–polymer hybrid nanoparticles (LPHNs) were prepared by double emulsification technology. The concentration of poloxamer 407 was optimized to ensure the high encapsulation efficiency of enoxaparin. Compared with traditional lipid nanoparticles, LPHNs possess not only higher encapsulation efficiency of enoxaparin, but also sustained release. In addition, optimized LPHNs could increase the concentration of enoxaparin in intestinal villi and facilitate enoxaparin penetration into the underlayer of enterocytes. Results of an in vivo pharmacokinetic study and an in vivo efficacy study further confirmed the superiority of LPHNs with regard to absorption-enhancing effects. In conclusion, rationally designed LPHNs could be excellent nanocarriers for oral delivery of enoxaparin.

Author Contributions: Conceptualization, G.F.; methodology, G.F.; software, B.T.; validation, G.F. and B.T.; formal analysis, G.F., B.T., and Y.Q.; investigation, G.F., B.T., and Y.Q.; data curation, B.T. and Y.Q.; writing—original draft preparation, G.F.; writing—review and editing, G.H.F.; funding acquisition, G.F. and B.T. All authors have read and agreed to the published version of the manuscript.

References

1. Hirsh, J.; Warkentin, T.E.; Shaughnessy, S.G.; Anand, S.S.; Halperin, J.L.; Raschke, R.; Granger, C.; Ohman, E.M.; Dalen, J.E. Heparin and Low-Molecular-Weight Heparin Mechanisms of Action, Pharmacokinetics, Dosing, Monitoring, Efficacy, and Safety. *Chest* **2001**, *119*, 64S–94S. [CrossRef] [PubMed]

2. Gray, E.; Mulloy, B.; Barrowcliffe, T.W. Heparin and low-molecular-weight heparin. *Thromb. Haemost.* **2008**, *99*, 807–818. [PubMed]
3. Fang, G.; Zhou, J.; Qian, Y.; Gou, J.; Yang, X.; Tang, B. Development and evaluation of thermo-sensitive hydrogel system with nanocomplexes for prolonged subcutaneous delivery of enoxaparin. *J. Drug Deliv. Sci. Technol.* **2018**, *48*, 118–124. [CrossRef]
4. Wang, L.; Li, L.; Sun, Y.; Tian, Y.; Li, Y.; Li, C.; Junyaprasert, V.B.; Mao, S. Exploration of hydrophobic modification degree of chitosan-based nanocomplexes on the oral delivery of enoxaparin. *Eur. J. Pharm. Sci. Off. J. Eur. Fed. Pharm. Sci.* **2013**, *50*, 263–271. [CrossRef] [PubMed]
5. Wang, L.; Li, L.; Sun, Y.; Ding, J.; Li, J.; Duan, X.; Li, Y.; Junyaprasert, V.B.; Mao, S. In vitro and in vivo evaluation of chitosan graft glyceryl monooleate as peroral delivery carrier of enoxaparin. *Int. J. Pharm.* **2014**, *471*, 391–399. [CrossRef]
6. Motlekar, N.A.; Youan, B.B. The quest for non-invasive delivery of bioactive macromolecules: A focus on heparins. *J. Control. Release Off. J. Control. Release Soc.* **2006**, *113*, 91–101. [CrossRef]
7. Neves, A.R.; Correia-da-Silva, M.; Sousa, E.; Pinto, M. Strategies to Overcome Heparins' Low Oral Bioavailability. *Pharmaceuticals* **2016**, *9*, 37. [CrossRef]
8. Fang, G.; Tang, B. Advanced delivery strategies facilitating oral absorption of heparins. *Asian J. Pharm. Sci.* **2020**. [CrossRef]
9. Valimaki, S.; Khakalo, A.; Ora, A.; Johansson, L.S.; Rojas, O.J.; Kostiainen, M.A. Effect of PEG-PDMAEMA Block Copolymer Architecture on Polyelectrolyte Complex Formation with Heparin. *Biomacromolecules* **2016**, *17*, 2891–2900. [CrossRef]
10. Ibrahim, S.S.; Osman, R.; Awad, G.A.; Mortada, N.D.; Geneidy, A.S. Low molecular weight heparins for current and future uses: Approaches for micro- and nano-particulate delivery. *Drug Deliv.* **2016**, *23*, 2661–2667. [CrossRef]
11. Ramadan, A.; Lagarce, F.; Tessier-Marteau, A.; Thomas, O.; Legras, P.; Macchi, L.; Saulnier, P.; Benoit, J.P. Oral fondaparinux: Use of lipid nanocapsules as nanocarriers and in vivo pharmacokinetic study. *Int. J. Nanomed.* **2011**, *6*, 2941–2951.
12. Kim, S.K.; Lee, E.H.; Vaishali, B.; Lee, S.; Lee, Y.K.; Kim, C.Y.; Moon, H.T.; Byun, Y. Tricaprylin microemulsion for oral delivery of low molecular weight heparin conjugates. *J. Control. Release Off. J. Control. Release Soc.* **2005**, *105*, 32–42. [CrossRef] [PubMed]
13. Paliwal, R.; Paliwal, S.R.; Agrawal, G.P.; Vyas, S.P. Biomimetic solid lipid nanoparticles for oral bioavailability enhancement of low molecular weight heparin and its lipid conjugates: In vitro and in vivo evaluation. *Mol. Pharm.* **2011**, *8*, 1314–1321. [CrossRef] [PubMed]
14. Rong, W.-T.; Lu, Y.-P.; Tao, Q.; Guo, M.; Lu, Y.; Ren, Y.; Yu, S.-Q. Hydroxypropyl-Sulfobutyl-β-Cyclodextrin Improves the Oral Bioavailability of Edaravone by Modulating Drug Efflux Pump of Enterocytes. *J. Pharm. Sci.* **2014**, *103*, 730–742. [CrossRef] [PubMed]
15. Lu, Y.; Liu, S.; Zhao, Y.; Zhu, L.; Yu, S. Complexation of Z-ligustilide with hydroxypropyl-beta-cyclodextrin to improve stability and oral bioavailability. *Acta Pharm.* **2014**, *64*, 211–222. [CrossRef]
16. Bagre, A.P.; Jain, K.; Jain, N.K. Alginate coated chitosan core shell nanoparticles for oral delivery of enoxaparin: In vitro and in vivo assessment. *Int. J. Pharm.* **2013**, *456*, 31–40. [CrossRef]
17. Meissner, Y.; Ubrich, N.; Ghazouani, F.E.; Maincent, P.; Lamprecht, A. Low molecular weight heparin loaded pH-sensitive microparticles. *Int. J. Pharm.* **2007**, *335*, 147–153. [CrossRef]
18. Fan, B.; Xing, Y.; Zheng, Y.; Sun, C.; Liang, G. pH-responsive thiolated chitosan nanoparticles for oral low-molecular weight heparin delivery: In vitro and in vivo evaluation. *Drug Deliv.* **2016**, *23*, 238–247. [CrossRef]
19. Yuan, H.; Chen, C.Y.; Chai, G.H.; Du, Y.Z.; Hu, F.Q. Improved transport and absorption through gastrointestinal tract by PEGylated solid lipid nanoparticles. *Mol. Pharm.* **2013**, *10*, 1865–1873. [CrossRef]
20. Wong, H.L.; Bendayan, R.; Rauth, A.M.; Li, Y.; Wu, X.Y. Chemotherapy with anticancer drugs encapsulated in solid lipid nanoparticles. *Adv. Drug Deliv. Rev.* **2007**, *59*, 491–504. [CrossRef]
21. Hirsh, J.; Anand Sonia, S.; Halperin Jonathan, L.; Fuster, V. Mechanism of Action and Pharmacology of Unfractionated Heparin. *Arterioscler. Thromb. Vasc. Biol.* **2001**, *21*, 1094–1096. [CrossRef] [PubMed]
22. Boushra, M.; Tous, S.; Fetih, G.; Korzekwa, K.; Lebo, D.B.; Xue, H.Y.; Wong, H.L. Development and evaluation of viscosity-enhanced nanocarrier (VEN) for oral insulin delivery. *Int. J. Pharm.* **2016**, *511*, 462–472. [CrossRef] [PubMed]

23. Lin, Z.; Gao, W.; Hu, H.; Ma, K.; He, B.; Dai, W.; Wang, X.; Wang, J.; Zhang, X.; Zhang, Q. Novel thermo-sensitive hydrogel system with paclitaxel nanocrystals: High drug-loading, sustained drug release and extended local retention guaranteeing better efficacy and lower toxicity. *J. Control. Release Off. J. Control. Release Soc.* **2014**, *174*, 161–170. [CrossRef] [PubMed]
24. Tang, X.; Huang, K.; Gui, H.; Wang, J.; Lu, J.; Dai, L.; Zhang, L.; Wang, G. Pluronic-based micelle encapsulation potentiates myricetin-induced cytotoxicity in human glioblastoma cells. *Int. J. Nanomed.* **2016**, *11*, 4991–5002. [CrossRef]
25. Wang, P.; Li, Y.; Jiang, M. Effects of the multilayer structures on Exenatide release and bioactivity in microsphere/thermosensitive hydrogel system. *Colloids Surf. B Biointerfaces* **2018**, *171*, 85–93. [CrossRef]
26. Fang, G.; Tang, B.; Chao, Y.; Xu, H.; Gou, J.; Zhang, Y.; Tang, X. Cysteine-Functionalized Nanostructured Lipid Carriers for Oral Delivery of Docetaxel: A Permeability and Pharmacokinetic Study. *Mol. Pharm.* **2015**, *12*, 2384–2395. [CrossRef]
27. Jiao, Y.; Ubrich, N.; Marchand-Arvier, M.; Vigneron, C.; Hoffman, M.; Lecompte, T.; Maincent, P. In Vitro and In Vivo Evaluation of Oral Heparin–Loaded Polymeric Nanoparticles in Rabbits. *Circulation* **2002**, *105*, 230–235. [CrossRef]
28. Hoffart, V.; Ubrich, N.; Lamprecht, A.; Bachelier, K.; Vigneron, C.; Lecompte, T.; Hoffman, M.; Maincent, P. Microencapsulation of Low Molecular Weight Heparin into Polymeric Particles Designed with Biodegradable and Nonbiodegradable Polycationic Polymers. *Drug Deliv.* **2003**, *10*, 1–7. [CrossRef]
29. Sherif, S.; Bendas, E.R.; Badawy, S. The clinical efficacy of cosmeceutical application of liquid crystalline nanostructured dispersions of alpha lipoic acid as anti-wrinkle. *Eur. J. Pharm. Biopharm. Off. J. Arb. Fur Pharm. Verfahr. e.V* **2014**, *86*, 251–259. [CrossRef]
30. Lakkireddy, H.R.; Urmann, M.; Besenius, M.; Werner, U.; Haack, T.; Brun, P.; Alie, J.; Illel, B.; Hortala, L.; Vogel, R.; et al. Oral delivery of diabetes peptides—Comparing standard formulations incorporating functional excipients and nanotechnologies in the translational context. *Adv. Drug Deliv. Rev.* **2016**, *106*, 196–222. [CrossRef]
31. Malhaire, H.; Gimel, J.-C.; Roger, E.; Benoît, J.-P.; Lagarce, F. How to design the surface of peptide-loaded nanoparticles for efficient oral bioavailability? *Adv. Drug Deliv. Rev.* **2016**, *106*, 320–336. [CrossRef] [PubMed]
32. Hansson, G.C. Mucus and mucins in diseases of the intestinal and respiratory tracts. *J. Intern. Med.* **2019**, *285*, 479–490. [CrossRef] [PubMed]

Hydrogel Formulations Incorporating Drug Nanocrystals Enhance the Therapeutic Effect of Rebamipide in a Hamster Model for Oral Mucositis

Noriaki Nagai [1,*], Ryotaro Seiriki [1], Saori Deguchi [1], Hiroko Otake [1], Noriko Hiramatsu [2], Hiroshi Sasaki [3] and Naoki Yamamoto [3]

1 Faculty of Pharmacy, Kindai University, 3-4-1 Kowakae, Higashi-Osaka, Osaka 577-8502, Japan; 1611610157u@kindai.ac.jp (R.S.); 2045110002h@kindai.ac.jp (S.D.); hotake@phar.kindai.ac.jp (H.O.)

2 Laboratory of Molecularbiology and Histochemistry, Fujita Health University Institute of Joint Research, 1-98 Dengakugakubo, Kutsukake, Toyoake, Aichi 470-1192, Japan; norikoh@fujita-hu.ac.jp

3 Department of Ophthalmology, Kanazawa Medical University, 1-1 Daigaku, Uchinada, Kahoku, Ishikawa 920-0293, Japan; sasaki-h@k5.dion.ne.jp (H.S.); naokiy@kanazawa-med.ac.jp (N.Y.)

* Correspondence: nagai_n@phar.kindai.ac.jp

Abstract: A mouthwash formulation of rebamipide (REB) is commonly used to treat oral mucositis, however, this formulation does not provide sufficient treatment or prevention in cases of serious oral mucositis. To improve treatment, we attempted to design a hydrogel incorporating REB nanocrystals (R-NPs gel). The R-NPs gel was prepared by a bead mill method using carbopol hydrogel, methylcellulose and 2-hydroxypropyl-β-cyclodextrin, and another hydrogel incorporating REB microcrystals (R-MPs gel) was prepared following the same protocol but without the bead mill treatment. The REB particle size in the R-MPs gel was 0.15–25 μm, and while the REB particle size was 50–180 nm in the R-NPs gel. Next, we investigated the therapeutic effect of REB nanocrystals on oral mucositis using a hamster model. Almost all of the REB was released as drug nanocrystals from the R-NPs gel, and the REB content in the cheek pouch of hamsters treated with R-NPs gel was significantly higher than that of hamsters treated with R-MPs gel. Further, treatment with REB hydrogels enhanced the healing of oral wounds in the hamsters. REB accumulation in the cheek pouch of hamsters treated with the R-NPs gel was prevented by an inhibitor of clathrin-dependent endocytosis (CME) (40 μM dynasore). In conclusion, we designed an R-NPs gel and found that REB nanocrystals are taken up by tissues through CME, where they provide a persistent effect resulting in an enhancement of oral wound healing.

Keywords: rebamipide; nanocrystals; oral mucositis; hydrogel; endocytosis

1. Introduction

Pain caused by serious oral mucositis affects food intake, nutrition, speaking, and swallowing, can cause life-threatening bacteremia, and ultimately leads to poor quality of life for patients [1,2]. Chemoradiotherapy for patients with head and neck cancer often causes serious oral mucositis, and the severe pain interferes with subsequent treatment and quality of life [3–5]. Previous studies have shown that reactive oxygen species cause cell apoptosis, DNA damage, and enhanced production of proinflammatory cytokines [6], and that these factors greatly impact mucositis. Therefore, topical granulocyte macrophage colony stimulating factors, anti-inflammatory agents and mucosal coating agents are widely used as medical therapies for oral mucositis [7]. In addition, Caphosol®, MuGard®, Mucotrol™, Gelclair®, Episil® and Palifermin have surfaced on the market. Caphosol® is a supersaturated calcium phosphate, electrolyte mouth rinse used as artificial saliva, and MuGard® (oral mucoadhesive) causes the formation of a protective coating over oral mucosa. Mucotrol™ is a mixture of herbal agents that is used as an oral gel wafer and includes sorbitol, *Cyamopsis tetragonolobus*, stearic acid, magnesium stearate and aloe. Gelclair® is a viscous gel that is used as a mouthwash and forms a protective film by adhering to the mucosa of the oropharyngeal cavity, helping to provide pain relief in mouth lesions. Episil® is a lipid-based fluid developed for the management and relief of pain associated with oral lesions of various aetiologies such as oral mucositis, a painful side effect of cancer therapies. Palifermin is a truncated human recombinant keratinocyte growth factor produced in *Escherichia coli*. The keratinocyte growth factor stimulates the growth of cells that line the surface of the mouth and intestinal tract. However, serious oral mucositis remains a frequent and critical complication of head and neck cancers [8–10].

Rebamipide (REB), 2-(4-chlorobenzoylamino)-3-[2(1H)-quinolinone-4-yl]-propionic acid, was developed by Otsuka Pharmaceutical Co., Ltd. (Tokyo, Japan) for the treatment of gastric ulcers, gastritis, and dry eye syndrome. It was reported that REB scavenges free radicals, exhibits an anti-inflammatory action and improves blood flow [11,12]. In addition, REB increases endogenous prostaglandins E2 and I2, leading to antibacterial effects, mucin secretagogue activity and anti-inflammatory action [13,14]. The efficacy of REB for the treatment of oral mucositis was first reported by Matsuda et al. in 1994, and a resulting mouthwash containing REB has been used as a therapy for mucositis caused by radiotherapy [15], chemotherapy [16] and Behcet's disease [7]. Furthermore, a pilot randomized controlled trial (RCT) reported that mouthwash containing REB reduces the onset of oral mucositis caused by chemoradiotherapy and radiotherapy [15,17,18]. The various pharmacological effects of REB include suppression of the induction of mucus secretion [19], promotion of endogenous prostaglandin production in the gastric mucosa [20,21], anti-free radical action [12], neutrophil activation [22,23], inhibition of inflammatory reactions [24–26] and up-regulation of epidermal growth factor and its receptor [27]. Pharmacokinetic studies using experimental animals have shown that REB acts directly on peptic ulcers and gastritis [28], and that a 4% REB liquid preparation is the optimal concentration for a mouthwash in terms of safety and efficacy profiles [18]. However, sufficient drug efficacy is difficult to obtain since the mouth-washing agent has a short residence time in the oral cavity, and a local concentration of REB on the oral mucosa cannot be maintained via a mouthwash containing liquid REB. We aimed to prepare mucoadhesive formulations, and focused to design the formulations incorporating drug nanocrystals into a hydrogel net. Moreover, we investigated the mucoadhesive properties, drug release and the uptake of REB into the cheek pouch tissue in the REB hydrogel.

It is important to consider the structure of the three-dimensional network in sputum to efficiently deliver REB particles to the oral mucosa. It has been reported that gastrointestinal mucus and cystic fibrosis sputum almost completely block the delivery of particles larger than 500 nm [29–31]. In addition, the mucoadhesive properties of a formulation are enhanced by decreasing their particle size, since this increases the relative surface area [32]. Therefore, we hypothesized that nanocrystals with a particle diameter smaller than 200 nm would be a suitable carrier of REB for the treatment of oral mucositis. We previously found that drug nanocrystals were taken up by cells, provided high efficiency, and showed that a hydrogel is suitable as a base for gel formulations, since the drug nanocrystals were easily released from the hydrogel base [33–35]. In this study, we attempted to design a hydrogel formulation containing REB nanocrystals smaller than 200 nm by incorporating the drug nanocrystals into a hydrogel net, and to demonstrate the usefulness of these REB nanocrystals as a therapy for oral mucositis.

2. Materials and Methods

2.1. Animals

Male golden or Syrian hamsters (*Mesocricetus auratus*, weight 98 ± 2.6 g) were purchased from Shimizu Laboratory Supplies Co., Ltd. (Kyoto, Japan). All animal experiments were approved by the animal experimental committee in Kindai University on 1 April 2019 (approval number KAPS-31-016).

2.2. Preparation of REB Hydrogel

Hydrogel formulations incorporating REB nanocrystals were prepared according to previous reports [33,34]. REB powder (0.4%; Wako Pure Chemical Industries, Ltd., Osaka, Japan), 0.5% methylcellulose (MC; Shin-Etsu Chemical Co., Ltd., Tokyo, Japan) and 5% 2-hydroxypropyl-β-cyclodextrin (HPβCD; Nihon Shokuhin Kako Co., Ltd., Tokyo, Japan) were added to distilled water containing 0.1 mm zirconia beads, and crushed at 5500 rpm for 1 min by a Micro Smash MS-100R (TOMY SEIKO Co. Ltd., Tokyo, Japan). The mill treatment was repeated 30 times, after which the dispersions were milled at 1500 rpm for 3 h with a Shake Master NEO (Bio-Medical Science Co., Ltd., Tokyo, Japan). The milled dispersions were incorporated into a Carbopol® 934 hydrogel net (Serva, Heidelberg, Germany) and used as hydrogel formulations incorporating REB nanocrystals (R-NPs gel) in this study. Hydrogel formulations incorporating REB microcrystals (R-MPs gel) were prepared by mixing the 0.4% REB powder, 0.5% MC and 5% HPβCD in the distilled water, and incorporated the REB microcrystals into Carbopol® 934 hydrogel net.

2.3. Characteristics of REB Hydrogels

The characteristics of the REB hydrogels were analyzed according to previous studies [33,34]. Briefly, the particle size distributions of the R-MPs gels were measured by a SALD-7100 (refractive index, 1.60-0.10i; Shimadzu Corp., Kyoto, Japan), and the particle size distribution and particle number of the R-NPs gel were determined using NANOSIGHT LM10 (viscosity, 1.27 mPa·s; QuantumDesign Japan, Tokyo, Japan). The atomic force microscopy (AFM) image of the REB nanocrystals was obtained using a SPM-9700 (Shimadzu Corp., Kyoto, Japan), and the crystal form was determined by a powder X-ray diffraction (XRD) Mini Flex II (Rigaku Co., Tokyo, Japan). The zeta potential of REB was analyzed by a model 502 zeta potential analyzer (Nihon Rufuto Co., Ltd., Tokyo, Japan). REB concentrations were measured on a HPLC LC-20AT system (Shimadzu Corp. Kyoto, Japan) with an Inertsil® ODS-3 column (GL Science Co., Inc., Tokyo, Japan) with detection at 287 nm. Methyl p-hydroxybenzoate was used as an internal standard, and the mobile phase was 50 mM phosphate buffer/acetonitrile (75/25 *v*/*v*) at a flow rate of 0.25 mL/min. The uniformity of the REB in the gels was determined as follows: 0.3 g of REB hydrogel was divided into 10 parts (0.03 g) and dissolved in *N*,*N*-dimethylformamide. The REB contents in the dissolved samples were measured by the HPLC method described above. In this study, the standard deviation (SD) of the REB levels in the 10 hydrogel divisions represents the non-uniformity of REB in the hydrogel.

2.4. Permeation Study from REB Hydrogels

Drug release from the REB hydrogels was analyzed according to the previous study using a Franz diffusion cell set on an MF™-MEMBRANE FILTER with a pore size of 220 nm (Merck Millipore, Tokyo, Japan) [33–35]. The reservoir chamber of the cell was filled with 12.2 mL of 10 mM phosphate buffer consist of sodium phosphate and potassium phosphate according to the Japanese Pharmacopoeia, 17th Edition (JP XVII), and the pH was adjusted by NaOH (pH 7.4). A total of 0.3 g of 0.4% REB hydrogels was added to the donor side. We collected 50 μL samples of phosphate from the reservoir chamber over time and replaced them with the same volume of 10 mM phosphate buffer. The nanoparticle size distribution, number, and released REB levels in the samples were measured by the NANOSIGHT and HPLC methods described in Section 2.3.

2.5. REB Contents in Hamsters Treated with REB Hydrogels

In this study, 10 μM cytochalasin D (phagocytosis inhibitor) [36], 2 μM rottlerin (MP—macropinocytosis inhibitor) [37], 40 μM dynasore (CME—clathrin-dependent endocytosis inhibitor) [38] and 54 μM nystatin (CavME—caveolae-dependent endocytosis inhibitor) [36] were used as inhibitors for each type of endocytosis. A total of 0.1 g of 0.4% REB hydrogel with or without endocytosis inhibitors was applied to the cheek pouch of hamsters and maintained for 2 or 8 h.

After that, the hamsters were euthanized under deep isoflurane anesthesia, and the cheek pouches were carefully collected. The collected cheek pouches were homogenized in *N,N*-dimethylformamide to extract the REB. Blood was collected from the vena cava, centrifuged at 20,400 g and a temperature of 4 °C for 20 min, and the supernatants were used as samples. REB levels in both the cheek pouch and blood samples were measured by HPLC, as described above.

2.6. Measurement of Wound Area in the Hamster Model for Oral Mucositis

Hamsters were anesthetized with isoflurane (3%, rate of flow 1 L/min), and 25 μL of 10% acetic acid was injected into the cheek pouch. After 2 days, the hamsters were used in experiments as a model for oral mucositis. A total of 0.1 g of REB hydrogel was applied once a day (10:00 a.m.) and the wound images were monitored by a digital camera. The wound size was measured daily with an image. The initial areas of the wound (0 days) were as follows: non-treated hamsters (None), 10.8 ± 0.76; vehicle-treated hamsters (Vehicle), 10.2 ± 3.3; R-MPs-treated hamsters, 10.3 ± 3.3; R-NPs-treated hamsters, 10.7 ± 1.9 (mm^2; means ± standard error of mean (SEM), n = 5–8). The values (%) were calculated as the ratio to the initial area of the respective wound.

2.7. Measurement of Wound Area in the Hamster Model for Oral Mucositis

The cheek pouches of euthanized hamsters were removed and fixed at room temperature using a tissue quick fixation solution (SUPER FIX, Kurabo Industries, Osaka, Japan). The fixed tissues were prepared in paraffin blocks by the general protocol, and serial sections with a thickness of 4 μm were prepared using a microtome. Hematoxylin and eosin (H&E) staining was performed for morphological observation, and immunostaining was performed with a multi-cytokeratin antibody to identify the oral mucosal epithelium; endogenous peroxidase treatment was performed with 0.3% hydrogen peroxide methanol; and microwave treatment was performed (90 °C, 20 min) in citric acid buffer (pH 6.0) for antigen activation. Samples were incubated with anti-multi-cytokeratin mouse monoclonal antibody (1:200, Clone: AE1/AE3, Leica Biosystems Nussloch GmbH) for 30 min at 37 °C. After three washes with phosphate buffer solution, samples were incubated with universal immune-peroxidase polymer (anti-mouse antibody, Histofine® Simple Stain MAX PO (M), Nichirei Biosciences, Tokyo, Japan) for 30 min at 37 °C. Samples were again washed three times with phosphate buffer solution, color washed with 3,3′-diaminobenzidine tetrahydrochloride (DAB) solution for 30 s, washed with water, and nuclear stained with Meyer's hematoxylin solution (Muto Chemical Co., Ltd., Tokyo, Japan) for 5 min. Specimens were observed using a biological upright microscope (Power BX-51, Olympus, Tokyo, Japan) with a digital camera (4× and 10× object lenses, DP-71, Olympus), and photographed at the central area of the oral wound.

2.8. Statistical Analysis

Data are shown as the mean ± SEM, and ANOVA, Student's *t*-test and Dunnett's multiple comparisons were used to analyze statistical differences.

3. Results

3.1. Design and Characteristics of the R-NPs Gel

Bead mill is a known method to prepare drug nanocrystals. We attempted to prepare REB nanocrystals using the bead mill method and investigated the characteristics of the hydrogel with REB nanocrystals. Figure 1 shows the particle size distribution of REB in the hydrogel. The aggregates of REB particles were observable in the R-MPs gel (Figure 1A,B) with the naked eye; however, bead mill treatment caused a decrease in REB particle size, after which aggregates were no longer visible in the R-NPs gel (Figure 1A,C). The particle size distribution was 50–180 nm after mill treatment (Figure 1C), and the AFM image also showed the REB particles crushed to nano-size (Figure 1D). In addition, we demonstrated the characteristics of the REB in the R-NPs gel (Figure 2). The REB content in R-NPs gel was uniform in comparison with the R-MPs gel (Figure 2A), and the REB solubility in the R-NPs gel was higher than that in the R-MPs gel (Figure 2B). On the other hand, the crystal form of REB was maintained in the R-NPs gel (Figure 2C), and the crystal structure of REB nanocrystals in the hydrogel was similar to that in the REB microcrystals. These results showed that the form did not affect the difference on its solubility. Moreover, we evaluated the stability of R-NPs gel. In this study the zeta potential of the REB nanocrystals was −11.9 mV, and no differences were observed in the size, content or form of the REB nanocrystals in hydrogel for one month.

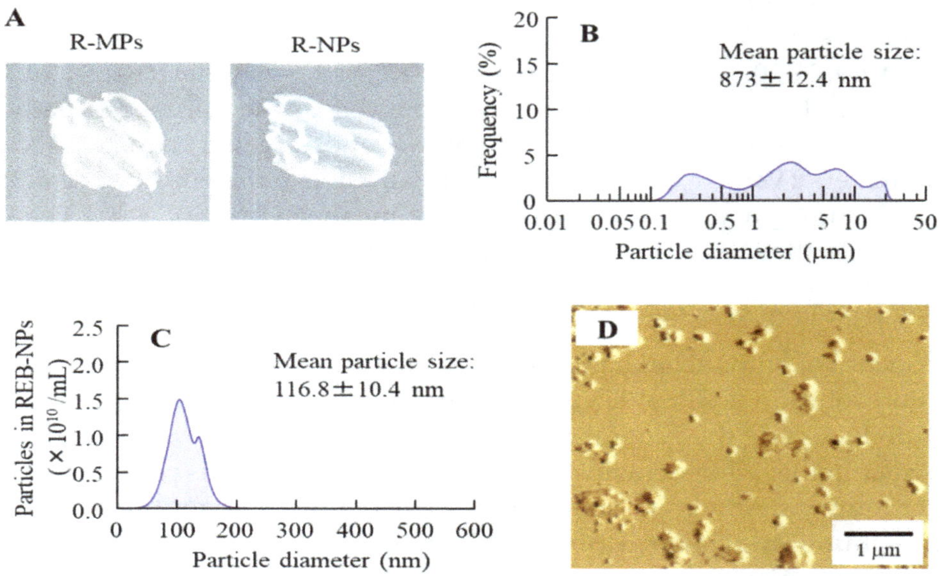

Figure 1. Condition of rebamipide (REB) in REB hydrogels. (**A**) Photographs of the R-MPs gel (hydrogel with incorporated rebamipide microcyrstals) and R-NPs gel (hydrogel with incorporated rebamipide nanocrystals). (**B**,**C**) Particle size in the R-MPs (**B**) and R-NPs (**C**) gels. (**D**) AFM image of the R-NPs gel. Bead mill treatment decreased the particle size of REB to the range of 50–180 nm.

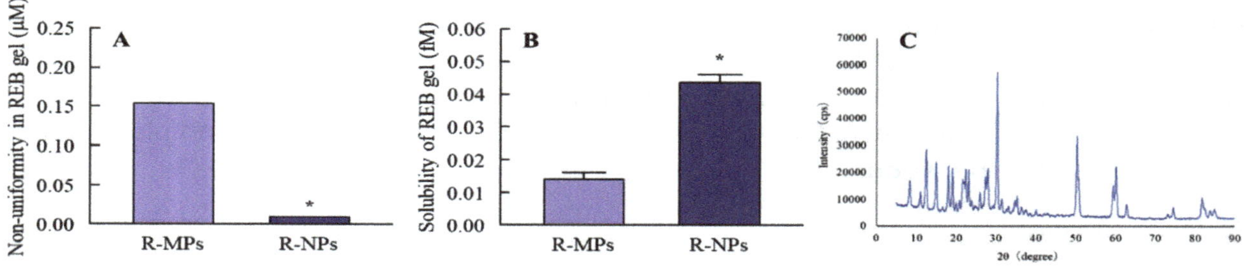

Figure 2. Characteristics of REB in the R-MPs and R-NPs gels. (**A**) Non-uniformity in REB particle distribution in the R-MPs and R-NPs gels. (**B**) Solubility of REB in the R-MPs and R-NPs gels. (**C**) XRD pattern of REB particles after bead mill treatment. $N = 7$. * $p < 0.05$ vs. R-MPs for each category. The mill-treated REB retained its crystal structure, but the uniformity of REB distribution in the R-NPs gel was higher than the non-milled REB in the R-MPs gel. Moreover, solubility of REB was increased by bead mill treatment.

3.2. Endocytic Uptake of REB Nanocrystals into Cheek Pouch Tissue

In the investigation of the mechanism for drug permeation in tissues, an evaluation of drug release from the hydrogel is necessary. Figure 3 shows the REB released from the hydrogel. The release of REB was observed for both the R-MPs and R-NPs gels, but the levels released from the R-NPs gel were significantly higher (Figure 3A). Almost all of the REB released from R-MPs gel was of the solution type, while drug nanocrystals were detected in the reservoir chamber after treatment with the R-NPs gel (Figure 3B,C). Next, we examined REB levels in the cheek pouch of hamsters treated with the R-MPs and R-NPs gels (Figure 4A). Eight hours after treatment, the REB levels in hamsters treated with the R-NPs gel were 25-fold higher than in hamsters treated with the R-MPs gel. We then investigated whether endocytosis is related to the uptake of REB into the cheek pouch tissue (Figure 4B,C). Co-treatment with nystatin, rottlerin or cytochalasin D did not affect REB levels in the cheek pouch of hamsters treated with the R-NPs gel. In contrast, co-treatment with dynasore resulted in a significant decrease in tissue REB levels, indicating that CME is related to the uptake of REB into the cheek pouch tissue. We also examined the REB levels in the blood of hamsters 0–8 h after treatment with REB hydrogels. No REB was detected in the plasma of hamsters treated with either the R-MPs or R-NPs gels.

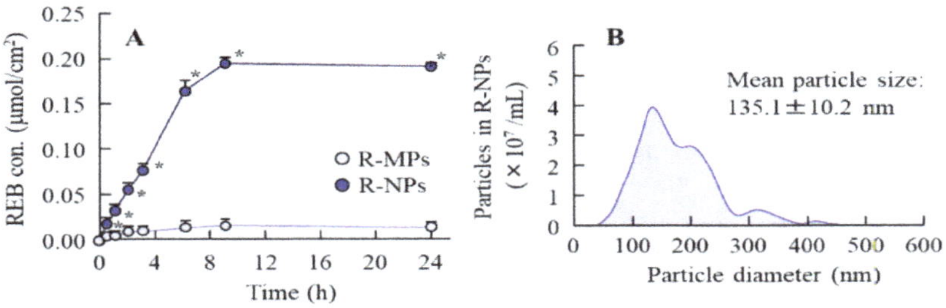

Figure 3. Drug release from R-MPs and R-NPs gels through a 220-nm pore membrane. (**A**) Release behavior of REB from R-MPs and R-NPs gels through a membrane. (**B**) and (**C**) Size distribution (**B**) and number (**C**) of REB nanocrystals in the reservoir chamber 24 h after R-NPs application. $n = 7$. N.D., not detectable. * $p < 0.05$ vs. R-MPs gel for each category. REB was released from the R-NPs gel in the form of nanocrystals.

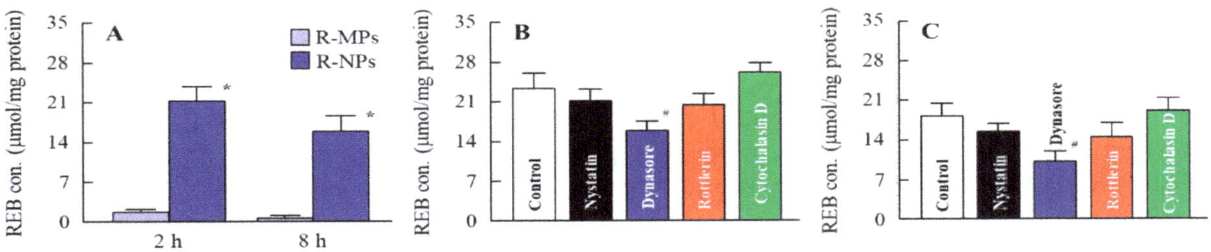

Figure 4. Changes in REB content in the cheek pouch of hamsters treated with REB hydrogels for oral mucositis. (**A**) REB contents in the cheek pouch of hamsters 2 and 8 h after treatment with R-MPs and R-NPs gels. (**B,C**) REB contents in the cheek pouch of hamsters treated with endocytosis inhibitors 2 h (**B**) and 8 h (**C**) after the application of R-MPs and R-NPs gels. Control—R-NPs-treated hamster. Nystatin—nystatin-treated hamster treated with R-NPs. Dynasore—dynasore-treated hamster treated with R-NPs. Rottlerin—rottlerin-treated hamster treated with R-NPs. Cytochalasin D—cytochalasin D-treated hamster treated with R-NPs. $n = 5$–7. * $p < 0.05$, vs. R-MPs for each category. # $p < 0.05$ vs. Control for each category. REB content in hamsters treated with R-NPs gel was higher than in those treated with R-MPs gel; the CME pathway appears to be related to the penetration of REB into the cheek pouch tissues from the hydrogel formulations.

3.3. Effect of REB Hydrogel on Oral Wound Healing in the Hamster Model

Figure 5 shows the therapeutic potential of the REB hydrogels for oral mucositis. The wounds in the hamsters injected with acetic acid remained uncured after three days with an area of 8.1 ± 0.5 mm^2. Although the oral wound in hamsters treated with vehicle also remained uncured after three days (8.0 ± 0.3 mm^2), hamsters treated with R-MPs gel showed a decrease in the oral wound area to 6.3 ± 0.4 mm^2. However, treatment with the R-NPs gel significantly enhanced healing of the wound, with the area reduced to 2.3 ± 0.3 mm^2 three days after the injection of acetic acid. Further, we examined wounds histologically by H&E staining and multi-cytokeratin immunostaining (Figure 6). The None and Vehicle group hamsters showed a degeneration and thickening of the oral mucosal epithelium, migration of inflammatory cells, (♠) and dilated blood vessels (black arrowheads) in the mucosal lamina propria. A regenerated oral mucosal epithelium (white arrowhead) was partially observed in the wounds of hamsters treated with the R-MPs or R-NPs gels, and inflammatory cell levels were reduced in the mucosal lamina propria (Figure 6A). A proliferation of basal cells in the regenerated oral mucosal epithelium was present in hamsters treated with the R-MPs and R-NPs gels (yellow arrowheads, Figure 6B). Oral mucosal epithelial cells containing multi-cytokeratin were stained brown by DAB. The multi-cytokeratin-positive cells in the None group were degenerated and necrotic, and the mucosal lamina propria underlying the mucosal epithelium was thickened (♣1). In the Vehicle group, the degenerated and necrotic mucosal epithelium was almost shedding, and the mucosal lamina propria was thickened as in the None group, with further migration of inflammatory cells (♣2). Regenerated oral mucosal epithelium was observed in the wounds of some of the hamsters treated with the R-MPs or R-NPs gels. The regenerated oral mucosal epithelium included basal cells (white arrowheads) and layers of multi-cytokeratin-positive cells (*) toward the surface of the mucosa (Figure 6C,D).

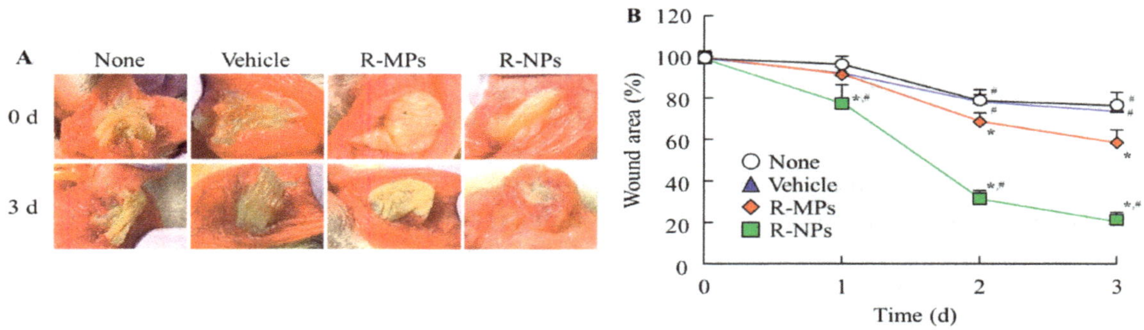

Figure 5. Therapeutic effect of R-NPs gel on wounds in the cheek pouch of hamsters. (**A**) Representative images of the cheek pouch of the hamster model for oral mucositis 0 and 3 d after treatment with REB hydrogels. (**B**), Wound area in the cheek pouch of the hamster model 0–3 d after treatment with REB hydrogels. $n = 5$–8. * $p < 0.05$, vs. Vehicle for each category. # $p < 0.05$ vs. R-MPs gel for each category. Treatment with REB hydrogel enhanced the therapeutic effect on oral mucositis. The wound areas in hamsters treated with R-NPs gel were significantly smaller than in hamsters treated with R-MPs gel.

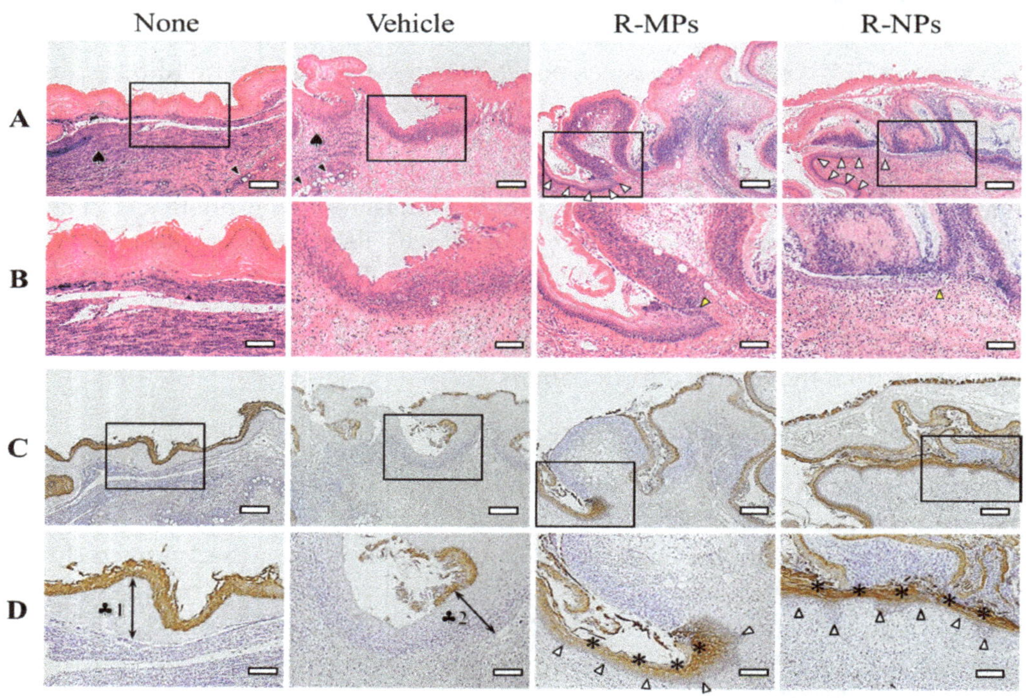

Figure 6. Microscopic effects of the R-NPs gel on oral mucositis. (**A**) Images of H&E-stained cheek

pouch tissue specimens from a hamster with oral mucositis three days after treatment with REB hydrogels (4× objective lens; bars indicate 200 μm). (**B**) High magnification images in the areas delineated by the squares in Figure A (10× objective lens; bars indicate 100 μm). (**C**) Images of immunostaining for multi-cytokeratin in the serial sections shown in Figure A (4× objective lens; bars indicate 200 μm). (**D**) High magnification images of the areas delineated by the squares in Figure C (10× objective lens; bars indicate 100 μm).

4. Discussion

Oral mucositis is the most common painful mucosal lesion, but traditional treatments, such as a mouthwash containing REB, do not provide sufficient treatment or prevention of this condition in serious cases [6,8,39]. Therefore, it is essential to look for effective treatments with few or no adverse effects. In this study, we developed a hydrogel formulation incorporating REB nanocrystals (R-NPs gel) and showed that CME is related to the uptake of REB nanocrystals into the cheek pouch tissue of hamsters. In addition, we found that R-NPs gel releases high levels of REB into tissues and provides a useful therapy for oral mucositis in the hamster model (Figure 7).

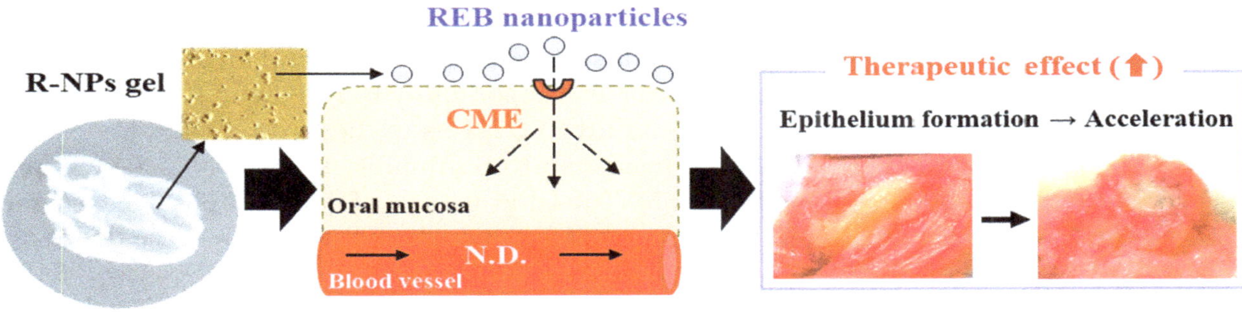

Figure 7. Drug delivery pathway and therapeutic effect of R-NPs gel in the cheek pouch of the hamster model for oral mucositis. N.D., not detectable.

Daniel et al. reported limited diffusion of particles larger than 0.5 μm through the mucin layer [31]. Szentkuti [30] showed that particles larger than 1 μm (1.09 μm diameter) do not accumulate on the surface of cell membranes and are undetectable 30 min after application, but the mucoadhesive properties of particles that are 415 nm in diameter are higher and they do accumulate on the apical membranes of surface epithelium cells and remain there for more than 30 min after treatment [30]. These reports suggest that the mucoadhesive properties of a drug increase as particle size decreases, and that the preparation of particles smaller than 400 nm in diameter is needed for application as a drug delivery system (DDS) for therapy of oral mucositis. Break down and build up methods have been used to prepare drug nanocrystals, and we previously succeeded in preparing drug nanocrystals of indomethachin and tranilast with an average particle diameter smaller than 100 nm by applying the bead mill method in the presence of various excipients, such as a cellulose compound and cyclodextrin [40,41]. Moreover, we showed that these drug nanocrystals show high mucoadhesive properties and bioavailability in the small intestine of rats [42,43]. Therefore, we tried to prepare nanocrystals of REB according to our previous protocol [40,41]. The particle size of the REB in the R-NPs gel was in the range of 50–180 nm (Figure 1C,D), so even the largest particle was smaller than 200 nm. Moreover, REB nanocrystals were dispersed uniformly in the hydrogel (Figure 1A) and were released from the R-NPs gel to a significantly greater extent than the R-MPs gel. In addition, REB was released from the hydrogel as drug nanocrystals, since REB nanocrystals were detected in the reservoir chamber of the Franz diffusion cell after passage through a 220 nm pore membrane (Figure 3).

The cheek pouches of a hamster represent a stable environment and drugs that are taken into them do not get washed away. Therefore, wounds in a hamster's cheek pouch are widely used as an animal model for the study of drug accumulation and the therapeutic effect on oral mucositis. We used this model in our study and found that the accumulation and persistence of REB in the cheek pouch of hamsters treated with the R-NPs gel were remarkably higher in comparison with treatment using the R-MPs gel (Figure 4A). This showed that the cellular uptake of REB nanocrystals was higher than microcrystals in the oral mucosa. In addition, R-NPs gel provided a significant increase in wound healing (Figure 5). The mucosal epithelium of acetic acid-denatured cheek pouch tissues underwent regeneration following treatment with R-MPs and R-NPs, and the number of inflammatory cells observed in the mucosal lamina propria were reduced in comparison with the None and Vehicle treatment groups. Treatment with both the R-MPs and R-NPs gels produced regeneration of the layered structure of the mucosal epithelium, but regeneration was greater in hamsters treated with the R-NPs gel (Figure 6). These results suggest that the REB particle size is suitable for use in a DDS to the oral mucosa, and show that treatment with the R-NPs gel can provide effective therapy for oral wound healing. On the other hand, no REB was detected in the plasma of hamsters treated with either hydrogel. The levels of blood flow and blood volume in the hamster cheek pouch may relate to the non-systemic distribution of REB. These results suggest that the therapeutic effect on oral wound healing by REB is local and not a systemic side effect in the hamster model.

It is important to clarify the mechanism for the enhancement of accumulation, persistence and therapeutic effect of REB in the cheek pouch of hamsters treated with R-NPs gel. In general, solubility is related to tissue penetration and cell uptake, and the solubility of REB in the R-NPs gel was increased by bead mill treatment. Cyclodextrin shows an inclusion ability for drugs, and inclusion enhances the solubility of poorly soluble drugs such as REB. In fact, the solubility of REB in an R-MPs gel without HPβCD is 0.0043 ± 0.0004 fM ($n = 5$), and the liquid REB levels in the hydrogel are lower than in the R-MPs gel containing 5% HPβCD. We also measured REB solubility in the R-NPs gel without 5% HPβCD and found it to be 0.016 ± 0.003 fM ($n = 5$). Thus, the amount of liquid REB is decreased when HPβCD is removed from the R-MPs gel formulation. However, the liquid REB level in the hydrogel formulation incorporating REB nanocrystals and 5% HPβCD was similar to that of the R-MPs gel These results suggest that the inclusion ability of the drug by HPβCD is enhanced with a decrease in particle size and is related to the increase in REB solubility. Both the liquid (solution) and crystalline types are mixed in the hydrogel formulations incorporating REB nanocrystals, and this enhancement of REB solubility may affect REB release from the hydrogel and uptake into the tissue. Otherwise, the amount of liquid REB in the hydrogel was small, with almost all REB existing as nanocrystals Therefore, we also investigated the mechanism for the accumulation of drug nanocrystals in the cheek pouch tissue.

The rate of mucosal absorption and retention of drug nanocrystals with a particle diameter smaller than 200 nm is high [29–32,43], and energy-dependent endocytosis is related to drug uptake in the cells and tissues of the small intestine [42]. Considering this, we investigated whether energy-dependent endocytosis is related to the uptake of REB nanocrystals into cheek pouch tissue by using various inhibitors of energy-dependent endocytosis. Energy-dependent endocytosis is classified into four pathways: Phagocytosis, MP, CME and CavME [44,45]. Large particles (0.5–5 μm) are taken up by phagocytosis, and somewhat smaller particles (100 nm–5 μm) are taken up by MP. CME and CavME relate to the uptake of particles smaller than those taken up by MP: <120 nm for CME and <80 nm for CavME [46]. Each of these energy-dependent endocytosis pathways can be specifically inhibited by different inhibitors: 10 μM cytochalasin D inhibits phagocytosis [36], 2 μM rottlerin inhibits MP [37], 40 μM dynasore inhibits CME [38] and 54 μM nystatin inhibits CavME [36]. Co-treatment of R-NPs gel and either cytochalasin D, rottlerin or nystatin had no effect of the amount of REB taken up by cheek pouch tissue. REB content in the cheek pouch of hamsters co-treated with R-NPs gel and dynasore were significantly decreased (Figure 4B,C). These results suggest that the REB nanocrystals are taken up into cheek pouch tissue by the CME pathway, resulting in the enhancement of wound healing (Figures 5 and 6).

5. Conclusions

We designed a hydrogel formulation incorporating REB nanocrystals (R-NPs gel) and found that most of the REB is released from the hydrogel as drug nanocrystals, which are taken up into the tissue through the CME pathway. REB provides a persistent effect, resulting in an enhancement of oral wound healing. It is possible that the R-NPs gel can provide useful therapy for serious oral mucositis. The development of formulations incorporating drug nanocrystals, such as hydrogels and mouthwashes, may be helpful when designing oral DDS for poorly soluble drugs.

Author Contributions: Conceptualization, N.N.; Data curation, R.S., S.D., H.O. and N.Y.; Formal analysis, R.S., S.D., H.O., N.H. and N.Y.; Funding acquisition, N.N.; Investigation, R.S., S.D., H.O., N.H. and N.Y.; Methodology, N.N., R.S., H.S. and N.Y.; Supervision, N.N.; Visualization, N.N.; Writing—original draft, N.N., H.S. and N.Y.; Writing—review & editing, N.N. All authors have read and agreed to the published version of the manuscript.

References

1. Sciubba, J.J.; Goldenberg, D. Oral complications of radiotherapy. *Lancet Oncol.* **2006**, *7*, 175–183. [CrossRef]
2. Rodríguez-Caballero, A.; Torres-Lagares, D.; Robles-García, M.; Pachón-Ibáñez, J.; González-Padilla, D.; Gutiérrez-Pérez, J.L. Cancer treatment-induced oral mucositis: A critical review. *Int. J. Oral Maxillofac. Surg.* **2012**, *41*, 225–238. [CrossRef]
3. Donnelly, J.P.; Blijlevens, N.M.; Verhagen, C.A. Can anything be done about oral mucositis? *Ann. Oncol.* **2003**, *14*, 505–507. [CrossRef]
4. Sonis, S.T. Oral mucositis in cancer therapy. *J. Support. Oncol.* **2004**, *2*, 3–8.
5. Trotti, A.; Bellm, L.A.; Epstein, J.B.; Frame, D.; Fuchs, H.J.; Gwede, C.K.; Komaroff, E.; Nalysnyk, L.; Zilberberg, M.D. Mucositis incidence, severity and associated outcomes in patients with head and neck cancer receiving radiotherapy with or without chemotherapy: A systematic literature review. *Radiother. Oncol.* **2003**, *66*, 253–262. [CrossRef]
6. Sonis, S.T.; Elting, L.S.; Keefe, D.; Peterson, D.E.; Schubert, M.; Hauer-Jensen, M.; Bekele, B.N.; Raber-Durlacher, J.; Donnelly, J.P.; Rubenstein, E.B. Perspectives on cancer therapy-induced mucosal injury: Pathogenesis, measurement, epidemiology, and consequences for patients. *Cancer* **2004**, *100*, 1995–2025. [CrossRef] [PubMed]
7. Prescribing Information: Mucosta®Tablets 100 mg, Ohtsuka Japan Inc. 2017. Available online: https://www.pmda.go.jp/PmdaSearch/iyakuDetail/GeneralList/2329021 (accessed on 20 May 2020). (In Japanese).
8. Lalla, R.V.; Bowen, J.; Barasch, A.; Elting, L.; Epstein, J.; Keefe, D.M.; McGuire, D.B.; Migliorati, C.; Nicolatou-Galitis, O.; Peterson, D.E.; et al. MASCC/ISOO clinical practice guidelines for the management of mucositis secondary to cancer therapy. *Cancer* **2014**, *120*, 1453–1461. [CrossRef] [PubMed]
9. Bensinger, W.; Schubert, M.; Ang, K.K.; Brizel, D.; Brown, E.; Eilers, J.G.; Elting, L.; Mittal, B.B.; Schattner, M.A.; Spielberger, R.; et al. NCCN Task Force Report. prevention and management of mucositis in cancer care. *J. Natl. Compr. Cancer Netw.* **2008**, *6*, S1–S21; quiz S22–S24.
10. Peterson, D.E.; Boers-Doets, C.B.; Bensadoun, R.J.; Herrstedt, J. ESMO Guidelines Committee Management of oral and gastrointestinal mucosal injury: ESMO Clinical Practice Guidelines for diagnosis, treatment, and follow-up. *Ann. Oncol.* **2015**, *26*, v139–v151. [CrossRef] [PubMed]
11. Murakami, K.; Okajima, K.; Uchiba, M.; Harada, N.; Johno, M.; Okabe, H.; Takatsuki, K. Rebamipide attenuates indomethacin-induced gastric mucosal lesion formation by inhibiting activation of leukocytes in rats. *Dig. Dis. Sci.* **1997**, *42*, 319–325. [CrossRef] [PubMed]
12. Yoshikawa, T.; Naito, Y.; Tanigawa, T.; Kondo, M. Free radical scavenging activity of the novel anti-ulcer agent rebsamipide studied by electron spin resonance. *Arzneimittelforschung* **1993**, *43*, 363–366. [PubMed]
13. Nanke, Y.; Kobashigawa, T.; Yago, T.; Kawamoto, M.; Yamanaka, H.; Kotake, S. Rebamipide, an Amino Acid Analog of 2(1H)-Quinolinone, Inhibits the Formation of Human Osteoclasts. *BioMed Res. Int.* **2016**, *2016*, 6824719. [CrossRef] [PubMed]
14. Tanaka, H.; Fukuda, K.; Ishida, W.; Harada, Y.; Sumi, T.; Fukushima, A. Rebamipide increases barrier function and attenuates TNFalpha-induced barrier disruption and cytokine expression in human corneal epithelial cells. *Br. J. Ophthalmol.* **2013**, *97*, 912–916. [CrossRef] [PubMed]

15. Yasuda, T.; Chiba, H.; Satomi, T.; Matsuo, A.; Kaneko, T.; Chikazu, D.; Miyamatsu, H. Preventive effect of rebamipide gargle on chemoradiotherpy-induced oral mucositis in patients with oral cancer: A pilot study. *J. Oral Maxillofac. Res.* **2011**, *2*, e3. [CrossRef] [PubMed]
16. Nabeta, I.; Nakamura, K.; Kimura, M.; Kaya, M.; Tsuneizumi, M.; Nakagami, K.; Kawarasaki, T.; Honma, M. The effect of rebamipide for prevention of mucositis associated with anthracycline chemotherapy for breast cancer. *J. Jpn. Soc. Hosp. Pharm.* **2010**, *46*, 1629–1634. (In Japanese)
17. Chaitanya, B.; Pai, K.M.; Yathiraj, P.H.; Fernandes, D.; Chhaparwal, Y. Rebamipide gargle in preventive management of chemo-radiotherapy induced oral mucositis. *Oral Oncol.* **2017**, *72*, 179–182. [CrossRef]
18. Yokota, T.; Ogawa, T.; Takahashi, S.; Okami, K.; Fujii, T.; Tanaka, K.; Iwae, S.; Ota, I.; Ueda, T.; Monden, N.; et al. Efficacy and safety of rebamipide liquid for chemoradiotherapy-induced oral mucositis in patients with head and neck cancer: A multicenter, randomized, double-blind, placebo-controlled, parallel-group phase II study. *BMC Cancer* **2017**, *17*, 314. [CrossRef]
19. Ishihara, K.; Komuro, Y.; Nishiyama, N.; Yamasaki, K.; Hotta, K. Effect of rebamipide on mucus secretion by endogenous prostaglandin-independent mechanism in rat gastric mucosa. *Arzneimittelforschung* **1992**, *42*, 1462–1466.
20. Yamasaki, K.; Kanbe, T.; Chijiwa, T.; Ishiyama, H.; Morita, S. Gastric mucosal protection by OPC-12759, a novel antiulcer compound, in the rat. *Eur. J. Pharmacol.* **1987**, *142*, 23–29. [CrossRef]
21. Kleine, A.; Kluge, S.; Peskar, B.M. Stimulation of prostaglandin biosynthesis mediates gastroprotective effect of rebamipide in rats. *Dig. Dis. Sci.* **1993**, *38*, 1441–1449. [CrossRef]
22. Nagano, C.; Azuma, A.; Ishiyama, H.; Sekiguchi, K.; Imagawa, K.; Kikuchi, M. Rebamipide suppresses formyl-methionyl-leucylphenylalanine (fMLP)-induced superoxide production by inhibiting fMLP-receptor binding in human neutrophils. *J. Pharmacol. Exp. Ther.* **2001**, *297*, 388–394.
23. Kobayashi, T.; Zinchuk, V.S.; del Saz, E.G.; Jiang, F.; Yamasaki, Y.; Kataoka, S.; Okada, T.; Tsunawaki, S.; Seguchi, H. Suppressive effect of rebamipide, an antiulcer agent, against activation of human neutrophils exposed to formyl-methionyl-leucyl-phenylalanine. *Histol. Histopathol.* **2000**, *15*, 1067–1076.
24. Masamune, A.; Yoshida, M.; Sakai, Y.; Shimosegawa, T. Rebamipide inhibits ceramide-induced interleukin-8 production in Kato III human gastric cancer cells. *J. Pharmacol. Exp. Ther.* **2001**, *298*, 485–492.
25. Kim, C.D.; Kim, H.H.; Hong, K.W. Inhibitory effect of rebamipide on the neutrophil adherence stimulated by conditioned media from helicobacter pylori-infected gastric epithelial cells. *J. Pharmacol. Exp. Ther.* **1999**, *288*, 133–138.
26. Arakawa, T.; Kobayashi, K.; Yoshikawa, T.; Tarnawski, A. Rebamipide: Overview of its mechanisms of action and efficacy in mucosal protection and ulcer healing. *Dig. Dis. Sci.* **1998**, *43*, 5S–13S.
27. Tarnawski, A.; Arakawa, T.; Kobayashi, K. Rebamipide treatment activates epidermal growth factor and its receptor expression in normal and ulcerated gastric mucosa in rats: One mechanism for its ulcer healing action? *Dig. Dis. Sci.* **1998**, *43*, 90S–98S.
28. Shioya, Y.; Kashiyama, E.; Okada, K.; Kusumoto, N.; Abe, Y. Metabolic fate of the anti-ulcer agent, (±)-2-(4-chlorobenzoylamino)-3-[2(1H)-quinolinon-4-yl]propionic acid (OPC-12759): Absorption, distribution, and excretion in rats and dogs. *Iyakuhin Kenkyu* **1989**, *20*, 522–533.
29. Sanders, N.N.; De Smedt, S.C.; Van Rompaey, E.; Simoens, P.; De Baets, F.; Demeester, J. Cystic fibrosis sputum: A barrier to the transport of nanospheres. *Am. J. Respir. Crit. Care Med.* **2000**, *162*, 1905–1911. [CrossRef]
30. Szentkuti, L. Light microscopical observations on luminally administered dyes, dextrans, nanospheres and microspheres in the pre-epithelial mucus gel layer of the rat distal colon. *J. Control. Release* **1997**, *46*, 233–242. [CrossRef]
31. Norris, D.A.; Sinko, P.J. Effect of size, surface charge and hydrophobicity on the translocation of polyestyrene microspheres through gastrointestinal mucin. *J. Appl. Polym. Sci.* **1997**, *63*, 1481–1492. [CrossRef]
32. Bravo-Osuna, I.; Vauthier, C.; Farabollini, A.; Palmieri, G.F.; Ponchel, G. Mucoadhesion mechanism of chitosan and thiolated chitosan-poly(isobutyl cyanoacrylate) core-shell nanoparticles. *Biomaterials* **2007**, *28*, 2233–2243. [CrossRef]
33. Nagai, N.; Ishii, M.; Seiriki, R.; Ogata, F.; Otake, H.; Nakazawa, Y.; Okamoto, N.; Kanai, K.; Kawasaki, N. Novel Sustained-Release Drug Delivery System for Dry Eye Therapy by Rebamipide Nanoparticles. *Pharmaceutics* **2020**, *12*, 155. [CrossRef]

34. Nagai, N.; Iwamae, A.; Tanimoto, S.; Yoshioka, C.; Ito, Y. Pharmacokinetics and Antiinflammatory Effect of a Novel Gel System Containing Ketoprofen Solid Nanoparticles. *Biol. Pharm. Bull.* **2015**, *38*, 1918–1924. [CrossRef]
35. Nagai, N.; Ogata, F.; Otake, H.; Nakazawa, Y.; Kawasaki, N. Design of a transdermal formulation containing raloxifene nanoparticles for osteoporosis treatment. *Int. J. Nanomed.* **2018**, *13*, 5215–5229. [CrossRef]
36. Mäger, I.; Langel, K.; Lehto, T.; Eiríksdóttir, E.; Langel, U. The role of endocytosis on the uptake kinetics of luciferin-conjugated cell-penetrating peptides. *Biochim. Biophys. Acta Biomembr.* **2012**, *1818*, 502–511. [CrossRef]
37. Hufnagel, H.; Hakim, P.; Lima, A.; Hollfelder, F. Fluid phase endocytosis contributes to transfection of DNA by PEI-25. *Mol. Ther.* **2009**, *17*, 1411–1417. [CrossRef]
38. Malomouzh, A.I.; Mukhitov, A.R.; Proskurina, S.E.; Vyskocil, F.; Nikolsky, E.E. The effect of dynasore, a blocker of dynamin-dependent endocytosis, on spontaneous quantal and non-quantal release of acetylcholine in murine neuromuscular junctions. *Dokl. Biol. Sci.* **2014**, *459*, 330–333. [CrossRef]
39. Nicolatou-Galitis, O.; Sarri, T.; Bowen, J.; Di Palma, M.; Kouloulias, V.E.; Niscola, P.; Riesenbeck, D.; Stokman, M.; Tissing, W.; Yeoh, E.; et al. Systematic review of anti-inflammatory agents for the management of oral mucositis in cancer patients. *Support. Care Cancer* **2013**, *21*, 3179–3189. [CrossRef]
40. Nagai, N.; Ito, Y.; Okamoto, N.; Shimomura, Y. A nanoparticle formulation reduces the corneal toxicity of indomethacin eye drops and enhances its corneal permeability. *Toxicology* **2014**, *319*, 53–62. [CrossRef]
41. Nagai, N.; Ito, Y. Therapeutic Effects of Gel Ointments containing Tranilast Nanoparticles on Paw Edema in Adjuvant-Induced Arthritis Rats. *Biol. Pharm. Bull.* **2014**, *37*, 96–104. [CrossRef]
42. Ishii, M.; Fukuoka, Y.; Deguchi, S.; Otake, H.; Tanino, T.; Nagai, N. Energy-Dependent Endocytosis is Involved in the Absorption of Indomethacin Nanoparticles in the Small Intestine. *Int. J. Mol. Sci.* **2019**, *20*, 476. [CrossRef] [PubMed]
43. Nagai, N.; Ito, Y. Effect of Solid Nanoparticle of Indomethacin on Therapy for Rheumatoid Arthritis in Adjuvant-Induced Arthritis Rat. *Biol. Pharm. Bull.* **2014**, *37*, 1109–1118. [CrossRef] [PubMed]
44. Wang, J.; Byrne, J.D.; Napier, M.E.; DeSimone, J.M. More effective nanomedicines through particle design. *Small* **2011**, *7*, 1919–1931. [CrossRef] [PubMed]
45. Rappoport, J.Z. Focusing on clathrin-mediated endocytosis. *Biochem. J.* **2008**, *412*, 415–423. [CrossRef]
46. Zhang, S.; Li, J.; Lykotrafitis, G.; Bao, G.; Suresh, S. Size-dependent endocytosis of nanoparticles. *Adv. Mater.* **2009**, *21*, 419–424. [CrossRef]

3

Assessing Drug Interaction and Pharmacokinetics of Loxoprofen in Mice Treated with CYP3A Modulators

Sanjita Paudel [1], Aarajana Shrestha [2], Piljoung Cho [1], Riya Shrestha [1], Younah Kim [1], Taeho Lee [1], Ju-Hyun Kim [2], Tae Cheon Jeong [2], Eung-Seok Lee [2] and Sangkyu Lee [1,*]

1 BK21 Plus KNU Multi-Omics based Creative Drug Research Team, College of Pharmacy, Research Institute of Pharmaceutical Sciences, Kyungpook National University, Daegu 41566, Korea; sanjitapdl99@gmail.com (S.P.); whvlfwjd@naver.com (P.C.); riya.shrestha07@gmail.com (R.S.); younah86@naver.com (Y.K.); tlee@knu.ac.kr (T.L.)

2 College of Pharmacy, Yeungnam University, Gyeongsan 38541, Korea; aarajanashrestha1@gmail.com (A.S.); jhkim@yu.ac.kr (J.-H.K.); taecheon@ynu.ac.kr (T.C.J.); eslee@ynu.ac.kr (E.-S.L.)

* Correspondence: sangkyu@knu.ac.kr

Abstract: Loxoprofen (LOX) is a non-selective cyclooxygenase inhibitor that is widely used for the treatment of pain and inflammation caused by chronic and transitory conditions. Its alcoholic metabolites are formed by carbonyl reductase (CR) and they consist of trans-LOX, which is active and cis-LOX, which is inactive. In addition, LOX can also be converted into an inactive hydroxylated metabolite (OH-LOXs) by cytochrome P450 (CYP). In a previous study, we reported that CYP3A4 is primarily responsible for the formation of OH-LOX in human liver microsomes. Although metabolism by CYP3A4 does not produce active metabolites, it can affect the conversion of LOX into trans-/cis-LOX since CYP3A4 activity modulates the substrate LOX concentration. Although the pharmacokinetics (PK) and metabolism of LOX have been well defined, its CYP-related interactions have not been fully characterized. Therefore, we investigated the metabolism of LOX after pretreatment with dexamethasone (DEX) and ketoconazole (KTC), which induce and inhibit the activities of CYP3A respectively. We monitored their effects on the PK parameters of LOX, cis-LOX, and trans-LOX in mice, and demonstrated that their PK parameters significantly changed in the presence of DEX or KTC pretreatment. Specifically, DEX significantly decreased the concentration of the LOX active metabolite formed by CR, which corresponded to an increased concentration of OH-LOX formed by CYP3A4. The opposite result occurred with KTC (a CYP3A inhibitor) pretreatment. Thus, we conclude that concomitant use of LOX with CYP3A modulators may lead to drug–drug interactions and result in minor to severe toxicity even though there is no direct change in the metabolic pathway that forms the LOX active metabolite.

Keywords: Loxoprofen; drug-drug interaction; CYP3A; Dexamethasone; Ketoconazole

1. Introduction

Loxoprofen (LOX) is an anti-inflammatory prodrug (NSAID) with potential antipyretic and analgesic properties, but its side effects are less defined when compared to other NSAIDs [1–3]. It is one of the most clinically prescribed NSAIDs in Japan, and it is also popular in Eastern Asia, the Middle East, Latin America, and Africa [1]. It is a well-known cyclo-oxygenase (COX1 and COX2) inhibitor that reduces the synthesis of inflammatory agents such as prostaglandins [2,4,5]. It is also widely used for the management of pain and inflammation in chronic and transient conditions (e.g., toothache, headache, menstrual cramps, common cold, etc.) [1,2,6].

Although LOX has fewer sides effects than other NSAIDs, many adverse effects have been reported such as GI disorders (erosive gastritis and bleeding), renal disorders, cardiovascular disorders, headaches, anaphylaxis, and abdominal pain [1,2,6,7]. Moreover, the use of LOX with drugs such as methotrexate, warfarin, aspirin, and valacyclovir is contraindicated [6,8–10]. Generally, the pharmacokinetic (PK) parameters of many drugs are influenced by the inhibition or induction of cytochrome P450 enzymes (CYPs) [11], which can result in various drug interactions, toxicity, and either an increase or decrease in drug activity [12].

Previous studies have extensively investigated the metabolic activities of LOX in various organisms such as rats, mice, monkeys, rabbits, and humans [1,13,14]. However, to the best of our knowledge, there is still a large gap in knowledge regarding the interactions of LOX with other drugs that may cause simple to severe adverse drug interactions. The alcoholic metabolites of LOX (cis-LOX and trans-LOX) are mainly produced by carbonyl reductase (CR), and trans-LOX is the only active metabolite derived from LOX, which LOX is a pharmacologically inactive drug unless it is metabolized to trans-LOX [1,5]. In addition to CR, LOX is also metabolized by CYP450. In our previous study, we reported that the CYP-mediated metabolism of LOX was catalyzed by CYP3A4 and CYP3A5 to form hydroxylated LOX (OH-LOX). We also found that an inactive metabolite of LOX catalyzed by CYP was significantly higher in dexamethasone (DEX)-induced liver microsomes [15].

It is well known that CYP3A4 is most abundant in the liver, and it can catalyze approximately 50% of commercially available drugs [16,17]. Many commercial drugs are known to regulate the activity of CYP3A, and they may be clinically administered with LOX. The CYP3A/LOX metabolic pathway produces an inactive metabolite and competes with another pathway for LOX that produces the active metabolite. If LOX is co-administered with a drug that modulates the activity of CYP3A, there may be possible drug interactions affecting the concentration of LOX or the active metabolite of LOX. Thus, we investigated the interaction of LOX with CYP3A by monitoring the effects of DEX (a CYP3A inducer) or ketoconazole (KTC, a CYP3A inhibitor) pretreatment on the PK parameters of LOX, cis-LOX, and trans-LOX in an ICR mouse model.

2. Materials and Methods

2.1. Materials

LOX (2-(4-((2-Oxocyclopentyl)methyl)phenyl)propanoic acid, $C_{15}H_{13}O_3$, CAS ID 68767-14-5) was procured from Tokyo Chemicals Industry (Tokyo, Japan). LOX was used to synthesize cis-LOX and trans-LOX ((2*S*)-2-[4-[[(1*R*,2*S*)-2-hydroxycyclopentyl]methyl]phenyl]propanoic acid, $C_{15}H_{20}O_3$, CAS ID 83648-76-4) with purities of 96.5% and 97.9%, respectively [18]. DEX, KTC, dextromethorphan, and phenacetin were purchased from Sigma-Aldrich Co., LLC. (St. Louis, MO, USA) while midazolam was procured from Bukwang Pharmaceutical Co., Ltd. (Seoul, Korea). Mass spectrometry (MS) grade water and acetonitrile (ACN) were obtained from Fischer Scientific (Pittsburgh, PA, USA).

2.2. Animal Treatments and Sample Preparations

Male ICR mice (36 mice of 5 weeks) were purchased from Orient Co. (Seongnam, Korea) andwere randomly divided into 4–6 mice per cage. Then, the mice were acclimatized for 1 week in a controlled environment (relative humidity: 60%, temperature: 25 °C) under a 12-h/12-h light/dark cycle and supplied standard rodent chow and tap water freely. All animal handling procedures followed protocols issued by the Society of Toxicology (USA, 1989) and were approved on March 21, 2019 by the Institutional Review Board of Kyungpook National University (project ID # 2019-41).

The acclimatized animals were divided into eight groups, with each group containing 3 mice: groups I and II, vehicle (corn oil); groups III and IV, DEX-treated; groups V and VI, vehicle (10% Ethanol); and groups VII and VIII, KTC-treated group. Briefly, groups I and II were intraperitoneally (*i.p.*) treated with corn oil for 3 days while DEX (dissolved in corn oil and administered at 40 mg/kg) was given to groups III and IV for 3 consecutive days [19]. Then, animals were fasted for 12 hours with free access to water before starting the experiment. After fasting, LOX (20 mg/kg) was administered orally to groups I, II, III, and IV. Ethanol (10%) and KTC (60 mg/kg) were administered *i.p.* to the vehicle-treated groups (V and VI) and KTC-treated groups (VII and VIII), respectively [20], and after 3 min, LOX was given orally (20 mg/kg).

After the oral administration of LOX, blood from groups I, III, V, and VII was collected from the tail at 0, 5, 10, 15, 30, 60, 120, and 240 min post-administration and placed into sodium heparin-containing tubes. After the last blood collection, the mice were sacrificed by cervical dislocation. Plasma was then prepared by centrifuging the blood at 4000× *g* for 15 min at 4 °C and stored at −80 °C until analysis. For analysis, each sample was prepared by mixing plasma (10 μL) and 90 μL of ACN containing 0.1% formic acid and 5 μM of tolbutamide as an internal standard (IS). The samples were then vortexed and centrifuged at 13,000× *g* for 10 min at 4 °C. Finally, 10 μL of sample supernatant was injected into the LC-MS/MS system. The PK parameters (the maximum plasma concentration [C_{max}], time to reach the maximum plasma concentration [T_{max}], elimination half-life [$T_{1/2}$], and area under the plasma concentrations [AUC]) were analyzed by WinNonlin software (Version 2.1, Scientific Consulting, Louisville, KY, USA).

Similarly, blood from groups II, IV, VI, and VIII was collected from the hepatic portal vein 10 min post-LOX administration to identify metabolites of LOX and to analyze drug–drug interactions. Plasma from these samples was prepared as explained above. Then, 300 μL of ACN having 0.1% formic acid and 5 μM of the IS were mixed with 100 μL of each plasma sample. Next, the samples were vortexed and centrifuged at 13,000× *g* for 10 min at 4 °C. Supernatants were transferred into tubes and dried using a Labconco Speed Vac (Labconco Corporation, Kansas City, MO, USA). The dried samples were reconstituted using 100 μL of 50% methanol and centrifuged at 13,000× *g* for 10 min at 4 °C. Each supernatant was transferred into an LCMS vial, and 5 μL were injected into a high-resolution mass spectrometer (HRMS).

2.3. CYP Activities in the Mouse Liver

Male ICR mice were divided into 4 groups with each group containing 3 mice: group I, vehicle (corn oil); group II, DEX-treated; group III, vehicle (10% Ethanol); and group IV, KTC-treated group. Group I was treated with corn oil for 3 days while DEX (dissolved in corn oil and administered at 40 mg/kg) was administered *i.p.* to group II for 3 consecutive days [19]. Similarly, group III and group IV were treated once with 10% ethanol or KTC (60 mg/kg), respectively [20]. Twenty-four hours after the last treatment, the liver was excised and homogenized with three volumes of ice-cold 0.1 M potassium phosphate buffer (pH 7.4). The supernatant fraction was then separated as the S9 fraction from the mixture by centrifugation at 9000× *g* at 4 °C and stored at −80 °C until use.

To characterize the CYP activities in the harvested livers, phenacetin *O*-demethylation (using 80 μM of phenacetin) for CYP1A, dextromethorphan *O*-demethylation (using 5 μM of dextromethorphan) for CYP2D, and midazolam 1′-hydroxylation (using 5 μM of midazolam) for CYP3A were used as cocktail probe reactions [21,22]. The level of protein in the S9 fraction was determined by Bradford assay [23]. The cocktail probes were then incubated with 10 μL of each S9 fraction, potassium phosphate buffer (pH 7.4), and an NADPH generating system (NGS) in a final volume of 100 μL. After incubation for 30 min at 37 °C, ice-cold ACN containing 0.1% formic acid and IS (5 μM) was added to stop the reaction. Samples were then vortexed and centrifuged at 13,000× *g* for 10 min at 4 °C. Finally, the supernatants were transferred to LC-MS/MS vials for analysis.

2.4. Instrument and Data Acquisition

A Shimadzu Prominence UFLC system (Kyoto, Japan) connected to a TSQ vantage triple quadrupole mass spectrometer with a HESI-II spray source incorporated with a DGU-20A$_5$ degasser, an LC-20AD pump, a SIL-20A autosampler, and a CTO-20A column oven was used for the analyses. A shim-pack GIS C18 column (150 × 3.0 mm, 3 μM) was used to separate analytes in the samples. Mobile phases A and B were composed of water with formic acid and ACN with 0.1% formic acid, respectively, and the flow rate was 0.50 mL/min at 40 °C. The gradient conditions were as follows: 20% of B between 0 and 0.25 min, 20–80% of B between 0.25 and 9.75 min, 80–20% of B between 9.75 and 10 min, and 20% of B between 10 and 13 min. The MS was operated under the following conditions: electrospray ionization in negative mode at 3.0 kV, capillary temperature at 350 °C, vaporizer temperature at 300 °C, sheath gas pressure at 35 Arb, and auxiliary gas pressure at 10 Arb. Finally, Xcalibur software (Thermo Fisher Scientific Inc., Waltham, MA, USA) was used for data analysis.

HRMS coupled with ultrahigh performance liquid chromatography (UHPLC) was used to detect hydroxy-LOX and other metabolites of LOX. The UHPLC system, Dionex Ultimate 3000 (Dionex Softron GmbH, Germering, Germany) consisted of an HPG-3200SD Standard binary pump, a WPS 3000 TRS analytical autosampler, and a TCC-3000 SD column compartment. In this experiment, the HRMS was a Q Exactive Focus quadrupole-Orbitrap MS (Thermo Fisher Scientific, Bremen, Germany) equipped with a heated electrospray ionization (HESI-II) ion probe.

LOX was detected as a deprotonated ion $[M\text{-}H]^-$ at m/z 245.1175 in negative ion mode. Therefore, negative ion mode was used with the following optimized conditions for LOX: spray voltage of 2.5 kV, capillary temperature of 320 °C, auxiliary gas at 12 aux unit, aux gas heater temperature of 200 °C, sheath gas at 35 aux units, and S-lens RF level of 50. LOX and its metabolites were separated using a 150 mm × 2.1 mm, 2.6-μm reverse-phase liquid chromatography column, Kinetex® C18 column (Phenomenex, CA, USA) at 40 °C. Furthermore, MS-grade solvents were used as the mobile phase in gradient elution mode: 0.1% aqueous formic acid as Solvent A and 0.1% formic acid in ACN as Solvent B. The flow was set to 0.22 mL/min with a gradient condition of Solvent B as 10% between 0 and 0.5 min, 10–50% between 0.5 and 21.5 min, 50–95% between 21.5 and 22.5 min, 95% between 22.5 and 25.5 min, 95–10% between 25.5 and 25.6 min, and 10% between 25.6 and 30 min.

2.5. Method Validation

Stock solutions of LOX, cis-LOX, and trans-Lox (40 mg/mL) were prepared in methanol to generate a calibration curve and linearity. The concentrations of LOX in plasma used to generate the calibration curve were 0.1, 0.2, 0.5, 1.0, 5.0, 10.0, 20.0, and 40.0 μg/mL. The concentrations of cis-LOX and trans-LOX used to generate their calibration curves were 0.2, 0.5, 1.0, 5.0, 10.0, 20.0, and 40.0 μg/mL. An amount of 10 μL of these samples was processed as mentioned above for LC-MS/MS analysis. Area peak ratios of analytes/IS versus concentration of samples were used to prepare the calibration curves. The calibration equation of LOX was $y = 8 \times 10^{-7}x + 0.0002$ ($R^2 = 0.997$). The calibration equations for cis-LOX and trans-LOX were $y = 2 \times 10^{-6}x + 0.0002$ ($R^2 = 0.996$) and $y = 1 \times 10^{-6}x - 0.0002$ ($R^2 = 0.997$), respectively.

To evaluate the accuracy and precision of LOX measurements, mouse plasma was spiked with a known concentration of LOX or QC samples at 0.2, 1.0, 10.0, 40.0 μg/mL ($n = 5$). Similarly, the accuracy and precision of cis-LOX and trans-LOX measurements were evaluated by spiking mouse plasma with a known concentration of either compound or QC samples at 0.5, 5.0, and 40.0 μg/mL ($n = 5$). Moreover, the accuracy and precision of intraday and interday were analyzed on the same day and five consecutive days at each concentration.

2.6. Statistical Analysis

The results are presented as the mean and the standard error of the mean. A Student's unpaired t-test was applied in the statistical analyses of the obtained results using Graph Pad Prism. Results with a p-value ≤ 0.05, ≤ 0.01 and ≤ 0.001 were considered statistically significant.

3. Results

3.1. Identification of Loxoprofen and Its Metabolites

To determine the plasma concentration of LOX and its metabolites via LC-MS/MS analysis, the produced product ions were checked and optimized for each compound. The ion intensities of LOX, cis-LOX, and trans-LOX were high in the negative mode of ionization; therefore, all the conditions for analysis used the negative mode for LC-MS/MS analysis. The MRM transitions chosen for LOX cis-LOX, and trans-LOX were m/z 245.0 → 83.1, 247.1 → 202.2, and 247.1 → 203.1, respectively [15] Representative MRM chromatograms of LOX, cis-LOX, trans-LOX, and the IS in mouse plasma are presented in Figure S1. LOX, cis-LOX, trans-LOX, and the IS were eluted at 8.5, 8.0, 8.2, and 8.9 min respectively. No endogenous sources of interference were observed. LOX and its two metabolites were evaluated for linearity, precision, and accuracy. The calibration curves calculated within the range of 0.1–40.0 μg/mL for LOX and within the range of 0.2–40.0 μg/mL for cis-LOX and trans-LOX were linear. The precision (RSD %) range of LOX, cis-LOX, and trans-LOX was 1.8–12.9%, and the accuracy (RE %) range was less than 14.7% (Table S1). Thus, the values were within the acceptable range and the method was accurate and precise.

3.2. *Evaluation Model for Determination of LOX–Drug Interaction*

To evaluate the CYP3A-induced LOX interaction, we prepared an experimental model that regulated CYP3A activity by administering an inducer (DEX) and an inhibitor (KTC) of CYP3A into mice. Briefly, DEX in corn oil was administered up to 3 consecutive days to induce CYP3A. Inhibition of CYP3A was induced by a single dose of KTC in 10% ethanol. Only vehicle groups were administered with their respective solvents without the addition of a CYP3A inducer or inhibitor. The induction and inhibition of CYP3A were confirmed with CYP assay using five different probe substrates (Figure S2)

DEX increased the metabolism of CYP3A substrate (midazolam) by approximately 10-fold when compared to the vehicle (VH) group. KTC significantly decreased the metabolism of CYP3A4 substrate (midazolam) when compared to the VH group (Figure S2). However, the metabolic activities of other CYP enzymes were unaffected between VH and treated groups. Thus, we validated our method of specifically regulating CYP3A activity via DEX and KTC.

3.3. *Pharmacokinetic Analysis*

The validated method was applied to determine the concentration of LOX, cis-LOX, and trans-LOX in mice pretreated with DEX or KTC. After pretreatment, LOX was orally administered to mice (20 mg/kg) after a 12-h fasting period. The plasma concentrations of LOX, cis-LOX, and trans-LOX were significantly decreased in the DEX pretreated group (Figure 1). In the KTC pretreated group, the plasma concentrations of cis-LOX, and trans-LOX were significantly increased and the plasma concentration of LOX was also increased but not significantly (Figure 1).

The PK parameters of LOX, cis-LOX, and trans-Lox in the VH- (corn oil) and DEX-treated groups are shown in Table 1. Although blood was collected for up to 240 min, LOX and its metabolites were not detected after 60 min. The C_{max}, $AUC_{(0–60)}$, and $AUC_{(0–\infty)}$ of all three compounds were significantly lowered in the DEX-pretreated group as opposed to the VH group. In the DEX-treated group, the C_{max} of LOX, cis-LOX, and trans-LOX was 2.5 ± 0.2, 1.1 ± 0.2, and 2.1 ± 0.2 μg/mL, respectively, and the $AUC_{(0–60)}$ of the three compounds was 53.5 ± 6.1, 29.9 ± 4.4, and 67.6 ± 5.7 μg·min/mL, respectively. However, the T_{max} from all three compounds did not show any statistical difference when compared to the VH group. In contrast to the VH group, $AUC_{(0–\infty)}$ of LOX, cis-LOX, and trans-Lox in the DEX-treated group indicated a lower area under plasma concentration (56.2 ± 6.9, 31.5 ± 4.4, and 85.8 ± 5.0, respectively) over an extended time period. Moreover, the elimination $T_{1/2}$ of LOX, cis-LOX, and trans-Lox in the VH group was 14.9 ± 0.6, 12.3 ± 0.3, and 18.2 ± 0.6 min, respectively, which is significantly different from the respective elimination $T_{1/2}$ (12.0 ± 0.7, 13.9 ± 0.6, and 26.4 ± 1.6 min) generated by the DEX-pretreated group.

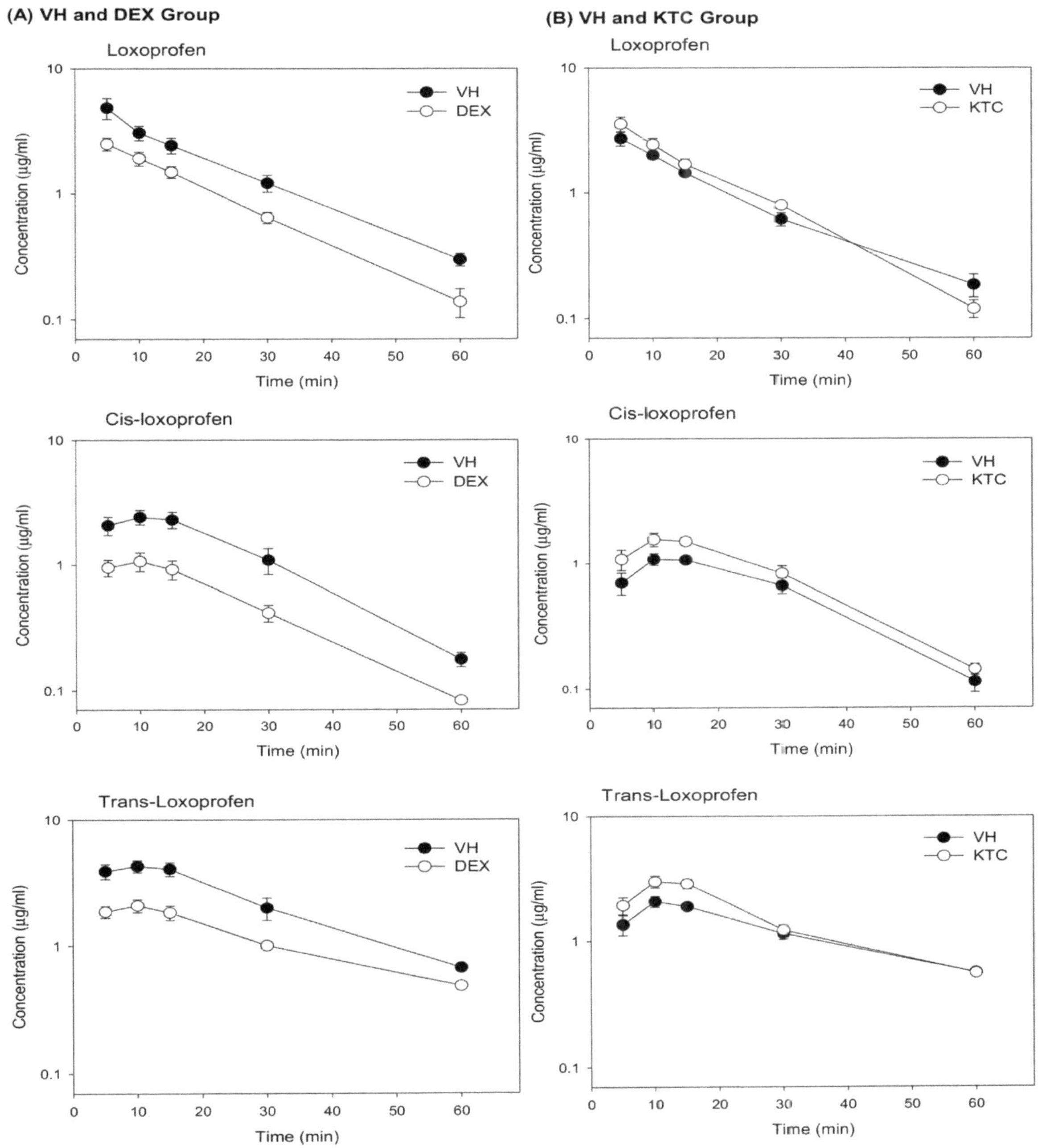

Figure 1. Mean plasma concentration versus time profiles of LOX, cis-LOX, and trans-LOX in either the presence of a CYP3A4 inducer (DEX) or inhibitor (KTC) with their respective vehicle. (**A**) Mean plasma concentration versus time profiles after *i.p.* administration of either VH (corn oil) or DEX (40 mg/kg) for 3 consecutive days. The plasma concentrations of all the compounds in the VH and DEX groups showed significant decrement up to 60 min in the DEX-treated group as compared to its VH group. The bars represent standard error (SE) ($n = 3$). (**B**) Mean plasma concentration versus time profiles after a single dose *i.p.* administration of either VH (10% ethanol) or KTC (60 mg/kg). In the KTC group, LOX, cis-LOX, and trans-LOX showed increased mean plasma concentrations as opposed to the VH group. The bars indicate standard error (SE) ($n = 3$).

Furthermore, the PK parameters for LOX, cis-LOX, and trans-LOX in the VH and KTC groups are represented in Table 2. The C_{max} of cis-LOX, and trans-LOX in the VH group (1.2 ± 0.1, and 2.1 ± 0.2 µg/mL, respectively) were significantly lower than those in the KTC-treated group (1.6 ± 0.1, and 3.1 ± 0.3 μg/mL, respectively). However, the T_{max} of these three compounds did not show significant variation between the VH and KTC groups. In contrast to the T_{max}, the elimination $T_{1/2}$ of trans-LOX in the VH group (26.0 ± 0.5 min) was statistically different from that in the KTC-treated group (19.8 ± 0.7 min). Moreover, The $AUC_{(0-60)}$ for, cis-LOX, and trans-LOX in the KTC-treated group was 49.0 ± 5.9, and 80.4 ± 9.6 μg·min/mL, respectively, which were higher than the respective values generated by the VH group. Altogether, the PK data generated by the DEX- and KTC-treated groups and their respective VH indicate that DEX and KTC significantly affected the PK of cis-LOX, and trans-LOX but PK of LOX was only affected by DEX, even though the formation of cis-LOX and trans-LOX was regulated by CR.

Table 1. Pharmacokinetic parameters of loxoprofen (LOX), cis-LOX, and trans-LOX in VH- (corn oil) and dexamethasone (DEX)-treated groups.

Analytes	Parameters	VH (Corn Oil)	DEX
LOX	C_{max} (μg/mL)	4.8 ± 0.9	2.5 ± 0.2 **
	T_{max} (min)	5.0 ± 0.0	5.0 ± 0.0
	$AUC_{(0-60)}$ (μg·min/mL)	95.7 ± 14.5	53.5 ± 6.1 **
	$T_{1/2}$ (min)	14.9 ± 0.6	12.0 ± 0.7 *
	$AUC_{(0-\infty)}$ (μg·min/mL)	102.2 ± 15.0	56.2 ± 6.9 ***
cis-LOX	C_{max} (μg/mL)	2.4 ± 0.3	1.1 ± 0.2 **
	T_{max} (min)	10.4 ± 0.7	10.0 ± 1.0
	$AUC_{(0-60)}$ (μg·min/mL)	72.7 ± 12.4	29.9 ± 4.4 **
	$T_{1/2}$ (min)	12.3 ± 0.3	13.9 ± 0.6 *
	$AUC_{(0-\infty)}$ (μg·min/mL)	75.8 ± 12.8	31.5 ± 4.4 **
trans-LOX	C_{max} (μg/mL)	4.4 ± 0.5	2.1 ± 0.2 **
	T_{max} (min)	9.1 ± 1.2	10.4 ± 0.9
	$AUC_{(0-60)}$ (μg·min/mL)	137.4 ± 19.0	67.6 ± 5.7 **
	$T_{1/2}$ (min)	18.2 ± 0.6	26.4 ± 1.6 **
	$AUC_{(0-\infty)}$ (μg·min/mL)	154.8 ± 19.2	85.8 ± 5.0 **

All data are expressed as the mean ± standard error (SE) (n = 3). C_{max}: maximum plasma concentration; $AUC_{(0-60)}$: area under the plasma concentration-time curve (AUC) from 0 to 60 min; T_{max}: time to reach maximum plasma concentration; $T_{1/2}$: elimination half-life; $AUC_{(0-\infty)}$: area under the plasma concentration-time curve from 0 to infinite time. * $p \leq 0.05$, ** $p \leq 0.01$ and *** $p \leq 0.001$.

Table 2. Pharmacokinetic parameters of LOX and its metabolites in 10% ethanol (VH) and KTC-treated groups.

Analytes	Parameters	VH (10% Ethanol)	KTC
LOX	C_{max} (μg/mL)	2.7 ± 0.3	3.5 ± 0.5
	T_{max} (min)	5.0 ± 0.0	5.0 ± 0.0
	$AUC_{(0-60)}$ (μg·min/mL)	54.7 ± 4.6	66.6 ± 6.6
	$T_{1/2}$ (min)	14.6 ± 1.1	12.2 ± 0.9
	$AUC_{(0-\infty)}$ (μg·min/mL)	59.1 ± 5.6	68.9 ± 6.5
cis-LOX	C_{max} (μg/mL)	1.2 ± 0.1	1.6 ± 0.1 *
	T_{max} (min)	13.3 ± 0.8	11.6 ± 0.8
	$AUC_{(0-60)}$ (μg·min/mL)	36.0 ± 3.9	49.0 ± 5.9 *
	$T_{1/2}$ (min)	13.3 ± 0.9	13.4 ± 0.6
	$AUC_{(0-\infty)}$ (μg·min/mL)	38.4 ± 4.4	51.9 ± 6.1 *
trans-LOX	C_{max} (μg/mL)	2.1 ± 0.2	3.1 ± 0.3 **
	T_{max} (min)	11.6 ± 0.8	11.7 ± 0.8
	$AUC_{(0-60)}$ (μg·min/mL)	69.9 ± 6.0	80.4 ± 9.6 *
	$T_{1/2}$ (min)	26.0 ± 0.5	19.8 ± 0.7 **
	$AUC_{(0-\infty)}$ (μg·min/mL)	90.9 ± 7.1	94.7 ± 11.0

All data are expressed as the mean ± standard error (SE) (n = 3). C_{max}: maximum plasma concentration; $AUC_{(0-60)}$: area under the plasma concentration-time curve (AUC) from 0 to 60 min; T_{max}: time to reach maximum plasma concentration; $T_{1/2}$: elimination half-life; $AUC_{(0-\infty)}$: area under the plasma concentration-time curve from 0 to infinite time. * $p \leq 0.05$, ** $p \leq 0.01$ and *** $p \leq 0.001$.

3.4. Metabolism and Metabolite Identification of LOX During DEX or KTC Treatment

The purpose of this study was to identify changes made by DEX and/or KTC on CR-mediated LOX metabolites (cis-LOX and trans-LOX) and also on CYP-mediated LOX metabolites (OH-LOX). During this PK study, OH-LOX could not be detected. Therefore, a full scan in Q Exactive Focus was used to identify all the metabolites present in plasma. A parallel reaction monitoring (PRM) mode was applied to confirm the metabolites through fragmentation patterns using collision induced dissociation (CID). Seven metabolites were confirmed after comparing the EICs of the test samples with blank plasma (Figures S3 and S4). LOX and all of its metabolites were detected in the negative ionization mode. To confirm the metabolites of LOX, their MS/MS fragmentation was checked (Figure S5). LOX ($C_{15}H_{17}O_3$) was detected at a retention time of 18 min with only one major fragment ion 83.0492 (C_5H_7O). Trans-LOX (M1, $C_{15}H_{19}O_3$) with an *m/z* ratio of 247.1339, eluted at 17.1 min with major fragment ions 233.1181 ($C_{14}H_{17}O_3$, $-CH_2$), 217.1230 ($C_{14}H_{17}O_2$, $-CH_2O$), 201.1279 ($C_{14}H_{17}O$), and 191.1071 ($C_{12}H_{15}O_2$, $-C_3H_4O$). Cis-LOX (M2, $C_{15}H_{19}O_3$), having the *m/z* ratio 247.1336, was detected at a retention time of 17.5 min. Its major fragments were 217.1230 ($C_{14}H_{17}O_2$, $-CH_2O$) and 191.1071 ($C_{12}H_{15}O_2$, $-C_3H_4O$). M3 and M4 are OH-LOX ($C_{15}H_{17}O_4$), having an *m/z* ratios of 261.1138 and 261.1133, and they were eluted at a retention time of 11.8 and 12.5 min, respectively. The MS/MS spectra of these metabolites were 99.0441 ($C_5H_7O_2$, $-C_{10}H_{10}O_2$) and 81.0335 (C_5H_5O, $-C_{10}H_{12}O_3$) for M3 and only a single major product ion 99.0441 ($C_5H_7O_2$) for M4. M5 is hydroxy trans-LOX ($C_{15}H_{19}O_4$), having an *m/z* ratio of 263.1288, and it was detected at a retention time of 11 min. Its major fragment ions were 233.1181 ($C_{14}H_{17}O_3$, $-CH_2O$), 207.1022 ($C_{12}H_{15}O_3$, $-C_3H_4O$), 133.0650 (C_9H_9O, $-C_6H_{10}O_3$), and 99.0442 ($C_5H_7O_2$, $-C_{10}H_{12}O_2$). M6 was identified as a taurine conjugate ($C_{17}H_{24}O_5NS$) whose *m/z* ratio was 354.1382, and it was detected at a retention time of 13.3 min. Its major fragments were 149.9859 ($C_3H_4O_4NS$, $-C_{14}H_{20}O$), 124.0065 ($C_2H_6O_3NS$, $-C_{15}H_{18}O_2$), and 106.9798 ($C_2H_3O_3S$, $-C_{15}H_{21}O_2N$). M7 was a glucuronide conjugate ($C_{21}H_{25}O_9$), having an *m/z* ratio 421.1514, and it eluted at a retention time of 14 min. Its major fragments were 245.1182 ($C_{15}H_{17}O_3$), 193.0348 ($C_6H_9O_7$), 175.0242 ($C_6H_7O_6$), and 83.0492 (C_5H_7O). Parent compounds and their fragments detected during the study are represented in Table 3.

Table 3. Identified metabolites of LOX in mouse plasma using HRMS.

Compounds	Parent Ions (*m/z*)	Elemental Composition	Error (ppm)	Product Ions (*m/z*)	Description
Lox	245.1179	$C_{15}H_{17}O_3$	0.4	83.0492	LOX
M1	247.1339	$C_{15}H_{19}O_3$	2.0	233.1181, 217.1230, 201.1279. 191.1071	Trans-LOX
M2	247.1336	$C_{15}H_{19}O_3$	0.5	217.1230, 191.1071	Cis-LOX
M3	261.1138	$C_{15}H_{17}O_4$	4.2	99.0441, 81.0335	OH-LOX
M4	261.1133	$C_{15}H_{17}O_4$	2.3	99.0441	OH-LOX
M5	263.1288	$C_{15}H_{19}O_4$	1.9	233.1181, 207.1022, 133.0650, 99.0442	OH-trans-LOX
M6	354.1382	$C_{17}H_{24}O_5NS$	2.0	149.9859, 124.0065, 79.9563	Taurine conjugate
M7	421.1514	$C_{21}H_{25}O_9$	3.6	245.1182, 193.0348, 175.0242, 83.0492	Glucuronide conjugate

We identified the effects of CYP3A induction and inhibition on seven different known metabolites of LOX. The general characteristics of LOX, its metabolites, and their concentration in different groups are described in (Table S2). In this study, we found that the concentration of LOX, trans-LOX (M1), and cis-LOX (M2) significantly decreased in the DEX-treated group (74.1 ± 6.3%, 80.1 ± 1.2%, and 61.9 ± 3.9%, respectively) and increased in the KTC-treated group (178.2 ± 8.3%, 158.9 ± 11.9%, and 173.1 ± 5.8%, respectively). Furthermore, the concentrations of M3, M4, and M5 significantly increased in the DEX-treated group (160.5 ± 4.1%, 440.4 ± 8.3%, and 286.3 ± 11.4%, respectively), and only the concentrations of M4 and M5 decreased in the KTC-treated group (93.6 ± 1.9% and 90.2 ± 2.7%, respectively). The taurine conjugate (M6) decreased in both the DEX- (65.3 ± 2.84%) and KTC-treated (91.2 ± 2.0%) groups. In contrast, the glucuronide conjugate increased in both the DEX- (174.4 ± 6.5%) and KTC-treated (275.7 ± 14.1%) groups. M6 and M7 are phase 2 metabolites, which indicates that

CYPs are not the main enzyme involved in the formation of these metabolites. The concentration of LOX and its metabolites in the VH, DEX-treated, and KTC-treated groups is represented graphically in Figure 2. DEX and KTC are well-known CYP3A modulators, and in this study, we found that the pretreatment of DEX or KTC had a significant effect on the concentration of both CYP-mediated and CR-mediated metabolites.

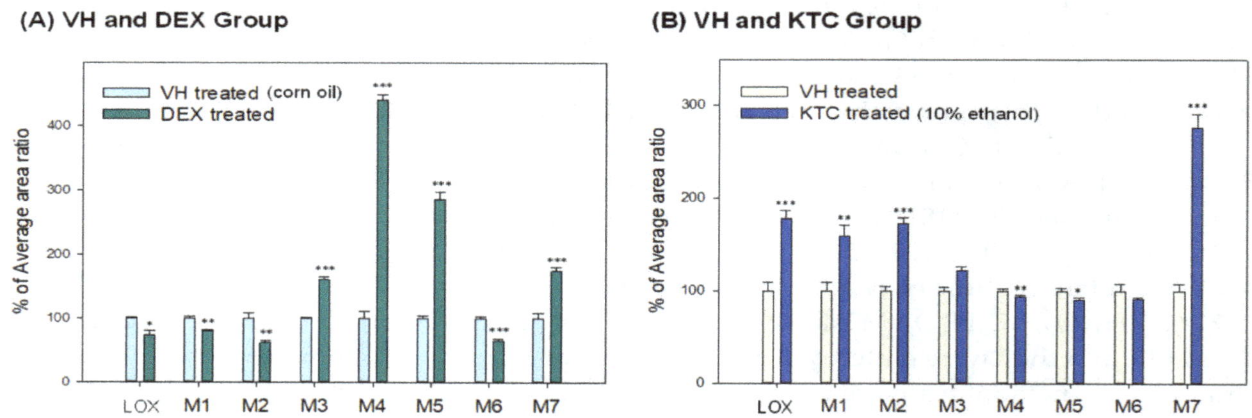

Figure 2. Comparison of loxoprofen (LOX) and its metabolites in male ICR mice treated with VH, DEX, or KTC. (**A**) The relative concentration of LOX and its metabolites after DEX administration (*i.p.* 40 mg/kg for consecutive 3 days, $n = 3$) compared to VH (*i.p.* corn oil for consecutive 3 days, $n = 3$). (**B**) The relative concentration of LOX and its metabolites after KTC administration (single dose *i.p.* 60 mg/kg, $n = 3$) compared to VH (10% ethanol, $n = 3$).

DEX and KTC affected the concentration and the PK of CYP-mediated metabolites, which, in turn, influenced the concentration and the PK of cis- and trans-LOX. The metabolites detected in this study are summarized in Figure 3.

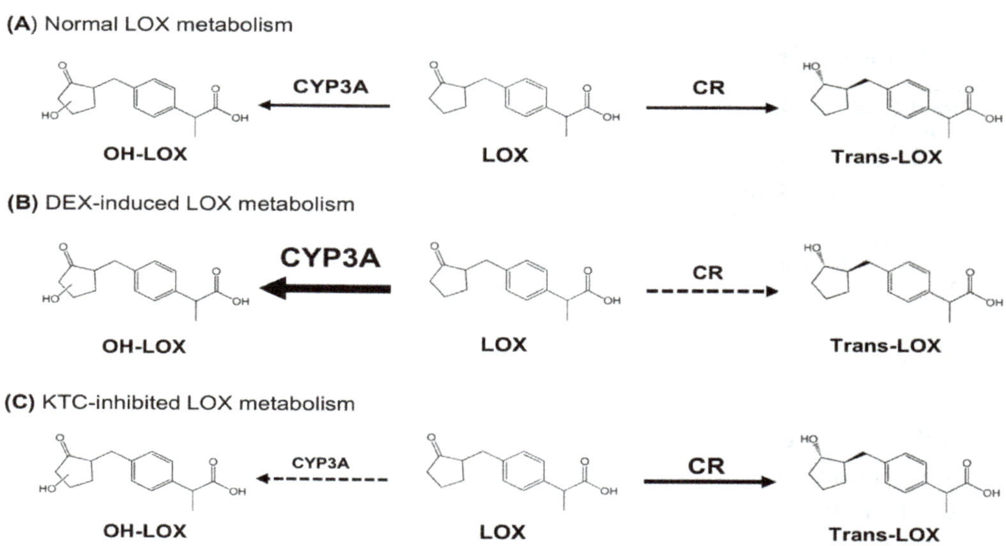

Figure 3. Metabolic pathway of loxoprofen and its metabolites.

4. Discussion

LOX is a nonselective COX inhibitor that is administered for the management of pain and inflammation, and it is well tolerated by patients [2,24,25]. Although the pharmacokinetics and metabolism of LOX are well defined, its interaction(s) with CYP enzymatic pathways have not been fully characterized [3,6–10,13,15,26–29]. However, CYP3A regulating commercial drugs are widely in clinical use [16,17] and there may be the chance to use CYP3A-regulating drugs and LOX together. Although CYP3A does not generate the LOX active metabolite, it may be possible to influence its generation by regulating CYP3A activity. To that end, we evaluated whether the rate of LOX active metabolite formation is influenced by CYP3A activity. We also investigated the effects of DEX and KTC, which are widely used CYP3A modulators, on the metabolism and PK of LOX, cis-LOX, and trans-LOX.

DEX is a steroidal drug used in the treatment of many conditions such as skin diseases, allergies, rheumatic disorder, asthma, and certain autoimmune diseases [30,31]. It is also effective in treating various cancers such as central nervous system tumors, brain metastases, advanced melanoma, leukemia, lymphoma, and multiple myeloma. Additionally, DEX is effective at combating the side effects of chemotherapy [32,33]. DEX is metabolized by CYP3A4 and CYP17A, but the CYP17A metabolic pathway plays no major role in its in vivo metabolism [34–36]. DEX has been used as a CYP3A4 inducer in clinical studies. Interestingly, rifampicin, rifabutin, phenytoin, phenobarbital, primidone, carbamazepine, etc., are strong CYP3A4 inducers [16]. It has also been reported that a single dose (50 mg/kg) of DEX can induce the activity of CYP3A. However, persistent administration of DEX could make stable induction of CYP3A activity, which was independent of inducer administration [37,38]. Moreover, chronic DEX administration likely leads to the autoinduction of CYP3A, which has a direct impact on the PK parameters of DEX [38]. Nevertheless, patients may suffer from an increase in substrate concentration after they stop using the CYP3A inducer if they take both the substrate (LOX) and the inducer (DEX) of CYP3A [37].

KTC is a broad-spectrum antifungal drug used in the treatment of many fungal infections such as blastomycosis, coccidioidomycosis, histoplasmosis, etc. [39,40]. KTC is a known reversible inhibitor of CYP3A4 [16] and displays hepatotoxicity through immune-allergic mechanisms, which limits its therapeutic use [41,42]. Usually, CYP3A4 inhibitors are divided into reversible inhibitors (such as KTC, itraconazole, terfenadine, astemizole, and quinidine) [43] and irreversible inhibitors (such as gestodene and levonorgestrel) [44]. Many studies also reported the biotransformation of KTC through oxidation, O-dealkylation, hydroxylation, and FMO (via the UGT1A4 metabolic pathway) [42,45]. Furthermore, one study revealed that KTC showed dose-dependent kinetics, indicating that its metabolism occurs in the liver [46]. A recent study also revealed that KTC metabolism is similar in humans and mice, which may help to resolve the issue regarding drug metabolism and toxicology [42]. Nevertheless, a sudden increase or decrease in the C_{max} of drugs and toxic metabolites could result from either the induction or inhibition of metabolizing enzymes [47].

CYP3A4 is the major CYP involved in LOX metabolism, but it does not form its active metabolite [15]. The active metabolite of LOX (trans-LOX) is formed via CR pathway [1,5]. Similarly to previous studies, we also found that DEX and KTC were strong CYP3A activity modulators [36,48,49]. In addition, we determined that the C_{max}, $AUC_{(0-60)}$, and $AUC_{(0-\infty)}$ of LOX, cis-LOX, and trans-LOX were significantly decreased in DEX-treated mice. However, the C_{max}, $AUC_{(0-60)}$, and $AUC_{(0-\infty)}$ of cis-LOX, and trans-LOX are significantly increased in KTC-treated mice. Furthermore, DEX increased the concentration of the OH-LOX metabolite and decreased the concentration of the active metabolite. This may lead to a decrease in the activity of trans-LOX during the subsequent administration of LOX and DEX. We also observed that changes in CYP pathway activity can modulate CR pathway activity regarding LOX, even though CYP3A4 does not participate in LOX active metabolite formation.

These results indicate that the co-administration of LOX and DEX may lead to a decrease in the pharmacological activity of LOX by decreasing the concentration of the active metabolite. We also observed that the concentration of active metabolites catalyzed by CR increased and that the concentration of inactive metabolites decreased during the co-administration of LOX and the CYP3A inhibitor, KTC. Therefore, if LOX and KTC are administered together, the pharmacological activity of LOX may be enhanced by increasing the active metabolite. Subsequently, this may also increase toxicity. In a previous study, LOX was associated with an increase in small bowel mucosal injury, erosive gastritis, gastroduodenal ulcers, etc., during concomitant use of a proton pump inhibitor such as lansoprazole [1,50,51]. Since lansoprazole is a known inhibitor of CYP3A and CYP2C19 [52,53], these side effects may have been caused by changes in the blood levels of LOX and its active metabolite caused by the concomitant use of LOX and lansoprazole. It has been reported that LOX slightly inhibited the metabolism of tacrolimus by interacting with CYP3A in human liver microsomes [54]. Similarly, tizanidine is typically used to manage muscle spasticity and pain [55]. However, it has been reported that combination therapy of tizanidine and LOX for neck pain increased the risk of irreversible symptomatic bradycardia via CYP inhibition [56].

These previous studies clearly show that LOX can interact with drugs that modulate CYP activity even though its active metabolite is not formed by CYP enzymes. Considering the pharmacokinetics and metabolism of LOX and its metabolites, the use of LOX with CYP modulators (e.g., DEX and KTC) may result in the decreased pharmacological action of LOX or may cause from minor toxicity to major toxicity by interacting with CYP3A.

5. Conclusions

The pharmacokinetic parameters of LOX and its active metabolite were significantly altered when LOX was co-administered with CYP3A activity modulators. In clinical practice, LOX is administered concurrently with many other drugs. Therefore, more studies are needed to assess the possible interactions of LOX with CYP enzymes. In this study, pharmacodynamic interactions were not evaluated; however, they will be evaluated in future studies.

Supplementary Materials:
Figure S1: Representative chromatograms: (A) blank plasma (B), standard loxoprofen (LOX), and its metabolites in plasma. LOX and its metabolites in plasma after administering 20 mg/mL LOX to the (C) VH (Corn oil) group ($n = 3$), (D) DEX-treated group ($n = 3$), (E) VH (10% Ethanol) group ($n = 3$), and (F) KTC-treated group ($n = 3$), Figure S2: CYP induction by dexamethasone ($n = 3$) (A), and CYP inhibition by ketoconazole ($n = 3$) (B), Figure S3: Representative EICs of Loxoprofen (LOX) and its metabolites in mouse plasma: VH (Corn oil) group ($n = 3$) (A), DEX-treated group ($n = 3$) (B), VH (10% Ethanol) group ($n = 3$) (C), and KTC-treated group ($n = 3$) (D), Figure S4: Representative EICs of loxoprofen (LOX) and its metabolites in mouse blank plasma (A) as well as standard LOX and tolbutamide (IS) (B), Figure S5: MS/MS spectra of Loxoprofen (A), M1 (B), M2 (C), M3 (D), M4 (E), M5 (F), M6 (G), and M7 (H), Table S1: Method validation table ($n = 3$), Table S2: Characterization of loxoprofen (LOX) metabolites identified in mouse plasma along with their average % of area ($n = 3$).

Author Contributions: Conceptualization, S.L.; Data Curation, S.P. and S.L.; Formal Analysis, S.P.; P.C.; R.S. and Y.K., Funding Acquisition, T.L. and S.L.; Methodology, S.P.; Resources, A.S., T.C.J., and E.-S.L., Writing – Original Draft Preparation, S.P.; Writing – Review & Editing, J.-H.K. and S.L.

References

1. Greig, S.L.; Garnock-Jones, K.P. Loxoprofen: A review in pain and inflammation. *Clin. Drug Investig.* **2016**, *36*, 771–781. [CrossRef] [PubMed]
2. Wan, D.; Zhao, M.; Zhang, J.; Luan, L. Development and In Vitro-In Vivo Evaluation of a Novel Sustained-Release Loxoprofen Pellet with Double Coating Layer. *Pharmaceutics* **2019**, *11*, 260. [CrossRef] [PubMed]
3. Helmy, S.A. Pharmacokinetics and Bioequivalence Evaluation of 2 Loxoprofen Tablets in Healthy Egyptian Male Volunteers. *Clin. Pharmacol. Drug Dev.* **2013**, *2*, 173–177. [CrossRef] [PubMed]
4. Yamakawa, N.; Suemasu, S.; Watanabe, H.; Tahara, K.; Tanaka, K.-I.; Okamoto, Y.; Ohtsuka, M.; Maruyama, T.; Mizushima, T. Comparison of pharmacokinetics between loxoprofen and its derivative with lower ulcerogenic activity, fluoro-loxoprofen. *Drug Metab. Pharmacok.* **2013**, *28*, 118–124. [CrossRef]
5. Kang, H.-A.; Cho, H.-Y.; Lee, Y.-B. Bioequivalence of hana loxoprofen sodium tablet to dongwha Loxonin® tablet (Loxoprofen Sodium 60 mg). *J. Pharm. Investig.* **2011**, *41*, 117–123. [CrossRef]
6. Moore, N.; Pollack, C.; Butkerait, P. Adverse drug reactions and drug–drug interactions with over-the-counter NSAIDs. *Ther. Clin. Risk. Manag.* **2015**, *11*, 1061–1075. [PubMed]
7. Sawamura, R.; Kazui, M.; Kurihara, A.; Izumi, T. Absorption, distribution, metabolism and excretion of loxoprofen after dermal application of loxoprofen gel to rats. *Xenobiotica* **2014**, *44*, 1026–1038. [CrossRef]
8. Takeda, M.; Khamdang, S.; Narikawa, S.; Kimura, H.; Hosoyamada, M.; Cha, S.H.; Sekine, T.; Endou, H. Characterization of methotrexate transport and its drug interactions with human organic anion transporters. *J. Pharmacol. Exp. Ther.* **2002**, *302*, 666–671. [CrossRef]

9. Yue, Z.; Shi, J.; Jiang, P.; Sun, H. Acute kidney injury during concomitant use of valacyclovir and loxoprofen: Detecting drug-drug interactions in a spontaneous reporting system. *Pharmacoepidemiol. Drug Saf.* **2014**, *23*, 1154–1159. [CrossRef]
10. Takahashi, H.; Kashima, T.; Kimura, S.; Murata, N.; Takaba, T.; Iwade, K.; Abe, T.; Tainaka, H.; Yasumori, T.; Echizen, H. Pharmacokinetic interaction between warfarin and a uricosuric agent, bucolome: Application of in vitro approaches to predicting in vivo reduction of (S)-warfarin clearance. *Drug Metab. Dispos.* **1999**, *27*, 1179–1186.
11. Dinger, J.; Meyer, M.R.; Maurer, H.H. Development of an in vitro cytochrome P450 cocktail inhibition assay for assessing the inhibition risk of drugs of abuse. *Toxicol. Lett.* **2014**, *230*, 28–35. [CrossRef] [PubMed]
12. Ab Rahman, N.S.; Abd Majid, F.A.; Wahid, A.; Effendy, M.; Zainudin, A.N.; Zainol, S.N.; Ismail, H.F.; Wong, T.S.; Tiwari, N.K.; Giri, S. Evaluation of Herb-Drug Interaction of Synacinn™ and Individual Biomarker through Cytochrome 450 Inhibition Assay. *Drug Metab. Lett.* **2018**, *12*, 62–67. [CrossRef] [PubMed]
13. Tanaka, Y.; Nishikawa, Y.; Hayashi, R. Species differences in metabolism of sodium 2-[4-(2-oxocyclopentylmethyl)-phenyl] propionate dihydrate (loxoprofen sodium), a new anti-inflammatory agent. *Chem. Pharm. Bull.* **1983**, *31*, 3656–3664. [CrossRef] [PubMed]
14. Jhee, O.H.; Lee, M.H.; Shaw, L.M.; Lee, S.E.; Park, J.H.; Kang, J.S. Pharmacokinetics and bioequivalence study of two brands of loxoprofen tablets in healthy volunteers. *Arzneimittelforschung* **2007**, *57*, 542–546. [CrossRef] [PubMed]
15. Shrestha, R.; Cho, P.; Paudel, S.; Shrestha, A.; Kang, M.; Jeong, T.; Lee, E.-S.; Lee, S. Exploring the Metabolism of Loxoprofen in Liver Microsomes: The Role of Cytochrome P450 and UDP-Glucuronosyltransferase in Its Biotransformation. *Pharmaceutics* **2018**, *10*, 112. [CrossRef]
16. Zhou, S.-F. Drugs behave as substrates, inhibitors and inducers of human cytochrome P450 3A4. *Curr. Drug Metab.* **2008**, *9*, 310–322. [CrossRef] [PubMed]
17. Basheer, L.; Kerem, Z. Interactions between CYP3A4 and dietary polyphenols. *Oxid. Med. Cell. Longev.* **2015**, *2015*. [CrossRef]
18. Naruto, S.; Terada, A. Synthesis of the eight possible optically active isomers of 2-[4-(2-hydroxycyclopentylmethyl) phenyl] propionic acid. *Chem. Pharm. Bull.* **1983**, *31*, 4319–4323. [CrossRef]
19. Seervi, M.; Lotankar, S.; Barbar, S.; Sathaye, S. Assessment of cytochrome P450 inhibition and induction potential of lupeol and betulin in rat liver microsomes. *Drug Metab. Pers. Ther.* **2016**, *31*, 115–122. [CrossRef]
20. Seneca, N.; Zoghbi, S.S.; Shetty, H.U.; Tuan, E.; Kannan, P.; Taku, A.; Innis, R.B.; Pike, V.W. Effects of ketoconazole on the biodistribution and metabolism of [^{11}C] loperamide and [^{11}C] N-desmethyl-loperamide in wild-type and P-gp knockout mice. *Nucl. Med. Biol.* **2010**, *37*, 335–345. [CrossRef]
21. Shrestha, R.; Kim, J.-H.; Nam, W.; Lee, H.S.; Lee, J.-M.; Lee, S. Selective inhibition of CYP2C8 by fisetin and its methylated metabolite, geraldol, in human liver microsomes. *Drug Metab. Pharmacok.* **2018**, *33*, 111–117. [CrossRef] [PubMed]
22. Sim, J.; Nam, W.; Lee, D.; Lee, S.; Hungchan, O.; Joo, J.; Liu, K.-H.; Han, J.Y.; Ki, S.H.; Jeong, T.C. Selective induction of hepatic cytochrome P450 2B activity by leelamine in vivo, as a potent novel inducer. *Arch. Pharmacal. Res.* **2015**, *38*, 725–733. [CrossRef] [PubMed]
23. Bradford, M.M. A rapid and sensitive method for the quantitation of microgram quantities of protein utilizing the principle of protein-dye binding. *Anal. Biochem.* **1976**, *72*, 248–254. [CrossRef]
24. Hamaguchi, M.; Seno, T.; Yamamoto, A.; Kohno, M.; Kadoya, M.; Ishino, H.; Ashihara, E.; Kimura, S.; Tsubakimoto, Y.; Takata, H. Loxoprofen sodium, a non-selective NSAID, reduces atherosclerosis in mice by reducing inflammation. *J. Clin. Biochem. Nutr.* **2010**, *47*, 138–147. [CrossRef] [PubMed]
25. Sekiguchi, H.; Inoue, G.; Nakazawa, T.; Imura, T.; Saito, W.; Uchida, K.; Miyagi, M.; Takahira, N.; Takaso, M. Loxoprofen sodium and celecoxib for postoperative pain in patients after spinal surgery: A randomized comparative study. *J. Orthop. Sci.* **2015**, *20*, 617–623. [CrossRef] [PubMed]
26. Nagashima, H.; Tanaka, Y.; Watanabe, H.; Hayashi, R.; Kawada, K. Optical inversion of (2R)-to (2S)-isomers of 2-[4-(2-oxocyclopentylmethyl)-phenyl] propionic acid (loxoprofen), a new anti-inflammatory agent, and its monohydroxy metabolites in the rat. *Chem. Pharm. Bull.* **1984**, *32*, 251–257. [CrossRef] [PubMed]
27. Foti, R.S.; Dalvie, D.K. Cytochrome P450 and non–cytochrome P450 oxidative metabolism: Contributions to the pharmacokinetics, safety, and efficacy of xenobiotics. *Drug Metab. Dispos.* **2016**, *44*, 1229–1245. [CrossRef]

28. Tanaka, Y.; Nishikawa, Y.; Matsuda, K.; Yamazaki, M.; Hayashi, R. Purification and some properties of ketone reductase forming an active metabolite of sodium 2-[4-(2-oxocyclopentylmethyl)-phenyl] propionate dihydrate (loxoprofen sodium), a new anti-inflammatory agent, in rabbit liver cytosol. *Chem. Pharm. Bull* **1984**, *32*, 1040–1048. [CrossRef]
29. Sawamura, R.; Kazui, M.; Kurihara, A.; Izumi, T. Pharmacokinetics of loxoprofen and its active metabolite after dermal application of loxoprofen gel to rats. *Pharm.* **2015**, *70*, 74–80.
30. Verhoef, C.M.; van Roon, J.A.; Vianen, M.E.; Lafeber, F.P.; Bijlsma, J.W. The immune suppressive effect of dexamethasone in rheumatoid arthritis is accompanied by upregulation of interleukin 10 and by differential changes in interferon γ and interleukin 4 production. *Ann. Rheum. Dis.* **1999**, *58*, 49–54. [CrossRef]
31. Liu, D.; Ahmet, A.; Ward, L.; Krishnamoorthy, P.; Mandelcorn, E.D.; Leigh, R.; Brown, J.P.; Cohen, A.; Kim, H A practical guide to the monitoring and management of the complications of systemic corticosteroid therapy *Allergy Asthma Clin. Immunol.* **2013**, *9*, 30. [CrossRef] [PubMed]
32. Cook, A.M.; McDonnell, A.M.; Lake, R.A.; Nowak, A.K. Dexamethasone co-medication in cancer patients undergoing chemotherapy causes substantial immunomodulatory effects with implications for chemo-immunotherapy strategies. *Oncoimmunology* **2016**, *5*, e1066062. [CrossRef] [PubMed]
33. Pufall, M.A. Glucocorticoids and Cancer. *Adv. Exp. Med. Biol.* **2015**, *872*, 315–333. [CrossRef] [PubMed]
34. Al Katheeri, N.; Wasfi, I.; Lambert, M.; Albo, A.G.; Nebbia, C. In vivo and in vitro metabolism of dexamethasone in the camel. *Vet. J.* **2006**, *172*, 532–543. [CrossRef] [PubMed]
35. Tomlinson, E.; Maggs, J.; Park, B.; Back, D. Dexamethasone metabolism in vitro: Species differences *J. Steroid. Biochem.* **1997**, *62*, 345–352. [CrossRef]
36. Tomlinson, E.; Lewis, D.; Maggs, J.; Kroemer, H.; Park, B.; Back, D. In vitro metabolism of dexamethasone (DEX) in human liver and kidney: The involvement of CYP3A4 and CYP17 (17, 20 LYASE) and molecular modelling studies. *Biochem. Pharmacol.* **1997**, *54*, 605–611. [CrossRef]
37. Iwanaga, K.; Honjo, T.; Miyazaki, M.; Kakemi, M. Time-dependent changes in hepatic and intestinal induction of cytochrome P450 3A after administration of dexamethasone to rats. *Xenobiotica* **2013**, *43*, 765–773 [CrossRef]
38. Li, J.; Chen, R.; Yao, Q.-Y.; Liu, S.-J.; Tian, X.-Y.; Hao, C.-Y.; Lu, W.; Zhou, T.-Y. Time-dependent pharmacokinetics of dexamethasone and its efficacy in human breast cancer xenograft mice A semi-mechanism-based pharmacokinetic/pharmacodynamic model. *Acta Pharmacol. Sin.* **2018**, *39* 472–481. [CrossRef]
39. Sohn, C.A. Evaluation of ketoconazole. *Clin. Pharm.* **1982**, *1*, 217–224.
40. Jones, H.E. Ketoconazole. *Arch. Dermatol.* **1982**, *118*, 217–219. [CrossRef]
41. Rodriguez, R.J.; Acosta, D. Metabolism of ketoconazole and deacetylated ketoconazole by rat hepatic microsomes and flavin-containing monooxygenases. *Drug Metab. Dispos.* **1997**, *25*, 772–777. [PubMed]
42. Kim, J.-H.; Choi, W.-G.; Lee, S.; Lee, H. Revisiting the metabolism and bioactivation of ketoconazole in human and mouse using liquid chromatography-mass spectrometry-based metabolomics. *Int. J. Mol. Sci* **2017**, *18*, 621. [CrossRef] [PubMed]
43. Zhou, S.; Chan, S.Y.; Goh, B.C.; Chan, E.; Duan, W.; Huang, M.; McLeod, H.L. Mechanism-based inhibition of cytochrome P450 3A4 by therapeutic drugs. *Clin. Pharmacok.* **2005**, *44*, 279–304. [CrossRef] [PubMed]
44. Thummel, K.; Wilkinson, G. In vitro and in vivo drug interactions involving human CYP3A. *Annu. Rev Pharmacol. Toxicol.* **1998**, *38*, 389–430. [CrossRef] [PubMed]
45. Bourcier, K.; Hyland, R.; Kempshall, S.; Jones, R.; Maximilien, J.; Irvine, N.; Jones, B. Investigation into UDP-glucuronosyltransferase (UGT) enzyme kinetics of imidazole-and triazole-containing antifungal drugs in human liver microsomes and recombinant UGT enzymes. *Drug Metab. Dispos.* **2010**, *38*, 923–929 [CrossRef] [PubMed]
46. Huang, Y.; Colaizzi, J.; Bierman, R.; Woestenborghs, R.; Heykants, J. Pharmacokinetics and dose proportionality of ketoconazole in normal volunteers. *Antimicrob. Agents Chemother.* **1986**, *30*, 206–210 [CrossRef]
47. Hukkanen, J. Induction of cytochrome P450 enzymes: A view on human in vivo findings. *Expert Rev. Clin. Pharmacol.* **2012**, *5*, 569–585. [CrossRef]
48. Gentile, D.M.; Tomlinson, E.S.; Maggs, J.L.; Park, B.K.; Back, D.J. Dexamethasone metabolism by human liver in vitro. Metabolite identification and inhibition of 6-hydroxylation. *J. Pharmacol. Exp. Ther.* **1996**, *277*, 105–112.

49. Kaeser, B.; Zandt, H.; Bour, F.; Zwanziger, E.; Schmitt, C.; Zhang, X. Drug-drug interaction study of ketoconazole and ritonavir-boosted saquinavir. *Antimicrob. Agents Chemother.* **2009**, *53*, 609–614. [CrossRef]
50. Fujimori, S.; Hanada, R.; Hayashida, M.; Sakurai, T.; Ikushima, I.; Sakamoto, C. Celecoxib Monotherapy Maintained Small Intestinal Mucosa Better Compared with Loxoprofen Plus Lansoprazole Treatment. *J. Clin. Gastroenterol.* **2016**, *50*, 218–226. [CrossRef]
51. Mizukami, K.; Murakami, K.; Yamauchi, M.; Matsunari, O.; Ogawa, R.; Nakagawa, Y.; Okimoto, T.; Kodama, M.; Fujioka, T. Evaluation of selective cyclooxygenase-2 inhibitor-induced small bowel injury: Randomized cross-over study compared with loxoprofen in healthy subjects. *Dig. Endosc.* **2013**, *25*, 288–294. [CrossRef] [PubMed]
52. Cascorbi, I. Drug interactions-principles, examples and clinical consequences. *Dtsch. Arztebl. Int.* **2012**, *109*, 546–556. [PubMed]
53. Li, X.-Q.; Andersson, T.B.; Ahlström, M.; Weidolf, L. Comparison of inhibitory effects of the proton pump-inhibiting drugs omeprazole, esomeprazole, lansoprazole, pantoprazole, and rabeprazole on human cytochrome P450 activities. *Drug Metab. Dispos.* **2004**, *32*, 821–827. [CrossRef] [PubMed]
54. Iwasaki, K. Metabolism of tacrolimus (FK506) and recent topics in clinical pharmacokinetics. *Drug Metab. Pharmacok.* **2007**, *22*, 328–335. [CrossRef]
55. Milanov, I.; Georgiev, D. Mechanisms of tizanidine action on spasticity. *Acta Neurol. Scand.* **1994**, *89*, 274–279. [CrossRef] [PubMed]
56. Li, X.; Jin, Y. Irreversible profound symptomatic bradycardia requiring pacemaker after tizanidine/loxoprofen combination therapy: A case report. *J. Int. Med.Res.* **2018**, *46*, 2466–2469. [CrossRef] [PubMed]

4

Solubility, Permeability, and Dissolution Rate of Naftidrofuryl Oxalate Based on BCS Criteria

Marta Kus-Slowinska [1,2], Monika Wrzaskowska [2], Izabela Ibragimow [2], Piotr Igor Czaklosz [2], Anna Olejnik [3,*] and Hanna Piotrowska-Kempisty [1,4,*]

1 Department of Toxicology, Poznan University of Medical Sciences, 30 Dojazd St., 60-631 Poznan, Poland; marta.kus-slowinska@ethifarm.pl

2 Research and Development Department of Ethifarm, Ethifarm Manufacturing Plant, 9 Stefana Zeromskiego St., 60-544 Poznan, Poland; monika.wrzaskowska@ethifarm.pl (M.W.); izabela.ibragimow@ethifarm.pl (I.I.); piotr.czaklosz@ethifarm.pl (P.I.C.)

3 Department of Biotechnology and Food Microbiology, Poznan University of Life Sciences, 48 Wojska Polskiego St., 60-627 Poznan, Poland

4 Department of Basic and Preclinical Sciences, Institute of Veterinary Medicine, Nicolaus Copernicus University in Toruń, 7 Gagarina St., 87-100 Torun, Poland

* Correspondence: anna.olejnik@up.poznan.pl (A.O.); hpiotrow@ump.edu.pl (H.P.-K.)

Abstract: The Biopharmaceutics Classification System (BCS) was conceived to classify drug substances by their in vitro aqueous solubility and permeability properties. The essential activity of naftidrofuryl oxalate (NF) has been described as the inhibition of the serotonin receptors (5-HT_2), resulting in vasodilation and decreasing blood pressure. Since the early 1980s, NF has been used to treat several venous and cerebral diseases. There is no data available on the BCS classification of NF. However, based on its physical-chemical properties, NF might be considered to belong to the 1st or the 3rd BCS class. The present study aimed to provide data concerning the solubility and permeability of NF through Caco-2 monolayers and propose its preliminary classification into BCS. We showed that NF is a highly soluble and permeable drug substance; thus, it might be suggested to belong to BCS class I. Additionally, a high dissolution rate of the encapsulated NF based on Praxilene® 100 mg formulation was revealed. Hence, it might be considered as an immediate-release (IR).

Keywords: naftidrofuryl oxalate; solubility; permeability; dissolution profiles; pharmaceutical availability; BCS drug classification

1. Introduction

Pharmacokinetics characterizes the drug's behavior in the body from its administration to excretion. It describes five major physical and chemical properties: liberation, absorption, distribution, metabolism, and elimination (LADME). The first two stages of LADME are characterized by the Biopharmaceutical Classification System (BCS), introduced by Amidon et al. in 1995 [1]. BCS is a scientific framework for classifying drug substances based on their aqueous solubility and intestinal permeability, which largely allows the prediction of a given drug substance bioavailability (BA) in human blood plasma. The BA of drugs depends mainly on their physicochemical properties (solubility, dissociation, and lipophilicity), dosage form (influence of excipients on active pharmaceutical ingredients (API) properties), and the route of administration (oral—liver metabolism) [2,3].

Naftidrofuryl hydrogen oxalate (NF, $C_{24}H_{33}NO_3$, $C_2H_2O_4$; synonym: nafronyl oxalate), as a pharmacologically active drug compound, is a mixture of four stereoisomers [4]. NF is a white powder freely soluble in water and ethanol (with pKa 8.2 at 30 °C) [5,6]. It selectively inhibits 5-hydroxytryptamine type 2A (serotonin; type 5-HT_{2A}) receptors present in vascular smooth muscle cells, platelets, and endothelial cells (in vascular and cerebral tissues). In vascular cells, NF causes vascular vasodilation (by preventing smooth muscle contraction) and decreases blood pressure [7]. Furthermore, it inhibits serotonin-induced platelet aggregation and platelet- induced vasospasm [8]. NF has also been shown to increase the ATP level in fibroblast and endothelial cells by improving the aerobic metabolism in the blood vessel wall [4]. As a drug product, NF has been mainly used for the treatment of intermittent claudication (since 80th) [9], less often also for stroke [10] and dementia [11].

A literature review of NF pharmacokinetics properties is detailed in Table 1. The main NF capsules manufacturer states that the peak plasma concentration (C_{max}) occurs about 30 min after oral dosing [12]. The relative BA of 100 mg NF administered orally was estimated 121% (oral solution containing 100 mg of NF as a reference was used) [6]. Furthermore, based on the pharmacokinetic data presented by Brodie et al., the high relative BA of NF (approx 100% following oral administration of 100 mg tablets) can be suggested [13]. However, the results of several studies about BA of NF are controversial. Nishigaki et al. showed that the relative bioavailability of 100 mg NF after its oral administration was within the 20–23% range. The authors concluded that this was due to the large first-pass elimination metabolism (80%) [14]. Additionally, the pharmacokinetic analysis performed in the dogs has also demonstrated a low absolute BA of 250 mg NF in the range of 0.3–2.7% due to presystemic and/or first-pass metabolism [15].

After absorption, NF is distributed and stored predominantly in fatty tissue [16]. NF is primarily biotransformed in hepatocytes to three acidic metabolites, among which NF free acid (3-(1-naphthyl)-2 tetrahydrofurfuryl propionic acid) is the main one [17,18]. Less than 1% of absorbed NF is excreted in urine within 48 h of administration, while most of it appears to be eliminated with the bile [19].

Table 1. Summary of literature data on the NF pharmacokinetics.

Dosage Form	Dosage [mg]	No. of Patients	$T_{1/2}$ [h]	T_{max} [h]	C_{max} [ng/mL]	AUC [ng/mL*h]	BA [%]	Reference
oral	nd	nd	nd	nd	nd	n.d	30	[20]
oral (gelatin capsules)	50	n/d	0.68	1.1	350	n.d	76	[21]
oral (capsules)	100	2	1.2	0.5	203	n.d	nd	[13]
intravenous	40	18	nd	nd	nd	n.d	nd	[16]
oral (gelatin capsules)	300	12	1.79	0.94	922	2022	nd	[21]
oral (fasted)	100	12	1.3	0.8	238	500	19.7	[14]
oral (nonfasted)			1.6	2	181	583	23.0	
	100			1	209	630	121	
oral (tablets)	300	9	nd	0.9	590	1271	77	[6]
	300			1.2	645	1955	114	
oral (tablets)	200	30	3.41	2.75	279	1797	nd	[22]
oral (tablets)	200	12	4.4	1.3	174	1504	nd	[23]

nd = no data; $T_{1/2}$ = half life; T_{max} = the time taken to reach the maximum concentration; C_{max} = the peak plasma concentration; AUC = area under curve; BA = bioavailability.

NF drug products are widely distributed all over the world. The clinical dose of naftidrofuryl is 100 or 200 mg for all its dosage forms (capsules and tablets).

To the best of the authors' knowledge, there is no data concerning the permeability of NF or its BCS classification. Hence, to fulfill the literature gap, the present study aimed to provide data concerning aqueous solubility and permeability of NF through Caco-2 monolayers and propose its preliminary classification into BCS. We performed three experiments concerning the solubility, permeability, and dissolution of NF largely based on the BSC guidelines for the pharmaceutical industry [24,25]. However, industry guidelines are mainly focused and directed for biowaiver approach applicants.

Hence, in the present study, several issues in experimental design and data evaluation differ from the formal requirements.

2. Materials and Methods

2.1. Reagents and References

The acetonitrile (ACN; VWR Chemicals, Fontenay-sous-Bois, France) and water (H_2O, VWR Chemicals, Fontenay-sous-Bois, France) for the HPLC assay were of chromatographic grade. Other reagents were of analytical grade: hydrochloric acid (HCl, Chempur, Piekary Slaskie Poland), disodium hydrogen phosphate (Na_2HPO_4; Chempur, Piekary Slaskie, Poland), ammonium acetate ($CH_3CO_2NH_4$; Chempur, Piekary Slaskie, Poland), sodium acetate (CH_3COONa; Chempur, Piekary Slaskie, Poland), glacial acetic acid (CH_3COOH; Chempur, Piekary Slaskie, Poland), and orthophosphoric acid (85%, H_3PO_4; Chempur, Piekary Slaskie, Poland). The media solutions used for solubility and dissolution tests were prepared according to European Pharmacopoeia (EP) Chapter 4–Reagents.

A British Pharmacopoeia Certificated Reference Standard of Naftidrofuryl oxalate (BPCRS, Cat no 362) was used for all the performed assays. Additionally, we used the Caffeine standard (CAF) (Sigma Aldrich–Merck Group, Darmstadt, Germany) for permeability tests as a reference. Praxilene® 100 mg Capsules (Merck Serono Ltd., Feltham, UK) was employed as a drug reference product. Each Praxilene capsule contained 100 mg of naftidrofuryl oxalate.

Naftidrofuryl oxalate (Sigma Aldrich–Merck Group, Darmstadt, Germany), magnesium stearate (Peter Greven Nederland C.V., Venlo, Netherland), and talc (C.H. Erbslöh, Krefeld, Germany) used for the in-house capsules were obtained from Ethifarm (Ethifarm, Poznan, Poland). Hard gelatin capsules, size 3 (Capsugel, Morristown, NJ, USA) used in the drug dosage manufacture were provided by Ethifarm (Ethifarm, Poznan, Poland).

2.2. Solubility Test

The solubility by equilibrium method was performed in three different media (0.1 M HCl, acetate buffer, and phosphate buffer), with a pH of 1.2, 4.5, and 6.8, respectively, based on European Medicines Agency (EMA) guideline [24]. Saturated solutions of NF in given media were prepared by adding an excessive amount of the drug until obtained a saturated solution (presence of visible precipitate on the tube). The samples were then incubated at 37 °C ± 0.5 (incubator chamber; Binder GmbH, Tuttlingen, Germany) for 24 h in an orbital agitation of 45 rpm (LLG-uniLOOPMIX 2 orbital shaker, LLG GmbH, Hamburg, Germany). After equilibration, the sample was filtered (0.45 μm) and diluted with the appropriate solution to the concentration within the linear calibration range. Drug concentration measurement was performed by a validated UV spectrophotometric method at $\lambda = 283$ nm with optical path 0.2 cm and spectrum recorded on 250–350 nm range (JASCO V-530 double-beam apparatus with Spectra Manager software, JASCO, Tokyo, Japan). The experiments were carried out in triplicate.

The dose number (D_0) for each pH buffer solution was calculated using the following equation:

$$D_0 = DOSE/V_0/S \quad (1)$$

where DOSE is the highest dose strength (mg), V_0 is the water volume (assumed to be 250 mL), and S is the aqueous solubility (mg/mL). Drug substances with $D_0 \leq 1$ are classified as high solubility drugs, while drugs with $D_0 \geq 1$ are assigned as low solubility drugs [26].

2.3. Cytotoxicity Analysis

The MTT (3-(4,5-dimethyl-2-thiazolyl)-2,5-diphenyl-2H-tetrazolium bromide) test (Sigma Aldrich–Merck Group, Darmstadt, Germany) was used to establish an appropriate concentration of analyzed substances NF and CAF in the Caco-2 cell line. To determine the effects of materials tested on cell viability, confluent stock cultures were detached using trypsin and seeded in 96-well plates at a density of 2×10^4 cells/well. They were allowed to attach overnight and then exposed for 2 h (time of transport across monolayer) for seven different NF/CAF concentrations in Hank's Balanced Salt Solution (HBSS, Sigma Aldrich–Merck Group, Darmstadt, Germany) pH 7.4 in the range of 0.0 mg/mL to 1.0 mg/mL. After NF/CAF discarding, the mixture of growth medium and MTT (5 mg/mL) was added. Cells were incubated for 3 h until intracellular purple formazan crystals were visible under a microscope, and then dimethyl sulfoxide (DMSO), (POCH-Avantor, Gliwice, Poland) was added to each well to dissolve purple crystals of formazan. The absorbance was measured using a spectrophotometric method (BioTek U.S., Winooski, VT, USA) at a wavelength of 540 nm.

2.4. *The Culture of Caco-2 Colon Cancer Cells*

The colon cancer Caco-2 cell line (ATCC® HTB-37™) was purchased from ATCC (American Type Culture Collection, Manassas, VA, USA) and used as the model of the epithelial intestinal permeability layer. Caco-2 cells were cultured in Dulbecco's Modified Eagle's Medium (DMEM, Merck Group, Darmstadt, Germany) supplemented with 1% nonessential amino acids mixture (MEM NON, Merck Group, Darmstadt, Germany), 20% fetal bovine serum (FBS, Merck Group, Darmstadt, Germany), and 2 mM L-glutamine, 100 U/mL penicillin and 0.1 mg/mL streptomycin solution (Merck Group, Darmstadt, Germany). For the transport monolayer preparation, the Caco-2 cells were seeded at $4 \times 10^5/cm^2$ into transparent membranes inserts with 0.4 μm pore size (Millipore–Merck Group, Darmstadt, Germany) in 6-wells plates (Corning-Life Science, Durham, NC, USA). The cells were cultured for 22 days at 37 °C in a humidified atmosphere containing 5% CO_2 and 95% air. The integrity of the Caco-2 monolayer was evaluated by measuring the Trans Epithelial Electrical Resistance (TEER) every 48 h. The cells were considered to be suitable for use in the permeability study if the average TEER value was >600 Ohm × cm^2 (Millicell ERS-2 Voltohmmeter, Millipore–Merck Group, Darmstadt, Germany).

2.5. *Permeability Test*

The permeability tests of NF and CAF solutions were performed in two directions: apical-to-basolateral (A–B) and basolateral-to-apical (B–A) in triplicate at 37 °C with shaking at 100 rpm for 2 h. For transport assay, drug substances (NF, CAF) were dissolved in the transport buffer solution (HBSS with 25 mM HEPES, pH 7.4) and applied in the apical or basolateral compartment in compliance with transport direction. At 15 min intervals, the sample from the acceptor compartment was taken during a 2-h transport experiment. Each sample volume (150 μL) was replaced with a fresh pre-heated (37 °C) transport buffer. The total solution volume in the apical and basolateral compartments was maintained at 2 mL and 4 mL, respectively. HPLC analysis was used to determine the concentration of the compound transported. Quantitative chromatographic analyses were performed using the reverse phase HPLC method and UV-VIS detector (Waters UPLC Acquity H-class apparatus with Empower 3.0 software, Waters Corporation, Milford, MA, USA). The analytical method of NF was based on British Pharmacopoeia monograph Naftydrofuryl capsules (with slight modifications) [27], while CAF was based on the European Pharmacopoeia monograph [5]. The chromatographic parameters for NF were set as follows: column (4.6 mm × 250 mm; 5 μm) filled with silica modified by phenyl groups (Spherisorb Phenyl columns, Waters Corporation, Milford, MA, USA). The liquid phase was a mixture of 55 volumes of ACN with 45 volumes of 0.05 M sodium acetate (pH 4.0 with 85% *v/v* orthophosphoric acid). The isocratic flow rate was set as 1 mL/min and the detection wavelength on $\lambda = 283$ nm. The retention time of Naftidrofuryl peak was about 10 min. Following the modifications, this chromatographic method was validated to be suitable for the assay. Transport data, including apparent permeability coefficient (P_{app}) that reflects the rate at which compounds pass the intestinal barrier, were calculated according to the protocols described by Tavelin et al. [28] and Hubatsch et al. [29].

2.6. In-House NF Capsules Preparation

In-house 100 mg capsules with Naftidrofuryl oxalate were prepared as a test product (laboratory scale) for the NF dissolution profile assay. The in-house NF capsules were made according to the Praxilene® 100 mg Capsules formulation, as presented in the Praxilene SPMC [12] in the proportions shown in Table 2.

Table 2. Composition of the developed in-house NF capsules.

Ingredients	Quantity (Per One Capsule)	Function
Naftidrofuryl oxalate	100 mg	active ingredient
Talc	rest of the unit filling weight	filler
Magnesium stearate	up to 0.5% of the unit filling weight	lubricant

2.7. In Vitro Dissolution Test and Data Evaluation

The release rate of NF (from in-house NF capsules vs. Praxilene® 100 mg Capsules) was determined by using automated dissolution apparatus (European Pharmacopoeia, Type II; Erweka DT 828/1000 LH; Erweka GmbH, Langen, Germany) with paddles operating at a rotation speed of 50 rpm in 37 °C (±0.5 °C). The parameters for the dissolution test: 900 mL of three different dissolution media (0.1 M HCl, acetate buffer, phosphate buffer) with pH of 1.2, 4.5, and 6.8 respectively were used. Twelve in-house NF capsules (and 12 Praxilene units) were tested in each dissolution medium. The concentration values of the released NF were recorded at the following time points: 5, 10, 15, 20, 30, and 45 min. Samples (10 mL) of the tested solutions were withdrawn, then filtered (0.2 μm nylon syringe filter), and subsequently subjected to quantitative assessment by validated spectrophotometric method (as described in Section 2.2—Solubility test). The dissolution data were statistically evaluated using the two factor (f_1, f_2) method, according to the United States Food and Drug Administration (FDA) guideline [25]. As the first step, the spectrophotometric results were qualitatively evaluated (% RSD—relative standard deviation percentage) to ensure that they are suitable for the two factors calculation stage and, subsequently, for the dissolution profiles comparison and evaluation. The aggregated % RSD was calculated based on all the three dissolution media timepoints results obtained. However, the % RSD not exceeding 20% of the results obtained in the early time points (up to 10 min) and 10% for the subsequent timepoints is mandatory in this approach. The difference factor (f_1) and similarity factor (f_2) were calculated according to the FDA guidelines [25,30]. The two curves are considered to be similar if the value for f_1 is not greater than 15% (0–15), while the value of f_2 is greater than 50% (50–100) [25,30].

3. Results

3.1. Solubility Test

The maximum dose strength for NF is 200 mg (according to data on https://www.drugs.com/international/naftidrofuryl.html). Using the equilibrium solubility method, we showed a high solubility of NF in all buffers pH range 1.2–6.8. The lowest value of solubility (about 169 mg/mL) was observed on acetic acid conditions (pH 4.5), and the highest value (about 290 mg/mL) was obtained in pH 6.8. Thus, the calculated minimum dose/solubility ratio (D/S) was lower than 250 mL, and the dose number (D_0) was less than 1 in each medium. The results of the equilibrium solubility are shown in Table 3.

Table 3. Solubility results of 200 mg NF in three different pH media at 37 °C. Results of the three replicates are presented as the mean ± SD.

Dose (D) (mg)	pH	Solubility (S) (mg/mL)	D/S Ratio (mL)	D_0
200	1.2	279.00 ± 15.69	0.69	0.003
	4.5	169.00 ± 6.79	1.19	0.005
	6.8	290.40 ± 19.83	0.67	0.003

3.2. Permeability Assay on Caco-2 Cell Line

To assess the permeability of NF across the Caco-2 monolayer, we selected CAF classified as the reference standard for highly permeable and BCS class I substances [24,25].

3.2.1. Effect of NF and CAF on Caco-2 Cells Viability

The concentrations of the drugs to be used for the permeability tests were established by using the MTT viability test. The highest concentration of the test compounds with no cytotoxic effect on Caco-2 cells was preferred. To evaluate the cytotoxic activity of NF and CAF, the Caco-2 cells were exposed for two hours to the concentration ranges of each compound from 0.0 mg/mL to 1.0 mg/mL. The MTT results (Figure 1) showed that NF caused a more cytotoxic effect, as compared to CAF since only the highest concentration of CAF (1.00 mg/mL) slightly decreased the viability of Caco-2 cells (~92%). In contrast, 0.250 mg/mL of NF concentration caused down-regulation of cell viability to ~67%. Hence, in the permeability study, we used 0.200 mg/mL and 0.125 mg/mL of NF concentrations as they were not cytotoxic in the Caco-2 cell line.

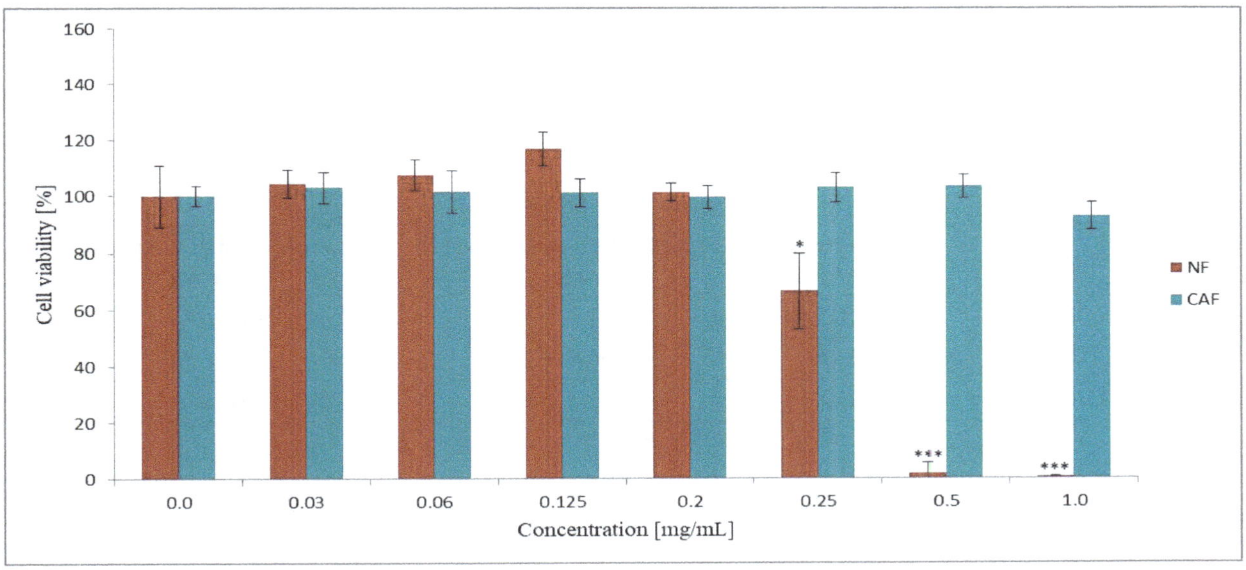

Figure 1. The effect of NF and CAF on Caco-2 cell viability. Results of the three independent replicates are presented as the mean ± SD. *** $p < 0.001$ and * $p < 0.05$.

3.2.2. Caco-2 Permeability Assay

The intestinal epithelial Caco-2 cell culture model was applied to determine the permeability of NF and CAF across the intestinal barrier. TEER value measurements monitored the integrity of the Caco-2 monolayers during 22-day cultivation. The TEER parameter stabilized at 614 ± 24 Ω cm^2 on the 7th day of culture. Only monolayers with TEER values beyond 600 Ω cm^2 were used in the transport experiments. Bidirectional transport was analysed at two NF concentrations (0.125 mg/mL and 0.200 mg/mL) to determine the drug dose permeability relationship. CAF, as a reference intestinal permeable compound, was transported across the Caco-2 barrier at a concentration of 0.500 mg/mL. No cytotoxicity of NF and CAF at the concentrations tested after 2-h transport was observed. The TEER measurement indicated the high integrity of Caco-2 cell monolayers before and after permeability experiments (data not shown).

Based on HPLC data, the NF and CAF transport kinetics and the apparent permeability coefficient (P_{app}) values were evaluated. The "weighted normalized cumulative amount of transported compound" for simplicity commonly named in the literature "cumulative fraction transported" (CFT) in the receiver compartment of the Caco-2 experimental model increased linearly with time, independently on transport direction (Figure 2). The time-course analysis of NF and CAF intestinal permeability showed that CFT was significantly higher in the absorptive direction (A-B transport) than in the secretory direction (B–A transport). This was also confirmed by the Papp values determined for NF and CAF transported in A–B and B–A direction (Table 4).

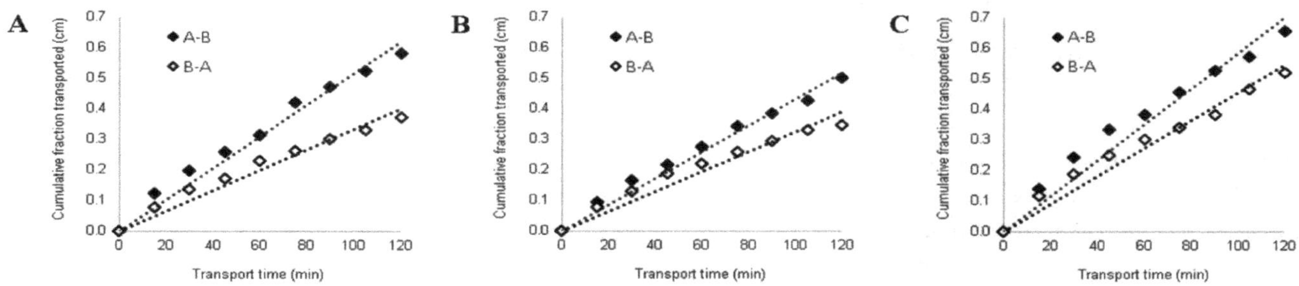

Figure 2. The experimentally (◇) and theoretically (········) determined "cumulative fraction transported" of naftidrofuryl oxalate (NF) and caffeine (CAF) versus time in bidirectional A–B and B–A transport across Caco-2 cell monolayer. NF concentrations in donor compartments were established at 0.125 mg/mL (**A**) and 0.200 mg/mL (**B**). CAF transport was analyzed at an initial concentration of 0.5 mg/mL (**C**).

Table 4. Apparent permeability coefficients (P_{app}) of naftidrofuryl oxalate (NF) and caffeine (CAF) determined in the Caco-2 intestinal barrier model (n = 3).

		$P_{app} \times 10^{-6}$ (cm/s)	
Drug Substance	**Concentration (mg/mL)**	**Apical-to-Basolaterial Transport**	**Basolaterial-to-Apical Transport**
NF	0.125	131.9 ± 34.8	84.1 ± 4.7
NF	0.200	100.8 ± 15.1	78.8 ± 1.0
CAF	0.500	161.3 ± 19.7	126.5 ± 2.4

The results obtained from transport experiments showed that in vitro permeability of NF across the Caco-2 intestinal barrier is relatively high. The P_{app} values estimated for A–B transport of NF at both concentrations were higher than 100×10^{-6} cm/s. Permeability coefficients for B–A transport were calculated at 84.1×10^{-6} cm/s and 78.8×10^{-6} cm/s for NF at concentrations of 0.125 mg/mL and 0.200 mg/mL, respectively (Table 4). The results obtained from transport studies confirmed high intestinal permeability of CAF in both transport directions.

3.3. Dissolution Profiles Comparison

The in vitro dissolution testing was performed based on EMA guideline [24]. NF was released from both products, Praxilene, and the in-house NF capsules, very rapidly > 85% in less than 15 min. The dissolution rate of NF capsules was independent of pH and buffer species of the dissolution media. We observed a slightly faster release NF from in-house NF capsules than a reference product (Praxilene). The results of dissolution profiles of NF from in-house NF capsules and Praxilene are shown in Figure 3.

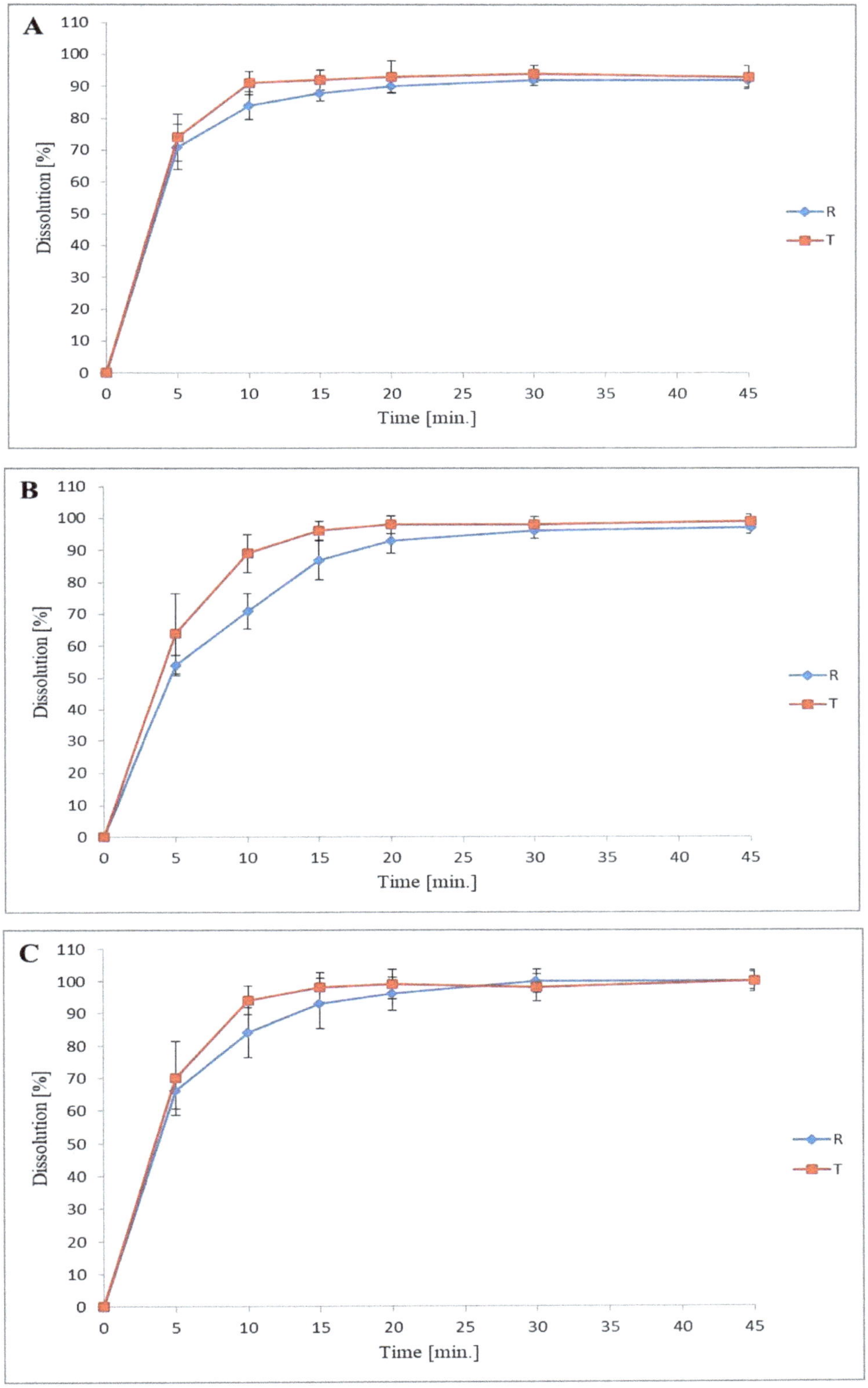

Figure 3. Comparative assessment of the in vitro release profiles of NF from in-house NF capsules (T, tested product) and Praxilene (R, reference product) in three different media 0.1 M HCl (**A**), acetate buffer (**B**), and phosphate buffer (**C**). Each time point on the curves shows the aggregated (n = 12) average percentage of NF release level from these products.

According to EMA, the confirmation of two curves (dissolution profiles) is not required for the IR product (≥85% in 15 min) [24]. Nevertheless, the mathematical estimation with standard statistical analysis was performed. The raw data (% RSD of the results in early dissolution time points, up to 10 min., of not more than 20%, and no more than of 10% in the subsequent time points) are consistent with the EMA guideline (Table 5) [24].

Table 5. The % RSD values for the in vitro release profiles of NF from in-house NF capsules (T, tested product) and Praxilene (R, reference product) in three different media 0.1 M HCl, acetate buffer, and phosphate buffer.

Time Point [min.]	0.1 M HCl pH 1.2 (%RSD)		Acetate Buffer pH 4.5 (%RSD)		Phosphate Buffer pH 6.8 (%RSD)	
	R	T	R	T	R	T
5	10.0	10.0	5.8	19.8	8.3	16.3
10	5.2	4.1	7.7	6.7	9.2	4.8
15	2.9	3.5	7.1	3.2	8.5	4.7
20	2.1	5.4	4.1	2.9	5.3	4.6
30	1.9	2.8	2.3	2.4	3.6	4.3
45	2.3	3.9	2.0	2.3	2.8	3.3

The statistical evaluation of the two profiles similarity was performed using the two factors (f_1, f_2) method. The summary of the results is presented in Table 6. Our results showed a mathematical similarity between the dissolution profiles of the test (in-house NF capsules) and the reference product (Praxilene) for each medium ($f_2 \geq 50$); the EMA guideline [24] was met. The release profiles showed the most significant similarity in pH 1.2 and 6.8 ($f_1 \leq 15$, $f_2 \geq 50$), while in pH 4.5, they were on the border of the accepted criteria ($f_2 = 51$, $f_1 = 11$).

Table 6. Summary of f_1 and f_2 values for dissolution profiles curves in three different media.

Requirement	0.1 M HCl pH = 1.2	Acetate Buffer pH = 4.5	Phosphate Buffer pH = 6.8
Difference factor f_1 (profiles are similar when $f_1 \leq 15$)	2	11	6
Similarity factor f_2 (profiles are similar when $f_2 \geq 50$)	71	51	65

4. Discussion

The BCS-based biowaiver guidelines take into account the rate of APIs release from the solid oral dosage forms, their solubility, and the in vitro transepithelial transport, thus describing the first stages of a drug LADME (liberation and absorption) [24,25]. To the best of the authors' knowledge, there is no data concerning the classification of NF to the BCS. NF is known to dissolve well in aqueous media and ethanol [5,27]. Based on this information, NF might be suggested to belong to BCS class I (high solubility, high permeability) or BCS class III (high solubility, low permeability). Thus, the present study aimed to determine the aqueous solubility of NF and its permeability through Caco-2 monolayers.

The determination of NF solubility was performed using the equilibrium solubility method. Based on EMA guideline, a substance is considered well soluble when the highest therapeutic dose dissolves in 250 mL or less of aqueous media within the pH range of 1.2–6.8 at 37 ± 1 °C [24]. According to FDA guideline, the solubility test should be evaluated based on the ionization characteristics of the tested substance in pH = pKa, pH = pKa + 1, and pH = pKa−1 [25]. The pKa value of NF has been reported as 8.2 [6,19], which is above the human gastrointestinal tract (GIT) physiological range. Therefore, we did not extend the pH condition above the physiological range. In the solubility studies, we used three media in ranges of gastrointestinal pH (1.2, 4.5, and 6.8) and the highest 200 mg NF dose strength. We showed that the minimum solubility of the NF highest single dose was 169.0 mg/mL at pH 4.5. The calculated D/S ratio was 1.2 mL, thus far below the critical value of 250 mL. Our results indicate that NF is a highly soluble substance in the entire examined pH range. The highest solubility value at pH 6.8 suggests that NF might be well soluble in intestinal pH conditions positively affecting drug absorption from the GIT.

According to BCS-based protocols, the permeability of a drug substance throughout the GIT can be assessed by in vitro methods using a monolayer of cultured epithelial cells [24,25]. Hence, to determine the absorption of NF, the permeability test using the Caco-2 cell line was performed, and permeability coefficients (P_{app}) were determined in both directions. In the present study, the permeability test of CAF was performed to confirm the suitability of the Caco-2 cell line system applied to determine transepithelial transport. CAF is recognized as a BCS reference substance [24,25] for which high permeability ($P_{app} = {\sim}50 \times 10^{-6}$ cm/s; concentration 0.06 mg/mL) has been well documented [31,32]. Since we observed high transepithelial transport of CAF in both directions, the usefulness of the Caco-2 cell model was confirmed. The permeability study of CAF was performed only at the highest concentration (0.5 mg/mL) without cytotoxic effects against Caco-2 cells. According to BCS requirements for permeability analysis, the concentration of drug substance should be used in the amount of 0.01, 0.1, and 1 times its highest strength dissolved in 250 mL [24,25]. Assuming the NF 200 mg as the highest dose dissolute in 250 mL, we obtained a concentration range as follows: 0.8 mg/mL, 0.08 and 0.008 mg/mL. We examined the cytotoxicity of NF starting on the highest 1.0 mg/mL concentration. The 0.250 mg/mL of NF concentration was observed to cause down-regulation of cell viability to ~67%. Therefore, the bidirectional transport of NF was investigated at the two highest non-cytotoxic concentrations (0.125 mg/mL and 0.200 mg/mL), in the order of magnitude close to 0.08 mg/mL. We did not perform the permeability study of NF in the lowest concentration (0.008 mg/mL) since the analytical range of the NF assay method was validated for 0.01–0.3 mg/mL concentrations. According to literature data, when P_{aap} is lower than 1×10^{-6}, the substance is considered as poorly permeable (0–20%). Concomitantly, the highly permeable drug is characterized by $P_{aap} > 10 \times 10^{-6}$ [29,33]. Our results showed that the permeability of NF across the cells barrier is quite high since the estimated values of P_{app} for A-B transport direction in both doses were larger than 100×10^{-6} cm/s. Furthermore, we observed that the P_{app} values of NF within its non-cytotoxic concentrations were almost as good as highly permeable CAF results. Hence, a rapid and total in vivo epithelial transport of NF might be suggested.

In general, we suggest that NF might be assigned to BCS I class due to its high solubility and high permeability. However, to fully comply with BCS requirements, the permeability tests should be validated using several additional reference substances that represent different levels of permeability (high, moderate, low, zero, and efflux substrates).

A drug product is eligible for biowaiver procedure when the substance belongs to BCS I or III class and is an immediate-release oral dosage form [24,25]. Thus, we also examined the in vitro dissolution rate of in-house prepared NF capsules in accordance with the Praxilene® 100 mg formulation as a reference drug. The Praxilene product has a relatively simple composition with only two excipients (talc and magnesium stearate) that allowed us to closely define the quantity of each excipient in the dosage form. In our study, we showed that both products fulfil the IR requirements (>85% in not less than 15 min). Additionally, the similarity of the curves was confirmed statistically ($f_1 \leq 15$; $f_2 \geq 50$) in all media used in the range of pH 1.2–6.8. Thus, we conclude that multisourced excipients used for NF capsules preparation had no or minimal effect on its release rate. Our observations are in agreement with Flangan et al. since the excipients used for BCS I class drugs have been generally shown not to affect the intestinal absorption rate [34]. Moreover, the IR status of analyzed products indicates high pharmaceutical availability of NF throughout the GIT. Thus, we suggest that NF oral dosage form in comparison with Praxilene as a reference product meets the pharmacological equivalence criteria.

5. Conclusions

NF is a highly soluble substance within a wide pH range of physiological GIT conditions and highly permeable across Caco-2 cell monolayer. Thus, in the present study, we suggest that NF might be classified into BCS class I. Furthermore, we showed high dissolution rate of encapsulated

NF based on Praxilene® 100 mg composition and, therefore, it might be considered as an IR. To the best of the authors' knowledge, this is the first attempt to classify NF based on BCS requirements The experimental design of this study was based mainly on the BSC guidelines for the pharmaceutical industry. Hence, our paper could be useful for further developmental studies on NF containing drugs

Author Contributions: Conceptualization, H.P.-K., A.O., and I.I.; formal analysis, M.K.-S. and M.W.; data curation M.W. and I.I.; writing—original draft preparation, M.K.-S.; writing—review and editing, H.P.-K., I.I., and A.O. supervision, H.P.-K., A.O., and I.I.; project administration, P.I.C.; funding acquisition, H.P.-K. and P.I.C. All authors have read and agreed to the published version of the manuscript.

References

1. Amidon, G.L.; Lennernäs, H.; Shah, V.P.; Crison, J.R. A Theoretical Basis for a Biopharmaceutic Drug Classification: The Correlation of in Vitro Drug Product Dissolution and in Vivo Bioavailability. *Pharm. Res* **1995**, *12*, 413–420. [CrossRef] [PubMed]
2. Manallack, D.T.; Prankerd, R.J.; Yuriev, E.; Oprea, T.I.; Chalmers, D.K. The significance of acid/base properties in drug discovery. *Chem. Soc. Rev.* **2013**, *42*, 485–496. [CrossRef] [PubMed]
3. Panakanti, R.; Narang, A.S. Impact of Excipient Interactions on Drug Bioavailability from Solid Dosage Forms. *Pharm. Res.* **2012**, *29*, 2639–2659. [CrossRef] [PubMed]
4. Hao, J.; Chen, B.; Yao, Y.; Hossain, M.; Nagatomo, T.; Yao, H.; Kong, L.; Sun, H. Practical access to four stereoisomers of naftidrofuryl and their binding affinity towards 5-hydroxytryptamine 2A receptor *Bioorganic Med. Chem. Lett.* **2012**, *22*, 3441–3444. [CrossRef]
5. European Directorate for the Quality of Medicines. *European Pharmacopoeia*, 10th ed.; European Directorate for the Quality of Medicines: Strasbourg, France, 2019; pp. 3322–3323.
6. Waaler, P.; Graffner, C.; Müller, B. Biopharmaceutical studies of naftidrofuryl in hydrocolloid matrix tablets *Int. J. Pharm.* **1992**, *87*, 229–237. [CrossRef]
7. Wiernsperger, N.F. Serotonin, 5-HT2 receptors, and their blockade by naftidrofuryl: A targeted therapy of vascular diseases. *J. Cardiovasc. Pharmacol.* **1994**, *23*, S37–S43. [CrossRef]
8. Verheggen, R.; Schrör, K. Effect of naftidrofuryl on platelet-induced vasospasm in vitro. Role of antiserotonergic actions. *Arzneimittelforschung* **1993**, *43*, 330–334.
9. Goldsmith, D.R.; Wellington, K. Naftidrofuryl. *Drugs Aging* **2005**, *22*, 967–977. [CrossRef]
10. Capon, A.; Lehert, P.; Opsomer, L. Naftidrofuryl in the treatment of subacute stroke. *J. Cardiovasc. Pharmacol* **1990**, *16*, 62–66.
11. Lu, D.; Song, H.; Hao, Z.; Wu, T.; Mccleery, J. Naftidrofuryl for dementia. *Cochrane Database Syst. Rev.* **2011** *12*, CD002955. [CrossRef]
12. Merck Serono Ltd. Praxilene 100 mg Capsules; Summary of Product Characteristics. Available online https://www.medicines.org.uk/emc/product/990/smpc#companyDetails (accessed on 12 November 2020).
13. Brodie, R.; Chasseaud, L.; Taylor, T.; Hunter, J.; Ciclitira, P. Determination of naftidrofuryl in the plasma of humans by high-performance liquid chromatography. *J. Chromatogr.* **1979**, *164*, 534–540. [CrossRef]
14. Nishigaki, R.; Umemura, K.; Okui, K.; Hayashi, T.; Yamamoto, T.; Sakurai, Y. The pharmacokinetical analysis of the fate of naphtidrofuryl oxalate (LS121) in human subjects. II. Estimation of the first-pass effect after oral administration. *Yakugaku Zasshi.* **1986**, *106*, 916–923. [CrossRef] [PubMed]
15. Garrett, E.R. Bioanalyses and Pharmacokinetics of Nafronyl in the Dog. *J. Pharm. Sci.* **1984**, *73*, 635–649 [CrossRef] [PubMed]
16. Platt, D.; Mühlberg, W.; Rieck, W.; Horn, H.J.; Schmitt-Rüth, R. Pharmacokinetics of naftidrofuryl in multimorbidity in geriatric patients. *Z. Gerontol.* **1984**, *17*, 246–250.
17. Roth, K.; Hildebrand, M.; Beyer, K.-H. Metabolism of nafronyl in man. *Eur. J. Drug Metab. Pharmacokinet.* **1989**, *14*, 133–138. [CrossRef]
18. Sabry, S.M.; Belal, T.S.; Barary, M.H.; Ibrahim, M.E.A. A validated HPLC method for the simultaneous determination of naftidrofuryl oxalate and its degradation product (metabolite), naftidrofuryl acid: Applications to pharmaceutical tablets and biological samples. *Drug Test. Anal.* **2012**, *5*, 500–508. [CrossRef]
19. Moffat, A.C.; Osselton, M.D.; Widdop, B.; Watts, J. *Clarke's Analysis of Drugs and Poisons*, 4th ed.; Pharmaceutical Press: London, UK; Gurnee, IL, USA, 2011; pp. 1746–1747.

20. Riederer, P.; Laux, G.; Pöldinger, W. *Neuro-Psychopharmaka Ein Therapie-Handbuch*; Springer: Wien, Austria, 1999; p. 660.
21. Walmsley, L.M.; Taylor, T.; Wilkinson, P.A.; Brodie, R.R.; Chasseaud, L.F.; Alun-Jones, V.; Hunter, J.O. Plasma concentrations and relative bioavailability of naftidrofuryl from different salt forms. *Biopharm. Drug Dispos.* **1986**, *7*, 327–334. [CrossRef]
22. Hulot, T.; Gamand, S.; Dupain, T.; Ahtoy, P.; Bromet, M. Influence of age on the pharmacokinetics of naftidrofuryl after single oral administration in elderly versus young healthy volunteers. *Arzneimittelforschung* **1998**, *48*, 900–904. [PubMed]
23. Legallicier, B.; Barbier, S.; Bolloni, L.; Fillastre, J.-P.; Godin, M.; Kuhn, T.; Porte, F.; Chretien, P.; Dupainc, T.; Bromet-Petitd, M. Pharmacokinetics of Naftidrofuryl in Patients with Renal Impairment. *Arzneimittelforschung* **2011**, *55*, 370–375. [CrossRef] [PubMed]
24. European Medicines Agency (EMA). ICH M9 Guideline on Biopharmaceutics Classification System-Based Biowaivers. Available online: https://www.ema.europa.eu/en/documents/scientific-guideline/ich-m9-biopharmaceutics-classification-system-based-biowaivers-step-5_en.pdf (accessed on 10 February 2020).
25. U.S. Food and Drug Administration (FDA). Waiver of In Vivo Bioavailability and Bioequivalence Studies for Immediate-Release Solid Oral Dosage Forms Based on a Biopharmaceutics Classification System Guidance for Industry. Available online: https://www.fda.gov/media/70963/download (accessed on 26 December 2017).
26. Dahan, A.; Miller, J.M.; Amidon, G.L. Prediction of Solubility and Permeability Class Membership: Provisional BCS Classification of the World's Top Oral Drugs. *AAPS J.* **2009**, *11*, 740–746. [CrossRef]
27. The British Pharmacopoeia Commission. *British Pharmacopoeia*; The British Pharmacopoeia Commission: London, England, 2020.
28. Tavelin, S.; Gråsjö, J.; Taipalensuu, J.; Ocklind, G.; Artursson, P.; Wise, C. Applications of Epithelial Cell Culture in Studies of Drug Transport. *Methods Mol Biol.* **2002**, *188*, 233–272. [CrossRef] [PubMed]
29. Hubatsch, I.; E Ragnarsson, E.G.; Artursson, P. Determination of drug permeability and prediction of drug absorption in Caco-2 monolayers. *Nat. Protoc.* **2007**, *2*, 2111–2119. [CrossRef] [PubMed]
30. U.S. Food and Drug Administration (FDA). Dissolution Testing of Immediate Release Solid Oral Dosage Forms. Guidance for Industry. Available online: https://www.fda.gov/media/70936/download (accessed on 25 August 1997).
31. Volpe, D.A.; Faustino, P.J.; Ciavarella, A.B.; Asafu-Adjaye, E.B.; Ellison, C.D.; Yu, L.X.; Hussain, A.S. Classification of Drug Permeability with a Caco-2 Cell Monolayer Assay. *Clin. Res. Regul. Aff.* **2007**, *24*, 39–47. [CrossRef]
32. Smetanová, L.; Stetinova, V.; Kholova, D.; Kvetina, J.; Smetana, J.; Svoboda, Z. Caco-2 cells and Biopharmaceutics Classification System (BCS) for prediction of transepithelial transport of xenobiotics (model drug: Caffeine). *Neuro Endocrinol. Lett.* **2009**, *30*, 101–105. [PubMed]
33. Yee, S. In Vitro Permeability across Caco-2 Cells (Colonic) Can Predict In Vivo (Small Intestinal) Absorption in Man—Fact or Myth. *Pharm. Res.* **1997**, *14*, 763–766. [CrossRef]
34. Flanagan, T.R. Potential for pharmaceutical excipients to impact absorption: A mechanistic review for BCS Class 1 and 3 drugs. *Eur. J. Pharm. Biopharm.* **2019**, *141*, 130–138. [CrossRef]

5

Strong and Selective Inhibitory Effects of the Biflavonoid Selamariscina A against CYP2C8 and CYP2C9 Enzyme Activities in Human Liver Microsomes

So-Young Park [1,2], Phi-Hung Nguyen [3], Gahyun Kim [2], Su-Nyeong Jang [1,2], Ga-Hyun Lee [1,2], Nguyen Minh Phuc [2,4], Zhexue Wu [2] and Kwang-Hyeon Liu [1,2,*]

1 BK21 Plus KNU Multi-Omics based Creative Drug Research Team, College of Pharmacy and Research Institute of Pharmaceutical Sciences, Kyungpook National University, Daegu 41566, Korea; soyoung561021@gmail.com (S.-Y.P.); wts1424@naver.com (S.-N.J.); lgh2710@gmail.com (G.-H.L.)

2 College of Pharmacy and Research Institute of Pharmaceutical Sciences, Kyungpook National University, Daegu 41566, Korea; hyunlove9137@naver.com (G.K.); phucnguyen0606@gmail.com (N.M.P.); wuzhexue527@gmail.com (Z.W.)

3 Institute of Natural Products Chemistry, Vietnam Academy of Science and Technology, 18-Hoang Quoc Viet, Cau Giay, Hanoi 100000, Vietnam; nguyenphihung1002@gmail.com

4 Vietnam Hightech of Medicinal and Pharmaceutical JSC, Group 11 Quang Minh town, Hanoi 100000, Vietnam

* Correspondence: dstlkh@knu.ac.kr

Abstract: Like flavonoids, biflavonoids, dimeric flavonoids, and polyphenolic plant secondary metabolites have antioxidant, antibacterial, antiviral, anti-inflammatory, and anti-cancer properties. However, there is limited data on their effects on cytochrome P450 (P450) and uridine 5′-diphosphoglucuronosyl transferase (UGT) enzyme activities. In this study we evaluate the inhibitory potential of five biflavonoids against nine P450 activities (P450s1A2, 2A6, 2B6, 2C8, 2C9, 2C19, 2D6, 2E1, and 3A) in human liver microsomes (HLMs) using cocktail incubation and liquid chromatography-tandem mass spectrometry (LC–MS/MS). The most strongly inhibited P450 activity was CYP2C8-mediated amodiaquine *N*-dealkylation with IC50 ranges of 0.019~0.123 μM. In addition, the biflavonoids—selamariscina A, amentoflavone, robustaflavone, cupressuflavone, and taiwaniaflavone—noncompetitively inhibited CYP2C8 activity with respective K_i values of 0.018, 0.083, 0.084, 0.103, and 0.142 μM. As selamariscina A showed the strongest effects, we then evaluated it against six UGT isoforms, where it showed weaker inhibition (UGTs1A1, 1A3, 1A4, 1A6, 1A9, and 2B7, IC50 > 1.7 μM). Returning to the P450 activities, selamariscina A inhibited CYP2C9-mediated diclofenac hydroxylation and tolbutamide hydroxylation with respective K_i values of 0.032 and 0.065 μM in a competitive and noncompetitive manner. However, it only weakly inhibited CYP1A2, CYP2B6, and CYP3A with respective K_i values of 3.1, 7.9, and 4.5 μM. We conclude that selamariscina A has selective and strong inhibitory effects on the CYP2C8 and CYP2C9 isoforms. This information might be useful in predicting herb-drug interaction potential between biflavonoids and co-administered drugs mainly metabolized by CYP2C8 and CYP2C9. In addition, selamariscina A might be used as a strong CYP2C8 and CYP2C9 inhibitor in P450 reaction-phenotyping studies to identify drug-metabolizing enzymes responsible for the metabolism of new chemicals.

Keywords: biflavonoid; cytochrome P450; drug interactions; selamariscina A; uridine 5′-diphosphoglucuronosyl transferase

1. Introduction

Flavonoids are polyphenolic secondary metabolites that are common in the plant kingdom and are ingested by humans in their food [1]. Flavonoids are grouped into various classes based on structure. These classes are: anthocyanidins, chalcones, flavanones, flavones, flavonols, isoflavonoids, and biflavonoids [2]. Many pharmacological benefits have been ascribed to flavonoids, including antioxidant, anti-inflammatory, anti-cancer, antiviral, and hepatoprotective effects [3,4].

Having flavonoids in your diet may reduce the risk of atherosclerosis, cardiovascular disease, diabetes mellitus, osteoporosis, and certain cancers [4,5]. Because of flavonoids' benefits and wide distribution, their intake has risen steadily in recent years in the West and Asia. Daily intake of flavonoids has been estimated at 100 mg/day in the Asian population because of the high consumption of soy products [6,7]. On the other hand, daily intake of flavonoids has been estimated to be in the range of 20–50 mg/day in Western populations [8]. Further intake of flavonoids through dietary supplements and plant extracts with prescribed drugs is common. The vast body of literature describes the significant interactions between flavonoid herbs and therapeutic drugs.

Several flavonoids are substrates for cytochrome P450 (P450) and uridine 5′-diphosphoglucuronosyl transferase (UGT) enzymes [2], suggesting that flavonoids could inhibit the activities of these enzymes. A number of studies have demonstrated that flavonoids are potent inhibitors of CYP1A2, CYP3A, and UGT1A1 in vitro [5,8]. For example, the flavone tangeretin competitively inhibits the activity of CYP1A2 with a *K*i value as low as 68 nM in human liver microsomes (HLMs) [9]. It also inhibits UGT1A1-mediated estradiol glucuronidation with an IC50 value of 1 μM [10]. The flavonols quercetin and kaempferol inhibit the metabolism of nifedipine and felodipine by CYP3A4 in HLMs at concentrations larger than 10 μM. [11]. Animal studies show that oral quercetin increases the bioavailability of oral doxorubicin [12]. These results can be attributed to the reduced first-pass metabolism of doxorubicin due to quercetin-induced inhibition of CYP3A and/or enhanced doxorubicin absorption in the gastrointestinal tract via quercetin-induced inhibition of P-glycoprotein (P-gp). Surya Sandeep et al. (2014) reported that naringenin significantly increases the bioavailability of orally administered felodipine, a P-glycoprotein and CYP3A4 substrate drug, in rats, through the inhibition of intestinal P-gp and CYP3A4 [13]. Alnaqeeb et al. (2019) reported that quercetin and guava leaf extracts in combination with warfarin exert a greater increase on warfarin's C_{max} and International Normalized Ratio values than when used alone, indicating the inhibition of CYP2C8, 2C9 and 3A4, major warfarin-metabolizing enzymes [14]. Biflavonoids, formed by the covalent bond between two monoflavonoids, are a subclass of flavonoid [15]. They are secondary metabolites, but are limited to several species in plants such as *Ginkgo biloba*, *Selaginella* species, *Hypericum perforatum*, and *Garcinia kola* [16]. Befitting their status as flavonoids, they have anti-cancer, anti-microbial, antiviral, and anti-inflammatory properties [16]. In contrast to the extensive studies on drug interaction with flavonoids, data on the inhibitory effects of biflavonoids on P450 and UGT enzymes are rare, though biflavonoids are taken in the form of dietary supplements (e.g., *Ginkgo biloba* extract [17]). The inhibitory potential of amentoflavone, the major biflavonoid in *Cupressus funebris*, against P450 and UGT enzymes was only recently reported [18,19].

In this study, we evaluate the inhibitory effects of five biflavonoids—selamariscina A, amentoflavone, robustaflavone, cupressuflavone, and taiwaniaflavone (Figure 1)—on nine P450 enzymes using HLMs. We further investigate the ability of selamariscina A, which most strongly inhibited CYP2C8 and CYP2C9 activities, to inhibit six UGT isoforms. Furthermore, the inhibition mechanism and kinetic parameters (K_i) were determined for selamariscina A and compared with those of montelukast, a well-known selective CYP2C8 inhibitor [20].

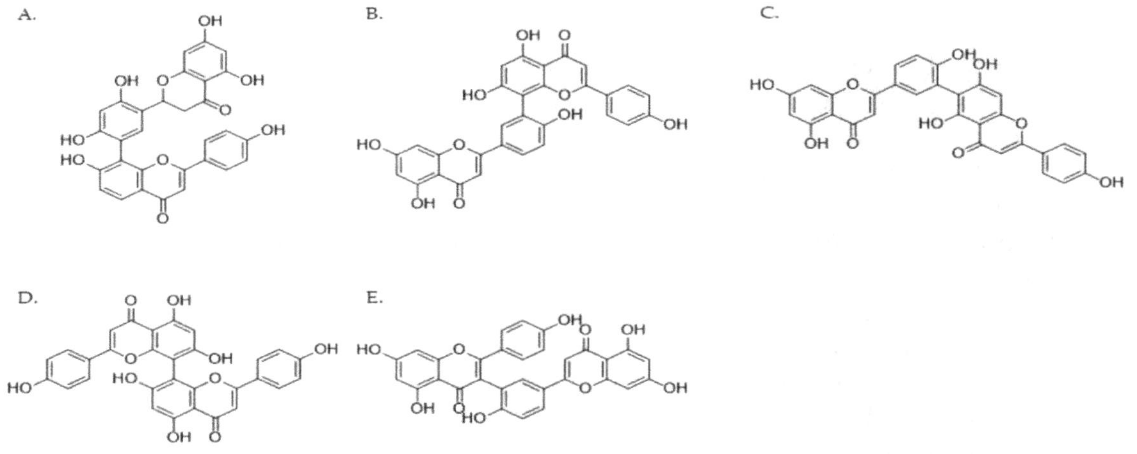

Figure 1. Chemical structures of biflavonoids from *Selaginella tamariscina*: selamariscina A (**A**), amentoflavone (**B**), robustaflavone (**C**), cupressuflavone (**D**) and taiwaniaflavone (**E**).

2. Materials and Methods

2.1. Chemicals and Reagents

We purchased acetaminophen, alamethicin, amodiaquine, bupropion, chenodeoxycholic acid chlorzoxazone, dextromethorphan, estrone glucuronide, glucose-6-phosphate (G6P), glucose- 6-phosphate dehydrogenase (G6PDH), hydroxybupropion, magnesium chloride (MgCl2), N-acetylserotonin β-nicotinamide adenine dinucleotide phosphate (NADP+), N-desethylamodiaquine, omeprazole phenacetin, trifluoperazine, trimipramine, and uridine 5′-diphosphoglucuronic acid (UDPGA) from Sigma-Aldrich (St. Louis, MO, USA). 4-Hydroxydiclofenac, 4-hydroxytolbutamide, 5-hydroxyrosiglitazone, coumarin, diclofenac, midazolam, montelukast, mycophenolic acid, rosiglitazone and tolbutamide came from Toronto Research Chemicals (Toronto, ON, Canada). We obtained 1′-hydroxymidazolam from Cayman Chemical (Ann Arbor, MI, USA), while 7-ethyl-10-hydroxycomptothecine (SN-38) was provided by Santa Cruz Biotechnology (Dallas, TX, USA). All solvents were LC–MS grade (Fisher Scientific, Pittsburgh, PA, USA). All the other reagents were of analytical or LC–MS grade and are commercially available. We purchased the pooled human liver microsomes (XTreme 200) from XenoTech (Lenexa, Kansas City, KS, USA). In this study, we used selamariscina A, amentoflavone, robustaflavone, cupressuflavone, and taiwaniaflavone identified from Selaginella tamariscina (Beauv.), which were collected at Yen Tu Mountain, Uong Bi town, Quang Nihn province Vietnam. The information regarding the identification of their chemical structures was described in our previously published paper [21,22].

We isolated selamariscina A, amentoflavone, robustaflavone, cupressuflavone, and taiwaniaflavone from Selaginella tamariscina (Beauv.), which were collected at Yen Tu Mountain, Uong Bi town, Quang Nihn province, Vietnam. The five compounds were purified and examined by HPLC to get 95% purity Their chemical structures were identified by analyzing their NMR data, which were in good agreement with those published in a previous report [21,22].

2.2. Inhibitory Effect of Five Biflavonoids against Human Cytochrome P450 Activity

The inhibitory potential of the five biflavonoids on the metabolism of nine P450 probe substrates was evaluated using previously developed methods with minor modifications [23,24]. Biflavonoids were dissolved in methanol. The final concentration of methanol in the incubation mixture was 1.0% (*v*/*v*). We used these P450 probe substrates: phenacetin for CYP1A2, coumarin for CYP2A6, bupropion for CYP2B6, amodiaquine for CYP2C8, diclofenac for CYP2C9, omeprazole for CYP2C19, dextromethorphan for CYP2D6, chlorzoxazone for CYP2E1 and midazolam for CYP3A (Table 1) The incubation mixtures containing pooled human liver microsomes (HLMs, XTreme 200, XenoTech),

P450 probe substrates, and inhibitor (0~20 μM) were pre-incubated at 37 °C for 5 min. The concentration range of the inhibitor varied (0, 0.002, 0.005, 0.02, 0.05, and 0.2 μM for CYP2C8; 0, 0.02, 0.05, 0.2, 0.5, and 2 μM for CYP2C9; 0, 0.5, 2, 5, 10, and 20 μM for other P450 isoforms). After pre-incubation, a reduced nicotinamide adenine dinucleotide phosphate (NADPH) generation system containing 1 unit/ml G6PDH, 1.3 mM β- nicotinamide adenine dinucleotide phosphate (β- $NADP^+$), 3.3 mM $MgCl_2$, and 3.3 mM G6P was added to initiate a reaction, and further incubated for 10 min at 37 °C. The reaction was stopped by adding 50 μL of ice-cold acetonitrile containing 7 nM trimipramine (internal standard, IS). After centrifugation at 18,000 g (5 min, 4 °C), aliquots of supernatants were analyzed by LC–MS/MS (Shimadzu LCMS 8060 system, Shimadzu, Kyoto, Japan). All microsomal incubations were conducted in triplicate.

Table 1. Selected reaction monitoring (SRM) condition for the major metabolites of the nine cytochrome P450 probe substrates and internal standard (IS).

P450 Enzyme	Substrates	Concentration (μM)	Metabolites	SRM Transition (*m/z*)	Polarity	Collision Energy (eV)
1A2	Phenacetin	100	Acetaminophen	152 > 110	ESI^+	25
2A6	Coumarin	5	7-Hydroxycoumarin	163 > 107	ESI^+	17
2B6	Bupropion	50	6-Hydroxybupropion	256 > 238	ESI^+	20
2C8	Amodiaquine	1	*N*-Desethylamodiaquine	328 > 283	ESI^+	17
	Rosiglitazone	5	*p*-Hydroxyrosiglitazone	374 > 151	ESI^+	17
2C9	Tolbutamide	100	4-Hydroxytolbutamide	287 > 89	ESI^+	60
	Diclofenac	10	4-Hydroxydiclofenac	312 > 231	ESI^+	15
2C19	Omeprazole	20	5-Hydroxyomeprazole	362 > 214	ESI^+	10
2D6	Dextromethorphan	5	Dextrorphan	258 > 157	ESI^+	35
2E1	Chlorzoxazone	50	6-Hydroxychlorzoxazone	184 > 120	ESI^-	18
3A	Midazolam	5	1′-Hydroxymidazolam	342 > 203	ESI^+	25
IS	Trimipramine	0.007		295 > 100	ESI^+	17

ESI: Electrospray ionization (ESI) interface to generate protonated ions $[M+H]^+$ or deprotonated ion $[M-H]^-$.

2.3. Kinetic Characterization of Five Biflavonoids on CYP2C8 in Human Liver Microsomes

To determine the inhibition mechanism and constants (Ki values) of the five biflavonoids against CYP2C8 activity, different concentrations of biflavonoids (0, 0.002, 0.005, 0.02, 0.05, and 0.2 μM for selamariscina A; 0, 0.05, 0.02, 0.05, 0.2 and 0.5 μM for the other four biflavonoids) were added to reaction mixtures containing different concentrations of amodiaquine (0.1, 0.4 and 1 μM). The other conditions were the same as in the cytochrome P450 inhibition study.

2.4. Kinetic Characterization of Selamariscina A on Five P450 Enzymes in Human Liver Microsomes

We used HLMs to determine the mechanisms and constants (Ki values) for selamariscina A inhibition of CYP1A2, CYP2B6, CYP2C8, CYP2C9 and CYP3A. The selamariscina A (0~50 μM) was added into the reaction mixtures, each of which contained concentrations of phenacetin (20, 50, and 100 μM), bupropion (20, 50, and 100 μM), amodiaquine (0.1, 0.4, and 1 μM), rosiglitazone (2, 5, and 10 μM), diclofenac (1, 4, and 10 μM), tolbutamide (50, 100, and 200 μM), and midazolam (0.5, 2, and 5 μM). The substrates were used at concentrations approximately near to their respective Km values [25–27]. The concentration range of selamariscina A varied (0, 0.002, 0.005, 0.02, 0.05, and 0.2 μM for CYP2C8; 0, 0.05, 0.02, 0.05, 0.2, and 0.5 μM for CYP2C9; 0, 0.2, 0.5, 2, 5, and 20 μM for CYP3A; 0, 0.5, 2, 5, 20, and 50 μM for CYP1A2 and CYP2B6). The other conditions were the same as in the cytochrome P450 inhibition study.

2.5. Time-Dependent Inhibition Assay

The time-dependent inhibition of selamariscina A against CYP2C8 and CYP2C9 enzymes was evaluated using an IC50 shift method. Selamariscina A was pre-incubated at six concentrations (0, 0.002, 0.005, 0.02, 0.05, and 0.2 μM) with HLMs in the presence of an NDAPH generation system for 30 min at 37 °C. The reaction was initiated by adding 1 μM amodiaquine or 10 μM diclofenac and further incubated for 10 min. Incubation was terminated by adding 50 μL of ice-cold acetonitrile containing 7 nM trimipramine. After centrifugation, aliquots of supernatants were analyzed by LC–MS/MS.

2.6. *Inhibitory Effect of Selamariscina A against Human UGT Activity*

The ability of selamariscina A to inhibit the metabolism of six UGT enzyme probe substrates was evaluated using previously developed methods with minor modifications [28]. The microsomal incubation was performed by dividing the non-interactive substrate cocktail sets (set A included SN-38 for UGT1A1, CDCA for UGT1A3 and TFP for UGT1A4 while set B included N-SER for UGT1A6, MPA for UGT1A9 and NX for UGT2B7) (Table 2). In brief, HLMs (0.25 mg/mL) were activated by incubation in the presence of alamethicin (25 μg/mL) for 15 min on ice. After the addition of UGT probe substrates and inhibitor (0, 0.5, 2, 5, 20 and 50 μM), the incubation mixtures were pre-incubated at 37 °C for 5 min. After pre-incubation, 5 mM UDPGA was added to initiate a reaction, and further incubated for 60 min at 37 °C. The reaction was stopped by adding 50 μL of ice-cold acetonitrile containing 250 nM estrone glucuronide (IS). After centrifugation at 18,000 g (5 min, 4 °C), aliquots of supernatants were analyzed by LC–MS/MS. All microsomal incubations were conducted in triplicate.

Table 2. Selected reaction monitoring (SRM) condition for the major metabolites of the six uridine 5′-diphosphoglucuronosyl transferase (UGT) enzyme substrates and internal standard (IS).

UGT Enzyme	Substrates	Concentration (μM)	Metabolites	SRM Transition (*m*/*z*)	Polarity	Collision Energy (eV)
1A1	SN-38	0.5	SN-38 glucuronide	569 > 393	ESI^+	30
1A3	Chenodeoxycholic acid (CDCA)	2	CDCA-24 glucuronide	567 > 391	ESI^-	20
1A4	Trifluoperazine (TFP)	0.5	TFP *N*-glucuronide	584 > 408	ESI^+	30
1A6	*N*-Acetylserotonin (*N*-SER)	1	*N*-SER glucuronide	395 > 219	ESI^+	10
1A9	Mycophenolic acid (MPA)	0.2	MPA 7-*O*-glucuronide	495 > 319	ESI^-	25
2B7	Naloxone (NX)	0.2	NX 3-glucuronide	504 > 310	ESI^+	30
IS	Estrone glucuronide	0.25		445 > 269	ESI^-	35

2.7. *LC–MS/MS Analysis*

All metabolites and the IS were separated on a Kinetex XB-C18 column (100 × 2.10 mm, 2.6 μm, 100 Å; Phenomenex, Torrance, CA, USA) and analyzed using a Shimadzu LCMS 8060 triple-quadrupole mass spectrometer coupled with a Nexera X2 ultra high-performance liquid chromatography system (Shimadzu, Kyoto, Japan) equipped with an electrospray ionization interface. The mobile phase consisted of 0.1% formic acid in water (A) and 0.1% formic acid in acetonitrile (B). The elution condition was set as 8% B (0–0.5 min), 8%→60% B (0.5–5 min), 60% B (5–6 min), 60%→8% B (6–6.1 min) and 8% B (6.1–9 min) for the analysis of metabolites of P450 probe substrates and set as 0%→40% B (0–1 min), 40%→50% B (1–5 min), 50%→0% B (5–5.1 min), and 0% B (5.1–8 min) for the analysis of metabolites of UGT probe substrates. The flow rate was 0.2 mL/min. Electrospray ionization was performed in positive-ion mode at 4000 V or in negative-ion mode at −3500 V. The optimum operating conditions were determined as follows: vaporizer temperature, 300 °C; capillary temperature, 350 °C; collision gas (argon) pressure, 1.5 mTorr. Quantitation was conducted in selected reaction monitoring (SRM) modes with the precursor-to-product ion transition for each metabolite (Tables 1 and 2).

2.8. *Data Analysis*

We analyzed the data with Shimadzu LabSolution LC–MS software. The IC50 values were calculated by WinNonlin software (Pharsight, Mountain View, CA, USA). The type of inhibition and the apparent kinetic parameters for inhibitory activity (*Ki*) were determined by following several criteria: visual inspection of Dixon plots, Lineweaver–Burk double reciprocal plots, and secondary plots of Lineweaver–Burk plots versus biflavonoid concentrations, the size of the sum of squares of the residuals, Akaike Information Criteria values, the S.E. and 95% confidence interval of the parameter estimates from the nonlinear regression analysis [29] using the WinNonlin software. The models tested included competitive, competitive partial, noncompetitive, noncompetitive partial, uncompetitive, uncompetitive partial, and mixed-type inhibition.

3. Results and Discussion

3.1. *Inhibition of Cytochrome P450 Enzymes Activities by Five Biflaovnoids*

The inhibitory potential of the five biflavonoids against cytochrome P450 enzyme activity was evaluated using HLMs (Table 3). We found selamariscina A, amentoflavone, robustaflavone, cupressuflavone, and taiwaniaflavone strongly inhibit CYP2C8 activity with respective IC50 values of 0.019, 0.084, 0.083, 0.083, and 0.12 μM. They also show strong inhibition on CYP2C9 activity with IC50 values of 0.047, 0.15, 0.15, 0.21, and 0.20 μM. Their inhibition of the other seven P450 isoforms was much lower (IC50 ≥ 1.2 μM) than on CYP2C8 and CYP2C9 (IC50 ≤ 0.21 μM). The IC50 value of the inhibition of diclofenac hydroxylase activity by amentoflavone that we found (0.15 μM) is 4.3 times higher than the 0.035 μM reported by von Moltke et al. (2004) [19]. The reason could be differences in incubation conditions, such as CYP2C19 probe substrate and concentrations (diclofenac 10 μM versus S-mephenytoin 25 μM) [30]. The inhibitory potential (IC50 = 1.3 μM) of amentoflavone on CYP3A was similar to the previously reported value (IC50 = 4.3 μM) [19].

Table 3. Inhibitory effects of five biflavonoids and montelukast against nine cytochrome P450 isoforms.

P450 Enzyme	Substrate	IC_{50} (μM)					
		Selamaris-Cina A	Amento-Flavone	Robusta-Flavone	Cupressu-Flavone	Taiwania-Flavone	Montelukast
1A2	Phenacetin	7.4	4.4	4.5	5.9	6.8	>50
2A6	Coumarin	11.6	11.9	11.8	>20	10.6	>50
2B6	Bupropion	5.3	7.1	5.7	6.7	6.4	>50
2C8	Amodiaquine	0.019	0.084	0.083	0.083	0.12	0.52
2C9	Diclofenac	0.047	0.15	0.15	0.21	0.20	9.73
2C19	Omeprazole	13.3	3.4	6.4	3.0	5.0	>50
2D6	Dextromethorphan	10.6	2.6	2.2	2.7	3.2	>50
2E1	Chlorzoxazone	>20	3.3	2.9	2.3	6.0	>50
3A	Midazolam	2.7	1.3	1.2	1.5	1.2	>50

As the five flavonoids strongly inhibited microsomal CYP2C8 activity, we sought to clarify the mechanism of inhibition. The Lineweaver–Burk plots, Dixon plots and secondary reciprocal plots indicated that selamariscina A, amentoflavone, robustaflavone, cupressuflavone, and taiwaniaflavone noncompetitively inhibited CYP2C8-mediated amodiaquine N-deethylation activity with Ki values of 0.018, 0.083, 0.084, 0.103, and 0.142 μM, respectively (Table 4), which are lower than those of the well-known CYP2C8 inhibitors zafirlukast (0.39 μM) [31] and quercetin (4.72 μM) [32].

Table 4. K_i values for inhibition of CYP2C8-catalyzed amodiaquine *N*-deethylation in human liver microsomes by five biflavonoids.

P450 Enzyme	Substrate	Inhibitor	K_i (μM) [a]	Mode of Inhibition
CYP2C8	Amodiaquine	Selamariscina A	0.018 ± 0.002	Noncompetitive
		Amentoflavone	0.083 ± 0.009	Noncompetitive
		Robustaflavone	0.084 ± 0.016	Noncompetitive
		Cupressuflavone	0.103 ± 0.017	Noncompetitive
		Taiwaniaflavone	0.142 ± 0.026	Noncompetitive

[a] Values represent the average ± standard error in triplicate.

Of the five biflavonoids, selamariscina A most strongly inhibited CYP2C8-mediated amodiaquine N-deethylation activity with a Ki value of 0.018 μM, which is similar to the IC50 value of the known strong CYP2C8 inhibitor montelukast (0.020 μM) [31]. Further, its inhibitory potential against CYP2C8 was much stronger than other known CYP2C8 inhibitors axitinib (Ki = 0.17 μM [33]) clotrimazole (IC50 = 0.78 μM [31]), felodipine (IC50 = 1.20 μM [31]), nilotinib (Ki = 0.10 μM [33]) and quercetin (Ki = 1.56 μM [34]). We further evaluated the inhibition mechanism of selamariscina A, which showed the strongest CYP2C8 inhibition, for the other P450 enzymes. The inhibitory potential (Ki) of selamariscina A against P450 enzyme activities was in the order: CYP2C8 > CYP2C9 > CYP1A2 > CYP3A > CYP2B6 (Table 5, Figure 2 and Figure S1). To determine whether inhibition by selamariscina A was substrate-specific, we evaluated its inhibitory effects on CYP2C8-mediated rosiglitazone 5-hydroxylation. We found that it showed strong inhibition with a Ki value of 0.010 μM in a substrate-independent manner. Selamariscina A also inhibited CYP2C9-mediated diclofenac and tolbutamide hydroxylation with Ki values of 0.032 and 0.065 μM, respectively, in a substrate-independent manner. Its inhibitory potential against CYP2C9 was much stronger than other known CYP2C8 inhibitors sulfaphenazole (Ki = 0.12–0.7 μM [35]), fluvoxamine (Ki = 0.63–16 μM [35]) fluconazole (Ki = 0.28 μM [36]), and fluoxetine (Ki = 19–87 μM [35]). Its inhibitory potential for CYP2C8 and CYP2C9 was much stronger than other P450s.

Table 5. K_i values for the inhibition of CYP1A2-catalyzed phenacetin *O*-deethylation, CYP2B6-catalyzed bupropion hydroxylation, CYP2C8-catalyzed amodiaquine *N*-deethylation, CYP2C8-catalyzed rosiglitazone 5-hydroxylation, CYP2C9-catalyzed diclofenac 4-hydroxylation, CYP2C9-catalyzed tolbutamide 4-hydroxylation, and CYP3A-catalyzed midazolam 1′-hydroxylation in human liver microsomes by selamariscina A.

P450 Enzyme	Substrate	K_i (μM) [a]	Mode of Inhibition
1A2	Phenacetin	3.1 ± 0.6	Competitive
2B6	Bupropion	7.9 ± 1.1	Noncompetitive
2C8	Amodiaquine	0.018 ± 0.002	Noncompetitive
	Rosiglitazone	0.010 ± 0.003	Noncompetitive, partial
2C9	Diclofenac	0.032 ± 0.007	Competitive
	Tolbutamide	0.065 ± 0.01	Noncompetitive
3A	Midazolam	4.5 ± 0.5	Noncompetitive

[a] Values represent the average ± standard error in triplicate.

In addition, several P450 inhibitors including azamulin, clopidogrel, methoxalene, and ticlopidine [37–39] have been shown to be time-dependent inhibitors of cytochrome P450. We investigated the effect of incubation time on IC50 values of selamariscina A using the CYP2C8 substrate amodiaquine and the CYP2C9 substrate diclofenac. The inhibitory potential of selamariscina A against CYP2C8-mediated amodiaquine O-deethylase activity and CYP2C9-mediated diclofenac hydroxylase activity in HLMs pre-incubated in the presence of an NADPH generation system (IC50 values of 0.031 and 0.092 μM, respectively) was a bit weaker than in untreated HLMs (IC50 values of 0.019 and 0.054 μM, respectively) This suggests that selamariscina A is not a time-dependent inhibitor (data are not shown).

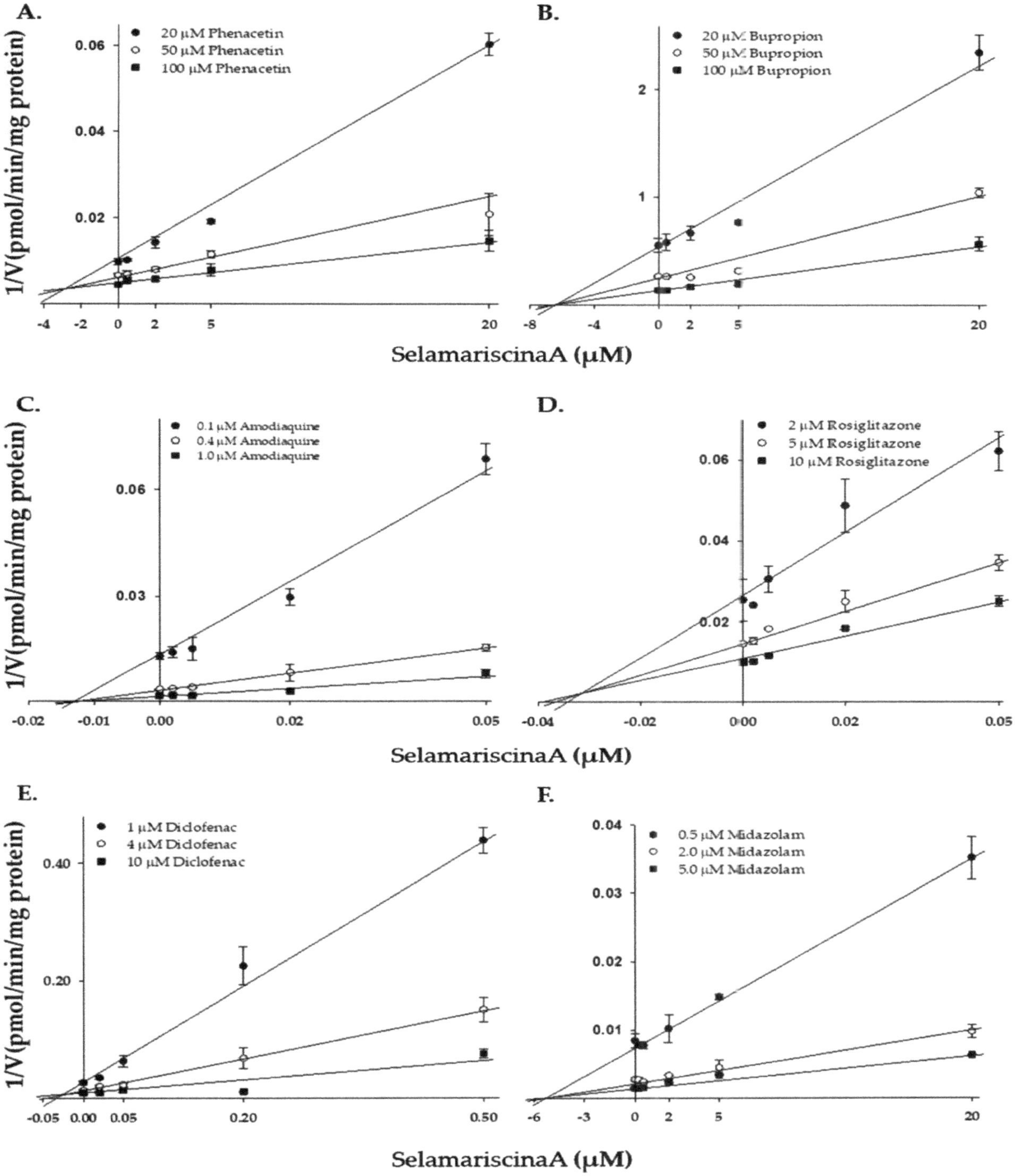

Figure 2. Representative Dixon plots obtained from a kinetic study of CYP1A2-catalyzed phenacetin *O*-deethylation (**A**), CYP2B6-catalyzed bupropion hydroxylation (**B**), CYP2C8-catalyzed amodiaquine N-deethylation (**C**), CYP2C8-catalyzed rosiglitazone 5-hydroxylation (**D**), CYP2C9-catalyzed diclofenac 4-hydroxylation (**E**), and CYP3A-catalyzed midazolam 1′-hydroxylation (**F**) in the presence of different concentrations of selamariscina A in pooled human liver microsomes (XTreme 200, XenoTech). Each data point shown represent the mean ± standard error in triplicate for the samples.

3.2. *Inhibition of UGT Enzymes Activities by Selamariscina A*

The inhibitory potential of selamariscina A against uridine 5′-diphosphoglucuronosyl transferase (UGT) activity was evaluated using HLMs (Table 6). Selamariscina A inhibited UGT1A1 and UGT1A4 activity with IC50 values of 1.7 and 7.7 μM, respectively. However, its inhibition of UGT1A1 and UGT1A4 isoforms was much weaker than that of CYP2C8 (IC50 = 0.019 μM). The inhibitory potential of selamariscina A for UGT1A3, UGT1A6, UGT1A9, and UGT2B6 was negligible (IC50 > 40 μM). The IC50 value of the inhibition of UGT1A1 activity by amentoflavone found in our study (1.7 μM) is similar to its previously reported value (IC50 = 0.78 μM) [18].

Table 6. Inhibitory effects of selamariscina A against six uridine 5′-diphosphoglucuronosyl transferase (UGT) isoforms.

UGT Enzyme	Substrate	IC50 (μM) [a]
1A1	SN-38 *	1.7 ± 0.5
1A3	Chenodeoxycholic acid	>50
1A4	Trifluoperazine	7.7 ± 1.9
1A6	*N*-Acetylserotonin	46.1 ± 11.7
1A9	Mycophenolic acid	40.4 ± 11.1
2B7	Naloxone	>50

* SN-38: 7-Ethyl-10-hydroxy camptothecin; [a] values represent the average ± standard error in triplicate.

3.3. *Comparison of the Selectivity of Selamariscina A and Montelukast for CYP2C8 Inhibition*

Montelukast has been used to inhibit CYP2C8 in reaction-phenotyping studies [20]. We re-evaluated its inhibitory potential against the nine P450 isoforms in this study using HLMs (XTreme 200, XenoTech). Montelukast strongly inhibited CYP2C8 activity with an IC50 value of 0.52 μM, but it showed weak inhibition on the other eight P450 enzymes (IC50 > 9.73 μM) (Table 3). The IC50 value for the CYP2C8 isoform (IC50 = 0.52 μM at 0.25 mg/mL microsomal protein concentration) was similar to previously reported values (IC50 = 0.18 μM at 0.3 mg/mL microsomal protein concentration) [20]. However, montelukast showed more than 25 times weaker inhibition than selamariscina A (IC50 = 0.019 μM at 0.25 mg/mL microsomal protein concentration). At 0.5 μM selamariscina A concentration, approximately 25 times greater than the Ki value, selamariscina A was found to inhibit CYP2C8 and CYP2C9 by 92.8% and 88.6% respectively, and only slightly affected the enzyme activities of the other P450 isoforms (Figure 3). Selamariscina A at 0.5 μM concentration inhibited none of the other P450 isoform-specific activities above 21.8% in HLMs, indicating that selamariscina A could be used as a selective CYP2C8 and CYP2C9 inhibitor in P450 phenotyping studies. Montelukast at 0.5 μM concentration, a well-known selective CYP2C8 inhibitor [20], showed moderate inhibition on CYP2C8 by 52.7% in pooled HLMs. At 5 μM concentration, montelukast inhibited CYP2C8 by 86.1% in HLMs; however, it also inhibited CYP2C9 and CYP2B6 activities by 31.0% and 20.4%, respectively in pooled HLMs. Montelukast (5 μM) showed negligible inhibition on the other six P450 isoforms. Selamariscina A could be useful as a strong CYP2C8 and CYP2C9 inhibitor in P450 reaction-phenotyping studies.

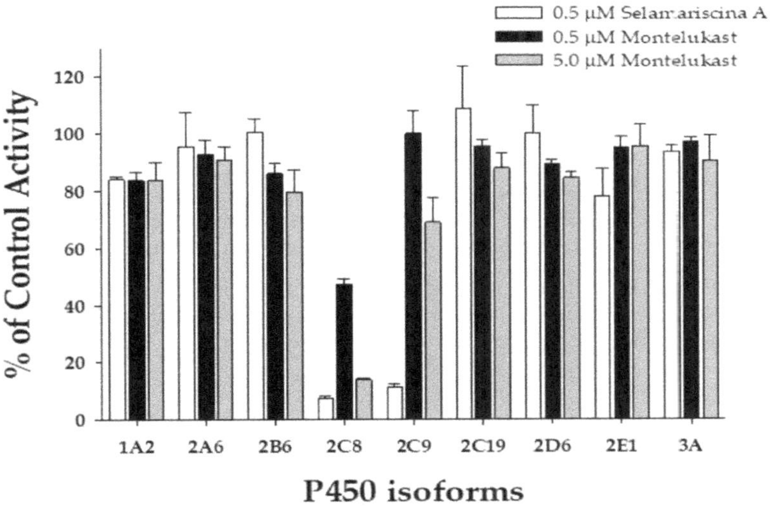

Figure 3. Inhibitory effects of selamariscina A (0.5 μM, □) and montelukast (0.5 μM, ■; 5 μM, ■) on the enzymatic activities of nine P450 isoforms in pooled human liver microsomes (0.25 mg/mL, XTreme 200, XenoTech). Phenacetin (100 μM), coumarin (5 μM), bupropion (50 μM), amodiaquine (1 μM), diclofenac (10 μM), omeprazole (20 μM), dextromethorphan (5 μM), chlorzoxazone (50 μM), and midazolam (5 μM) were used as the respective substrates of P450s 1A2, 2A6, 2B6, 2C8, 2C9, 2C19, 2D6, 2E1, and 3A. The data are means of the average ± standard error in triplicate.

3.4. *Evaluation of Drug Interaction Potential of Selamariscina A*

It was estimated that an in vivo interaction potential via the inhibition of P450 would likely occur if the ratio of inhibitor C_{max}/K_i exceeded one and would be possible if it was between 0.1 and 1.0 [40,41]. Based on amentoflavone's maximum concentrations (0.041 and 0.063 μM) in rat blood after a single oral dose of *Selaginella doderleinii* Hieron extracts (200 mg/kg; contents: 103.82 mg/g amentoflavone, 37.52 mg/g robustaflavone, 44.4 mg/g 2,″3′-dihydro-3′,3″-biapigenin, 53.4 mg/g 3′,3″-binaringenin, and 35.1 mg/g delicaflavone) [42] and *Selaginella doderleinii* Hieron extracts (600 mg/kg) [43], the respective values of C_{max}/K_i were 0.49 and 0.76 from the data of pooled HLMs (K_i = 0.083 μM), indicating that amentoflavone has possible drug interaction potential with CYP2C8 substrate drugs [44]. Recently, nanotechnology-based delivery systems such as liposomes have been developed for improving oral bioavailability [42]. The values of C_{max} (0.22 μM) of amentoflavone after administration of liposome-based *Selaginella doderleinii* Hieron extracts (200 mg/kg) were 5.4 times higher than those of the control [42], resulting in a C_{max}/K_i value of 2.65, indicating that amentoflavone has drug interaction potential. In the case of selamariscina A, the present study provides the first published data on its pharmacokinetics in animals and humans. Therefore, it is difficult to estimate the drug interaction potential of selamariscina A for humans. However, selamariscina A might have drug interactions with CYP2C8 substrate drugs such as cerivastatin [45], paclitaxel [46], and rosiglitazone [47] because its CYP2C8 inhibitory potential was more than 4.5 times stronger than that of amentoflavone. Therefore, in vivo studies are necessary to determine whether drug interactions between selamariscina A and CYP2C8 or CYP2C9 substrates have clinical relevance.

4. Conclusions

In conclusion, we report that selamariscina A is a strong CYP2C8 and CYP2C9 inhibitor. When evaluated for amodiaquine *O*-deethylation and diclofenac hydroxylation inhibitory activity against CYP2C8 and CYP2C9, as well as seven other P450s, it exhibited above 50-fold selectivity. Like montelukast and sulfaphenazole, selamariscina A could be useful as a strong CYP2C8 and CYP2C9 inhibitor in P450 phenotyping studies when HLMs are the enzyme source. Additionally, selamariscina A might cause clinically relevant pharmacokinetic drug interactions with other co-administered drugs metabolized by CYP2C8 or CYP2C9. These in vitro findings provide primary data for future in vivo animal and clinical studies on risk prediction related to the interaction of drugs with herbs.

Supplementary Materials:
Figure S1: Representative Lineweaver–Burk plots obtained from a kinetic study of CYP1A2-catalyzed phenacetin *O*-deethylation (A), CYP2B6-catalyzed bupropion hydroxylation (B), CYP2C8-catalyzed amodiaquine *N*-deethylation (C), CYP2C8-catalyzed rosiglitazone 5-hydroxylation (D), CYP2C9-catalyzed diclofenac 4-hydroxylation (E), and CYP3A-catalyzed midazolam 1′-hydroxylation (F) in the presence of different concentrations of selamariscina A. Each data point shown represent the mean ± standard error in triplicate samples

Author Contributions: S.-Y.P. and K.-H.L. conceived and designed the experiments; S.-Y.P., P.-H.N., G.K., S.-N.J. G.-H.L., and N.M.P. performed experiments; S.-Y.P., Z.W., and K.-H.L. analyzed the data; S.-Y.P. and K.-H.L. wrote the paper. All authors have read and agreed to the published version of the manuscript.

References

1. Bravo, L. Polyphenols: Chemistry, dietary sources, metabolism, and nutritional significance. *Nutr. Rev.* **1998** *56*, 317–333. [CrossRef] [PubMed]
2. Cermak, R.; Wolffram, S. The potential of flavonoids to influence drug metabolism and pharmacokinetics by local gastrointestinal mechanisms. *Curr. Drug Metab.* **2006**, *7*, 729–744. [CrossRef] [PubMed]
3. Kumar, S.; Pandey, A.K. Chemistry and biological activities of flavonoids: An overview. *Sci. World J.* **2013** *2013*, 162750. [CrossRef]
4. Miron, A.; Aprotosoaie, A.C.; Trifan, A.; Xiao, J. Flavonoids as modulators of metabolic enzymes and drug transporters. *Ann. N. Y. Acad. Sci.* **2017**, *1398*, 152–167. [CrossRef] [PubMed]
5. Kopecna-Zapletalova, M.; Krasulova, K.; Anzenbacher, P.; Hodek, P.; Anzenbacherova, E. Interaction of isoflavonoids with human liver microsomal cytochromes P450: Inhibition of CYP enzyme activities *Xenobiotica* **2017**, *47*, 324–331. [CrossRef] [PubMed]
6. Manach, C.; Scalbert, A.; Morand, C.; Remesy, C.; Jimenez, L. Polyphenols: Food sources and bioavailability *Am. J. Clin. Nutr.* **2004**, *79*, 727–747. [CrossRef] [PubMed]
7. Tikkanen, M.J.; Adlercreutz, H. Dietary soy-derived isoflavone phytoestrogens. Could they have a role in coronary heart disease prevention? *Biochem. Pharm.* **2000**, *60*, 1–5. [CrossRef]
8. Cermak, R. Effect of dietary flavonoids on pathways involved in drug metabolism. *Expert Opin. Drug Metab Toxicol.* **2008**, *4*, 17–35. [CrossRef]
9. Obermeier, M.T.; White, R.E.; Yang, C.S. Effects of bioflavonoids on hepatic P450 activities. *Xenobiotica* **1995** *25*, 575–584. [CrossRef]
10. Williams, J.A.; Ring, B.J.; Cantrell, V.E.; Campanale, K.; Jones, D.R.; Hall, S.D.; Wrighton, S.A. Differential modulation of UDP-glucuronosyltransferase 1A1 (UGT1A1)-catalyzed estradiol-3-glucuronidation by the addition of UGT1A1 substrates and other compounds to human liver microsomes. *Drug Metab. Dispos.* **2002** *30*, 1266–1273. [CrossRef]
11. Miniscalco, A.; Lundahl, J.; Regardh, C.G.; Edgar, B.; Eriksson, U.G. Inhibition of dihydropyridine metabolism in rat and human liver microsomes by flavonoids found in grapefruit juice. *J. Pharmacol. Exp. Ther.* **1992**, *261* 1195–1199. [PubMed]
12. Choi, J.S.; Piao, Y.J.; Kang, K.W. Effects of quercetin on the bioavailability of doxorubicin in rats: Role of CYP3A4 and P-gp inhibition by quercetin. *Arch. Pharm. Res.* **2011**, *34*, 607–613. [CrossRef] [PubMed]
13. Surya Sandeep, M.; Sridhar, V.; Puneeth, Y.; Ravindra Babu, P.; Naveen Babu, K. Enhanced oral bioavailability of felodipine by naringenin in Wistar rats and inhibition of P-glycoprotein in everted rat gut sacs in vitro *Drug Dev. Ind. Pharm.* **2014**, *40*, 1371–1377. [CrossRef] [PubMed]
14. Alnaqeeb, M.; Mansor, K.A.; Mallah, E.M.; Ghanim, B.Y.; Idkaidek, N.; Qinna, N.A. Critical pharmacokinetic and pharmacodynamic drug-herb interactions in rats between warfarin and pomegranate peel or guava leaves extracts. *BMC Complement. Altern. Med.* **2019**, *19*, 29. [CrossRef] [PubMed]
15. Tabares-Guevara, J.H.; Lara-Guzman, O.J.; Londono-Londono, J.A.; Sierra, J.A.; Leon-Varela, Y.M. Alvarez-Quintero, R.M.; Osorio, E.J.; Ramirez-Pineda, J.R. Natural Biflavonoids Modulate Macrophage Oxidized LDL Interaction In Vitro and Promote Atheroprotection In Vivo. *Front. Immunol.* **2017**, *8*, 923 [CrossRef] [PubMed]

16. Kim, H.P.; Park, H.; Son, K.H.; Chang, H.W.; Kang, S.S. Biochemical pharmacology of biflavonoids: Implications for anti-inflammatory action. *Arch. Pharm. Res.* **2008**, *31*, 265–273. [CrossRef]
17. Liu, H.; Ye, M.; Guo, H. An updated review of randomized clinical trials testing the improvement of cognitive function of ginkgo biloba extract in healthy people and Alzheimer's patients. *Front. Pharmacol.* **2019**, *10*, 1688. [CrossRef]
18. Lv, X.; Zhang, J.B.; Wang, X.X.; Hu, W.Z.; Shi, Y.S.; Liu, S.W.; Hao, D.C.; Zhang, W.D.; Ge, G.B.; Hou, J.; et al. Amentoflavone is a potent broad-spectrum inhibitor of human UDP-glucuronosyltransferases. *Chem. Biol. Interact.* **2018**, *284*, 48–55. [CrossRef]
19. Von Moltke, L.L.; Weemhoff, J.L.; Bedir, E.; Khan, I.A.; Harmatz, J.S.; Goldman, P.; Greenblatt, D.J. Inhibition of human cytochromes P450 by components of *Ginkgo biloba*. *J. Pharm. Pharmacol.* **2004**, *56*, 1039–1044. [CrossRef]
20. Walsky, R.L.; Obach, R.S.; Gaman, E.A.; Gleeson, J.P.; Proctor, W.R. Selective inhibition of human cytochrome P4502C8 by montelukast. *Drug Metab. Dispos.* **2005**, *33*, 413–418. [CrossRef]
21. Nguyen, P.H.; Ji, D.J.; Han, Y.R.; Choi, J.S.; Rhyu, D.Y.; Min, B.S.; Woo, M.H. Selaginellin and biflavonoids as protein tyrosine phosphatase 1B inhibitors from *Selaginella tamariscina* and their glucose uptake stimulatory effects. *Bioorg. Med. Chem.* **2015**, *23*, 3730–3737. [CrossRef] [PubMed]
22. Zhang, Y.X.; Li, Q.Y.; Yan, L.L.; Shi, Y. Structural characterization and identification of biflavones in Selaginella tamariscina by liquid chromatography-diode-array detection/electrospray ionization tandem mass spectrometry. *Rapid Commun. Mass Spectrom.* **2011**, *25*, 2173–2186. [CrossRef] [PubMed]
23. Heo, J.K.; Nguyen, P.H.; Kim, W.C.; Phuc, N.M.; Liu, K.H. Inhibitory effect of selaginellins from *Selaginella tamariscina* (Beauv.) spring against cytochrome p450 and uridine 5′-diphosphoglucuronosyltransferase isoforms on human liver microsomes. *Molecules* **2017**, *22*, 1590. [CrossRef] [PubMed]
24. Kim, H.J.; Lee, H.; Ji, H.K.; Lee, T.; Liu, K.H. Screening of ten cytochrome P450 enzyme activities with 12 probe substrates in human liver microsomes using cocktail incubation and liquid chromatography-tandem mass spectrometry. *Biopharm. Drug Dispos.* **2019**, *40*, 101–111. [CrossRef] [PubMed]
25. Perloff, E.S.; Mason, A.K.; Dehal, S.S.; Blanchard, A.P.; Morgan, L.; Ho, T.; Dandeneau, A.; Crocker, R.M.; Chandler, C.M.; Boily, N.; et al. Validation of cytochrome P450 time-dependent inhibition assays: A two-time point IC50 shift approach facilitates kinact assay design. *Xenobiotica* **2009**, *39*, 99–112. [CrossRef]
26. Kim, S.J.; You, J.; Choi, H.G.; Kim, J.A.; Jee, J.G.; Lee, S. Selective inhibitory effects of machilin A isolated from *Machilus thunbergii* on human cytochrome P450 1A and 2B6. *Phytomedicine* **2015**, *22*, 615–620. [CrossRef]
27. Krishnan, S.; Moncrief, S. An evaluation of the cytochrome p450 inhibition potential of lisdexamfetamine in human liver microsomes. *Drug Metab. Dispos.* **2007**, *35*, 180–184. [CrossRef]
28. Joo, J.; Lee, B.; Lee, T.; Liu, K.H. Screening of six UGT enzyme activities in human liver microsomes using liquid chromatography/triple quadrupole mass spectrometry. *Rapid Commun. Mass Spectrom.* **2014**, *28*, 2405–2414. [CrossRef]
29. Shin, J.G.; Soukhova, N.; Flockhart, D.A. Effect of antipsychotic drugs on human liver cytochrome P-450 (CYP) isoforms in vitro: Preferential inhibition of CYP2D6. *Drug Metab. Dispos.* **1999**, *27*, 1078–1084. [PubMed]
30. Lee, E.; Wu, Z.; Shon, J.C.; Liu, K.H. Danazol Inhibits Cytochrome P450 2J2 Activity in a Substrate-independent Manner. *Drug Metab. Dispos.* **2015**, *43*, 1250–1253. [CrossRef]
31. Walsky, R.L.; Gaman, E.A.; Obach, R.S. Examination of 209 drugs for inhibition of cytochrome P450 2C8. *J. Clin. Pharmacol.* **2005**, *45*, 68–78. [CrossRef] [PubMed]
32. Cao, L.; Kwara, A.; Greenblatt, D.J. Metabolic interactions between acetaminophen (paracetamol) and two flavonoids, luteolin and quercetin, through in-vitro inhibition studies. *J. Pharm. Pharmacol.* **2017**, *69*, 1762–1772. [CrossRef] [PubMed]
33. Wang, Y.; Wang, M.; Qi, H.; Pan, P.; Hou, T.; Li, J.; He, G.; Zhang, H. Pathway-dependent inhibition of paclitaxel hydroxylation by kinase inhibitors and assessment of drug-drug interaction potentials. *Drug Metab. Dispos.* **2014**, *42*, 782–795. [CrossRef] [PubMed]
34. Li, X.Q.; Bjorkman, A.; Andersson, T.B.; Ridderstrom, M.; Masimirembwa, C.M. Amodiaquine clearance and its metabolism to N-desethylamodiaquine is mediated by CYP2C8: A new high affinity and turnover enzyme-specific probe substrate. *J. Pharmacol. Exp. Ther.* **2002**, *300*, 399–407. [CrossRef] [PubMed]

35. Khojasteh, S.C.; Prabhu, S.; Kenny, J.R.; Halladay, J.S.; Lu, A.Y. Chemical inhibitors of cytochrome P450 isoforms in human liver microsomes: A re-evaluation of P450 isoform selectivity. *Eur. J. Drug Metab. Pharmacol.* **2011**, *36*, 1–16. [CrossRef] [PubMed]
36. Brown, H.S.; Galetin, A.; Hallifax, D.; Houston, J.B. Prediction of in vivo drug-drug interactions from in vitro data: Factors affecting prototypic drug-drug interactions involving CYP2C9, CYP2D6 and CYP3A4. *Clin. Pharmacol.* **2006**, *45*, 1035–1050. [CrossRef]
37. Richter, T.; Murdter, T.E.; Heinkele, G.; Pleiss, J.; Tatzel, S.; Schwab, M.; Eichelbaum, M.; Zanger, U.M. Potent mechanism-based inhibition of human CYP2B6 by clopidogrel and ticlopidine. *J. Pharmacol. Exp. Ther.* **2004**, *308*, 189–197. [CrossRef]
38. Palacharla, R.C.; Molgara, P.; Panthangi, H.R.; Boggavarapu, R.K.; Manoharan, A.K.; Ponnamaneni, R.K.; Ajjala, D.R.; Nirogi, R. Methoxsalen as an in vitro phenotyping tool in comparison with 1-aminobenzotriazole. *Xenobiotica* **2019**, *49*, 169–176. [CrossRef]
39. Stresser, D.M.; Broudy, M.I.; Ho, T.; Cargill, C.E.; Blanchard, A.P.; Sharma, R.; Dandeneau, A.A.; Goodwin, J.J.; Turner, S.D.; Erve, J.C.; et al. Highly selective inhibition of human CYP3Aa in vitro by azamulin and evidence that inhibition is irreversible. *Drug Metab. Dispos.* **2004**, *32*, 105–112. [CrossRef]
40. Bjornsson, T.D.; Callaghan, J.T.; Einolf, H.J.; Fischer, V.; Gan, L.; Grimm, S.; Kao, J.; King, S.P.; Miwa, G.; Ni, L.; et al. The conduct of in vitro and in vivo drug-drug interaction studies: A Pharmaceutical Research and Manufacturers of America (PhRMA) perspective. *Drug Metab. Dispos.* **2003**, *31*, 815–832. [CrossRef]
41. Lee, H.; Heo, J.K.; Lee, G.H.; Park, S.Y.; Jang, S.N.; Kim, H.J.; Kwon, M.J.; Song, I.S.; Liu, K.H. Ginsenoside rc is a new selective ugt1a9 inhibitor in human liver microsomes and recombinant human ugt isoforms. *Drug Metab. Dispos.* **2019**, *47*, 1372–1379. [CrossRef] [PubMed]
42. Chen, B.; Wang, X.; Lin, D.; Xu, D.; Li, S.; Huang, J.; Weng, S.; Lin, Z.; Zheng, Y.; Yao, H.; et al. Proliposomes for oral delivery of total biflavonoids extract from Selaginella doederleinii: Formulation development, optimization, and in vitro-in vivo characterization. *Int. J. Nanomed.* **2019**, *14*, 6691–6706. [CrossRef] [PubMed]
43. Chen, B.; Wang, X.; Zou, Y.; Chen, W.; Wang, G.; Yao, W.; Shi, P.; Li, S.; Lin, S.; Lin, X.; et al. Simultaneous quantification of five biflavonoids in rat plasma by LC-ESI-MS/MS and its application to a comparatively pharmacokinetic study of *Selaginella doederleinii* Hieron extract in rats. *J. Pharm. Biomed. Anal.* **2018**, *149*, 80–88. [CrossRef] [PubMed]
44. Liu, D.; Wu, J.; Xie, H.; Liu, M.; Takau, I.; Zhang, H.; Xiong, Y.; Xia, C. Inhibitory effect of hesperetin and naringenin on human udp-glucuronosyltransferase enzymes: Implications for herb-drug interactions. *Biol. Pharm. Bull.* **2016**, *39*, 2052–2059. [CrossRef]
45. Wang, J.S.; Neuvonen, M.; Wen, X.; Backman, J.T.; Neuvonen, P.J. Gemfibrozil inhibits CYP2C8-mediated cerivastatin metabolism in human liver microsomes. *Drug Metab. Dispos.* **2002**, *30*, 1352–1356. [CrossRef]
46. Vaclavikova, R.; Horsky, S.; Simek, P.; Gut, I. Paclitaxel metabolism in rat and human liver microsomes is inhibited by phenolic antioxidants. *Naunyn. Schmiedebergs Arch. Pharmacol.* **2003**, *368*, 200–209. [CrossRef] [PubMed]
47. Baldwin, S.J.; Clarke, S.E.; Chenery, R.J. Characterization of the cytochrome P450 enzymes involved in the in vitro metabolism of rosiglitazone. *Br. J. Clin. Pharmacol.* **1999**, *48*, 424–432. [CrossRef]

6

Evaluation of the Effect of CYP2D6 Genotypes on Tramadol and *O*-Desmethyltramadol Pharmacokinetic Profiles in a Korean Population Using Physiologically-Based Pharmacokinetic Modeling

Hyeon-Cheol Jeong [1], Soo Hyeon Bae [2], Jung-Woo Bae [3], Sooyeun Lee [3], Anhye Kim [4], Yoojeong Jang [1] and Kwang-Hee Shin [1,*]

1 College of Pharmacy, Research Institute of Pharmaceutical Sciences, Kyungpook National University, Daegu 41566, Korea; houkiboshi01@knu.ac.kr (H.-C.J.); kersy@daum.net (Y.J.)

2 Korea Institute of Radiological & Medical Sciences, Seoul 01812, Korea; shbae@kirams.re.kr

3 College of Pharmacy, Keimyung University, Daegu 42601, Korea; jwbae11@kmu.ac.kr (J.-W.B.); sylee21@kmu.ac.kr (S.L.)

4 Department of Clinical Pharmacology and Therapeutics, CHA Bundang Medical Center, CHA University, Seongnam 13496, Korea; ahkim1@cha.ac.kr

* Correspondence: kshin@knu.ac.kr

Abstract: Tramadol is a μ-opioid receptor agonist and a monoamine reuptake inhibitor. *O*-desmethyltramadol (M1), the major active metabolite of tramadol, is produced by CYP2D6. A physiologically-based pharmacokinetic model was developed to predict changes in time-concentration profiles for tramadol and M1 according to dosage and CYP2D6 genotypes in the Korean population. Parallel artificial membrane permeation assay was performed to determine tramadol permeability, and the metabolic clearance of M1 was determined using human liver microsomes. Clinical study data were used to develop the model. Other physicochemical and pharmacokinetic parameters were obtained from the literature. Simulations for plasma concentrations of tramadol and M1 (after 100 mg tramadol was administered five times at 12-h intervals) were based on a total of 1000 virtual healthy Koreans using SimCYP® simulator. Geometric mean ratios (90% confidence intervals) (predicted/observed) for maximum plasma concentration at steady-state ($C_{max,ss}$) and area under the curve at steady-state ($AUC_{last,ss}$) were 0.79 (0.69–0.91) and 1.04 (0.85–1.28) for tramadol, and 0.63 (0.51–0.79) and 0.67 (0.54–0.84) for M1, respectively. The predicted time–concentration profiles of tramadol fitted well to observed profiles and those of M1 showed under-prediction. The developed model could be applied to predict concentration-dependent toxicities according to CYP2D6 genotypes and also, CYP2D6-related drug interactions.

Keywords: CYP2D6; *O*-desmethyltramadol; pharmacokinetics; physiologically-based pharmacokinetics; tramadol

1. Introduction

Tramadol is an orally available, centrally acting, weak-opioid analgesic drug [1]. The anti-nociceptive effect of tramadol is due to two mechanisms: an opioid mechanism, and a non-opioid mechanism [2]. Tramadol acts as a μ-opioid receptor agonist, like traditional opioids. It also has analgesic effects by inhibiting reuptake of monoamine neurotransmitters, such as 5-hydroxytryptamine (5-HT) and noradrenaline [3,4]. These mechanisms lead to reduced pain signal conduction and analgesic effects. Tramadol is a racemate, and analgesic mechanisms differ depending on the isomer:

(−)-tramadol exhibited ≈ 10-fold higher noradrenaline reuptake inhibitory activity than (+)-tramadol and (+)-tramadol showed ≈ 4-fold higher 5-HT reuptake inhibitory activity than (−)-tramadol [5].

Tramadol is predominantly metabolized in the liver. Approximately 10%–30% of administered tramadol is excreted, unmetabolized, in the urine. The well-known metabolic pathway of tramadol is divided into three major pathways: *O*-desmethyltramadol (M1) is produced by cytochrome P450 (CYP) 2D6, and *N*-desmethyltramadol (M2) is produced by CYP2B6 and CYP3A4. These metabolites are converted to either *N*,*O*-didesmethyltramadol (M5) and other inactive metabolites by CYP2D6, CYP2B6, and CYP3A4, or converted to glucuronides by UDP-glucuronosyltransferase (UGT) 1A8 and UGT2B7 [6]. M1, a major active metabolite of tramadol, has about 700-fold higher affinity for μ-opioid receptors than tramadol [7]. M5 also has 24-fold higher affinity for μ-opioid receptors than tramadol [3]. Tramadol is mainly considered to inhibit monoamine reuptake, while M1 and M5 bind to μ-opioid receptors and exhibit analgesic effects. Thus, genetic polymorphism of CYP2D6 could have an effect on the risk of adverse events during tramadol administration [4].

A physiologically-based pharmacokinetic (PBPK) approach is a bottom-up approach that requires data about the physicochemical properties and pharmacokinetic (PK) parameters (i.e., absorption, distribution, metabolism, and excretion; ADME) of the target drug [8,9]. In addition, the PBPK model considers bodyweight, height, organ volume, blood flow, and inter-individual variation for metabolizing enzymes and transporters [10]. Therefore, the PBPK model can be used to predict plasma concentration–time profiles more closely than traditional compartmental PK models [11]. In this regard, PBPK modeling can predict human PK profiles using in vitro or preclinical study data from drug development. Further, such modeling is also used to investigate the interaction potential with other drugs or food, and to predict PK profiles in special populations, such as pregnant women, geriatric patients, or children [9,12].

Studies predicting the PK profile of tramadol using PK modeling have been reported previously. Many articles used a population PK approach with nonlinear mixed-effects modeling (NONMEM), however a PBPK approach was rarely used to predict the PK profile of tramadol [13–15]. When tramadol was administered, M1 also had impact on efficacy and toxicity [16]. Therefore, M1 should be integrated for PBPK model of tramadol for better interpretation.

The aims of this study were to develop a PBPK model that could predict the concentration–time profiles of tramadol and M1 in Koreans, and to investigate effects of the CYP2D6 genotype on PK profiles at routinely administered doses. The developed PBPK model was applied to predict the effects of CYP2D6 genotype and tramadol dosage on the plasma concentration profiles of tramadol and M1 in a healthy Korean population.

2. Materials and Methods

2.1. Clinical Study Design

The clinical study was approved by the Institutional Review Board of Keimyung University (Deagu, Republic of Korea, approval number: 40525-201509-BR-70-02, 23 February 2016) and Kyungpook National University Hospital (Daegu, Republic of Korea, approval number of clinical trial: 2016-08-005, 24 August 2016) and carried out at the Kyungpook National University Hospital Clinical Trial Center (Daegu, Republic of Korea). A total of 23 subjects participated who voluntarily agreed to take part in the clinical study and signed their informed consent. Subject characteristics are presented in Table 1. All subjects received a 100-mg tramadol hydrochloride tablet (Tridol® extended-release (ER); Yuhan Pharmaceutical, Seoul, Korea) five times at 12-h intervals. Whole blood was collected in an anticoagulant tube at pre-dose, and at 0.5, 1, 1.5, 2, 2.5, 4, 6, 8, 10, 12, 24, 48, and 72 h after administration. The obtained whole blood was used for CYP2D6 genotyping, and the plasma was separated for determination of tramadol and M1 [17].

Table 1. Demographic characteristics ($n = 23$).

Characteristic	Mean (SD)
Age (years)	24.78 (4.30)
Height (cm)	176.51 (5.64)
Weight (kg)	71.61 (8.37)
CYP2D6 genotypes (no. of subjects)	
Wild-type	14
*5/*5	1
*10/*10	8

SD, standard deviation.

2.2. CYP2D6 Genotyping

The determination of CYP2D6 genotype was performed for *CYP2D6*2* (normal function), *CYP2D6*5* (no function), and *CYP2D6*10* (decreased function). Genotyping for *CYP2D6*2* and *CYP2D6*10* was performed using pyrosequencing. *CYP2D6*5* was sequenced by long polymerase chain reaction (PCR) because of deletion of a specific sequence. Pyrosequencing was performed using Pyromark Q96 ID and Pyromark Gold Q96 reagents (Qiagen, Hilden, Germany). The conditions of PCR (total 35 cycles) were: denaturation (94 °C for 30 s), annealing (56 °C for 30 s), and polymerization (72 °C for 30 s). The processes were finished by extension at 72 °C for 5 min. *CYP2D6*5* and duplication were determined by long-PCR, as previously described [18,19]. The *CYP2D6* phenotype was determined based on genotype and activity score [20–23]. *CYP2D6**5 was a non-functional allele and homozygous *CYP2D6**5 was classified as a poor metabolizer (PM). Homozygous *CYP2D6**10 was classified as an intermediate metabolizer (IM).

2.3. Determination of Tramadol and O-Desmethyltramadol (M1) Using LC-MS/MS

The obtained whole blood samples were immediately centrifuged at 4 °C, 3000 rpm for 10 min. The isolated plasma samples were transferred to a new microcentrifuge tube and kept at −70 °C until analysis. The plasma samples were completely thawed, then 10 μL of internal standard (tramadol ^{13}C-d_3 for tramadol, and M1-d_6 for M1) were added to 100 μL samples and mixed briefly. A total of 300 μL of acetonitrile was added, and then samples were mixed thoroughly for 30 s prior to centrifugation at 2500 rpm for 10 min. The organic solvent layer was transferred to a new polypropylene tube and evaporated under nitrogen gas at 40 °C. Methanol 200 μL was added into tubes containing pellets for reconstitution, and 5 μL of reconstituted sample were analyzed. Analyses were carried out on API3200 tandem mass spectrometry system (AB SCIEX, Framingham, MA, USA) equipped with an Agilent 1260 series HPLC system (Agilent Technologies, Santa Clara, CA, USA). Separation of tramadol and M1 was conducted using a Luna C18 column (5.0 μm, 2.0 × 50 mm; Phenomenex, Torrance, CA, USA). Five millimoles ammonium formate and 0.1% formic acid in methanol (A), and 5 mM ammonium formate solution (B), were used for the mobile phase. The used gradient method was as follows: 0–2 min (97%–5% B), 2–4 min (5% B), 4–5 min (5%–97% B), and 5–8 min (97% B). Electrospray ionization-positive ion mode was used for mass detection. The mass transitions (m/z) used were 264.2→58.1 for tramadol, 268.2→58.1 for tramadol internal standard (IS), 250.2→58.2 for M1, and 256.2→64.1 for M1 IS. To obtain pharmacokinetic parameters, non-compartmental analysis (NCA) was performed using Phoenix (Certara Inc., Princeton, NJ, USA).

2.4. Parallel Artificial Membrane Permeability Assay (PAMPA)

To determine the permeability of tramadol, a parallel artificial membrane permeability assay (PAMPA) was performed [24]. Gentest™ Pre-coated PAMPA Plate System (Corning, Tewksbury, MA, USA) was used for the permeability assay. All the processes were followed according to the manufacturer's protocol. Tramadol hydrochloride, dimethyl sulfoxide (DMSO), phosphate-buffered saline (PBS), and acetonitrile were purchased from Sigma-Aldrich (St. Louis, MO, USA). Tramadol stock solution (1 mM) was prepared using 100% DMSO and diluted to 15 μM using PBS (pH 7.4). The PAMPA plate was equilibrated for 30 min at room temperature before performing the permeability assay. PBS 200 μL was dispensed on the acceptor side and 300 μL of working solution was dispensed on the donor side. Incubation was carried out at room temperature for 5 h, and the acceptor and donor side buffers were analyzed using liquid chromatography-tandem mass spectrometry (LC-MS/MS). A total of 12 replicated samples were assayed and mean permeability was calculated and applied to the model.

2.5. *Assessment of Intrinsic Clearance of M1*

For the experiments, *O*-desmethyltramadol HCl (M1), glucose 6-phosphate, glucose 6-phosphate dehydrogenase, $MgCl_2$, β-nicotinamide adenine dinucleotide phosphate (NADP), chlorpropamide, Trizma® base, Trizma® hydrochloride, DMSO and formic acid were obtained from Sigma-Aldrich (St. Louis, MO, USA). To evaluate the intrinsic clearance of M1 by CYPs, metabolic stability studies under NADPH system were conducted in human liver microsoms (HLM) [25,26]. For details, NADPH-generating system (1.3 mM $NADP^+$, 3.3 mM glucose 6-phosphate, 3.3 mM $MgCl_2$, and 0.4 unit/mL glucose-6-phosphate dehydrogenase) and HLM 0.25 mg/mL were added and preincubated at 37 °C for 5 min. Then, 20 μM M1 was added and reacted at 37 °C for 0, 1, 5, 10, 20, 30, and 40 min, respectively. The total volume of the reaction mixture was 100 μL. After each reaction, the reaction was terminated by addition of 150 μL of acetonitrile containing an internal standard (100 ng/mL chlorpropamide). All experiments were repeated duplicated and the samples were vortexed for 5 min and centrifuged (13,000 rpm, 4 °C) for 15 min. Then, supernatants were injected into LC-MS/MS and M1 were analyzed. The concentration of M1 (20 μM) at 0 min was used to evaluate the metabolism of CYP through the change of drug concentration over time.

2.6. *Qunatitaion Methods of M1 in In Vitro Experiments Using LC-QTOF*

High-performance liquid chromatography (HPLC)-grade acetonitrile and deionized water were obtained from Berdick and Jackson (Muskegon, MI, USA). HLM (50 donors pooled) were purchased from Corning. Analyses were carried out on Sciex QTOF 5600 plus (AB SCIEX, Framingham, MA, USA) equipped with an Agilent 1260 series HPLC system (Agilent Technologies, Santa Clara, CA, USA). For quantitation of M1, the compounds were separated on a Poroshell 120 (4.6 × 50 mm, 2.7 μm; Agilent Technologies) with an isocratic mobile phase consisting of acetonitrile and 0.1% aqueous formic acid (70:30 *v*/*v*) at a flow rate of 0.5 mL/min. The overall run time was 5 min per sample. The column and autosampler temperatures were maintained at 40 °C and 4 °C, respectively. Time-of-flight mass spectrometry analysis was selected in positive ion mode for the sample analysis. The quantitative analytical data were processed using PeakView® (Version 2.2.0; AB SCIEX, Framingham, MA, USA) and MultiQuant® (Version 3.0.2; Framingham, MA, USA), and the formulas $C_{15}H_{23}NO_2$ (M1), and $C_{10}H_{13}ClN_2O_3S$ (chlorpropamide) were used for quantitation.

2.7. *Development of PBPK Model for Tramadol and M1*

PBPK model development was performed using SimCYP® simulator version 18 (Certara, Sheffield, UK). Most of the parameters for tramadol and M1 were entered with reference to the literature. According to previous reports, tramadol was not substrate for P-glycoprotein (P-gp) (ABCB1) and the role of proton-based pumps such as OATP for tramadol permeability was unclear [27,28]. Therefore, in this study, the permeability of tramadol was determined by PAMPA assay. The advanced drug absorption and metabolism model was used to consider the ER formulation, and the dissolution profiles of Tridol® ER 100 mg (Yuhan Pharmaceutical, Seoul, Korea) were applied. The elimination profile for M1 applied the intrinsic clearance by HLM. Kp scalar of tramadol was set to match the observed Vss and the predicted V_{ss} value in the model, and Kp scalar of M1 was obtained from parameter estimation. In clinical study, the V_{ss} of tramadol was calculated to 2.6 L/kg by non-compartmental analysis. That of M1 was not calculated because the exact dose of M1 is unknown. Intrinsic clearance involved in tramadol metabolism was estimated using retrograde model option, and human liver microsomal intrinsic clearance was applied to M1 library. The renal clearance of tramadol and M1 were applied for the predicted value which is the closest to the observed blood concentration–time profile by parameter estimation. The PBPK model was evaluated so that it could effectively predict PK profiles for tramadol and M1 when observed mean plasma concentrations fitted to the predicted plasma concentration–time profile and its 90% confidence interval (CI). The other evaluation criteria were geometric mean ratio for peak plasma concentration at steady-state ($C_{max,ss}$), and area under the plasma concentration–time curve at last observation at steady-state ($AUC_{last,ss}$), and the 90% CI for these values. If the geometric mean ratio and its 90% CI were within the range 0.7–1.43, the model was considered to fit well.

2.8. Prediction of Changes in Concentration–Time Profiles for Tramadol and M1 According to CYP2D6 Genotype and Dosing Regimen

The therapeutic range and toxic range of tramadol and M1 were determined by reference to the literature. Because the manufacturer's recommended acceptable maximum dose of Tridol® ER was 400 mg per day, the tramadol ER tablet was administered to a virtual healthy Korean population at 100 and 200 mg (5 times at 12-h intervals) to simulate the change of concentration–time profiles for tramadol and M1. This simulation assumes linear PK properties for multiple doses of tramadol 100 mg and 200 mg [29]. The effect of CYP2D6 genotype was also simulated for tramadol 100 mg and 200 mg for populations consisting of CYP2D6 poor metabolizers (PM), intermediate metabolizers (IM), extensive metabolizers (EM), and ultra-rapid metabolizers (UM).

3. Results

3.1. Clinical Study

A total of 23 subjects, aged 20–34 years, were enrolled in the clinical study. The average plasma concentration–time profiles for tramadol and M1 are shown in Figure 1. The allele (phenotype) frequencies for *CYP2D6* were: Wild-type (EM, 14 subjects), *10/*10 (IM, 8 subjects), and *5/*5 (PM, 1 subject).

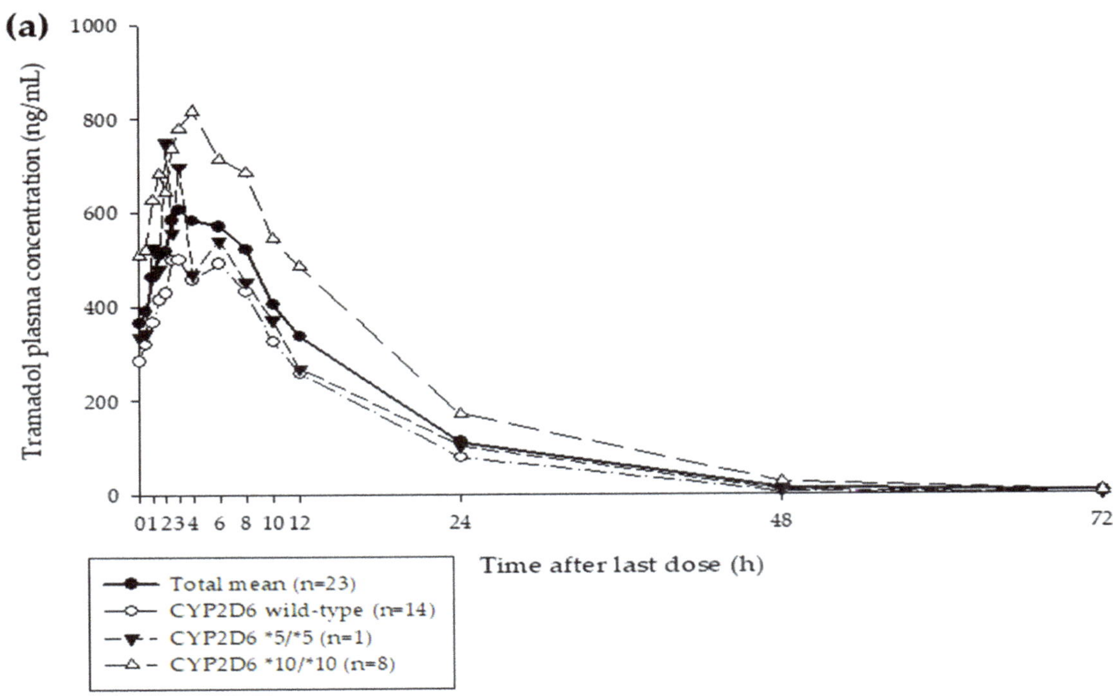

Figure 1. *Cont.*

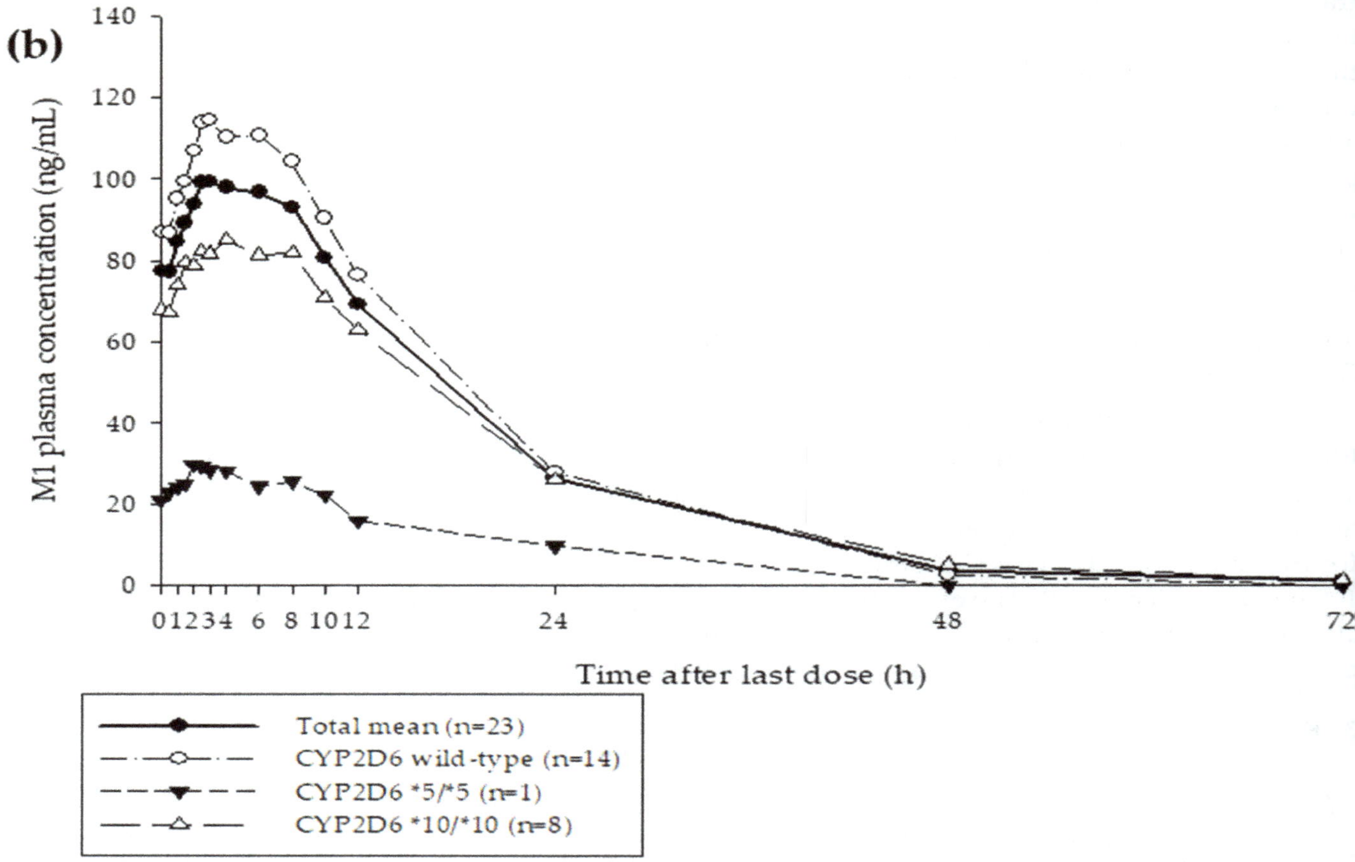

Figure 1. The average plasma concentration–time profiles after five times oral administration (τ = 12 h) of 100 mg tramadol for (**a**) tramadol and (**b**) *O*-desmethyltramadol (M1). Solid blue line, average for all subjects (n = 23); solid black line, *CYP2D6* wild-type subjects (n = 14); short dashed black line, *CYP2D6* *5/*5 subject (n = 1); long dashed black line, *CYP2D6* *10/*10 (n = 8).

3.2. Metabolism Assay for O-Desmethyltramadol (M1)

We conducted metabolic stability study of M1 and confirmed that M1 was metabolized mainly by CYPs and partially by UGTs. In control sample without NADPH or HLM, more than 96% of tramadol and M1 remained during the incubation time, indicating that the disappearance of tramadol and M1 were mainly caused by CYP enzymes. Metabolic stability of M1 by CYP was assessed using results of the disappearance test for M1. The slope of linear regression was calculated and intrinsic clearance (CL_{int}) of the drug in the in vitro microsome system was calculated:

$$CL_{int,mic}\ (\mu L/min/mg\ protein) = k \times V_{incubation}/C_{incubation} \quad (1)$$

where $V_{incubation}$ is incubation volume, $C_{incubation}$ is concentration of microsomal protein.

To apply the elimination profile to *O*-desmethyltramadol (M1), an HLM assay was performed The M1 disappearance test showed an HLM intrinsic clearance ($CL_{int,HLM}$) of 52.95 μL/min/mg protein (Figure 2). $CL_{int,HLM}$ for M1 was applied to the M1 PBPK model.

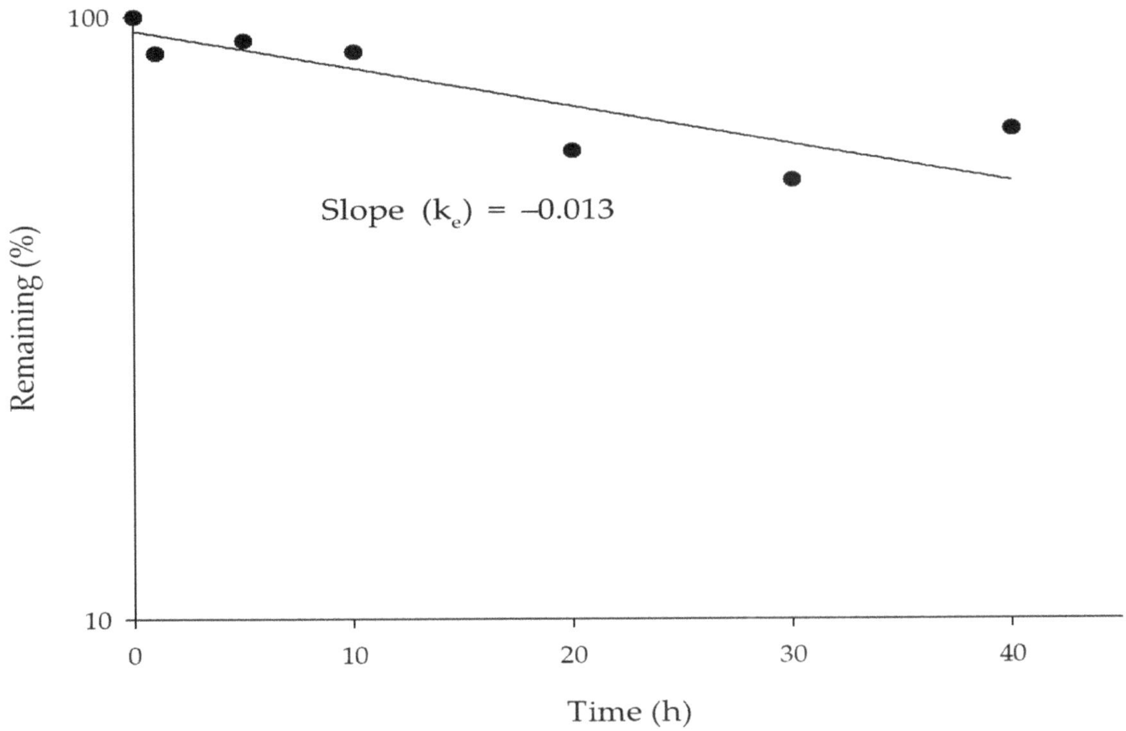

Figure 2. The plot of remaining rate of *O*-desmethyltramadol (M1) after incubation with human liver microsoms (HLM). Each point (obtained by duplicate measurements) represents the mean value. The intrinsic clearance by HLM ($CL_{int,mic}$) was calculated as 52.92 μL/min/mg protein.

3.3. PAMPA Results

Results of the PAMPA assay for 12 tramadol samples diluted to 15 μM showed permeability ranges from 9.14×10^{-6} cm/s to 11.5×10^{-6} cm/s. The mean ± standard deviation permeability was calculated as $10.4 \times 10^{-6} \pm 0.056$ cm/s. The calculated mean PAMPA permeability was applied to the tramadol PBPK model.

3.4. Development of the PBPK Model for Tramadol and M1

The input parameters for tramadol and M1 and demographic characteristics for virtual population in the PBPK model are presented in Tables 2 and 3. Data for the healthy Korean population were obtained from the Certara repository. Ten virtual trials, including 100 virtual subjects in each virtual trial (total 1000 subjects), were performed for tramadol and M1. In the tramadol model, most of the observation profiles were within the 5th and 95th percentile range, and the predicted mean tramadol concentration in plasma was similar to the observed profile (Figure 3a). The geometric mean ratios of $C_{max,ss}$ and $AUC_{last,ss}$ for tramadol were 0.79 and 1.04, respectively (Table 4). Most observed concentration–time profiles were included in the 5th and 95th percentiles of the predicted concentration–time profiles. In addition, the mean predicted plasma tramadol concentration was well fitted to the observed tramadol concentration. In the concentration–time profiles for M1, most of the observations were also within the 5th and 95th percentile range of the predicted profile (Figure 3b). The range of 90% CI for $C_{max,ss}$ and $AUC_{last,ss}$ were included in the range of 0.7–1.43 (30% range of geometric mean ratio); however, the geometric mean ratio was predicted to be relatively low (Table 4). Both tramadol and M1 were predominantly distributed in the liver. The second most common distributio sites were the spleen (tramadol) and heart (M1; Table 5).

Table 2. Input parameters for tramadol and *O*-desmethyltramadol (M1) in the physiologically-based pharmacokinetic (PBPK) model.

Parameters	Tramadol		M1 *	
	Value	Source	Value	Source
Physicochemical properties and blood binding				
Molecular weight (g/mol)	263.4	[30]	249.354	[31]
Log *P*	1.35	[30]	2.26	[32]
pKa	9.41 (Monoprotic base)	[30]	9.62 (Monoprotic base)	[32]
fu_p	0.8	[33]	0.525	Predicted in SimCYP
Absorption				
Absorption type	PAMPA	-	n/a	-
P_{app} ($\times 10^{-6}$ cm/s)	10.2	Experimental data	n/a	-
Distribution				
Kp scalar	0.946	Adjusted using V_{ss}	0.107	Estimated
V_{ss} (L/kg)	2.6	Observed data	0.628	Estimated
Elimination				
CL_{int} (μL/min/pmol or mg protein)	CYP2D6: 0.447; CYP2B6: 0.028; CYP3A4: 0.020	Retrograde model	52.92 (WOMC–HLM)	Experimental data
CL_R	1.850	Estimated	0.481	Estimated

CL_{int}: intrinsic clearance; CL_R: renal clearance; CYP: cytochrome P450 superfamily; fu_p: unbound fraction in plasma; HLM: human liver microsomes; Kp: plasma-tissue partition coefficient; PAMPA: parallel artificial membrane permeability assay; P_{app}: apparent permeability; V_{ss}: volume of distribution in steady-state; WOMC: whole organ metabolic clearance, n/a: not applicable. * Metabolite model does not take account of absorption.

Table 3. The demographic characteristics of the participated subjects for virtual Korean population ($n = 1000$).

Parameters	Mean (Range)
Age (years)	28.9 (20.2–40.0)
Height (cm)	166.2 (147.6–188.0)
Weight (kg)	62.3 (42.9–93.9)
The percentage of female	50%

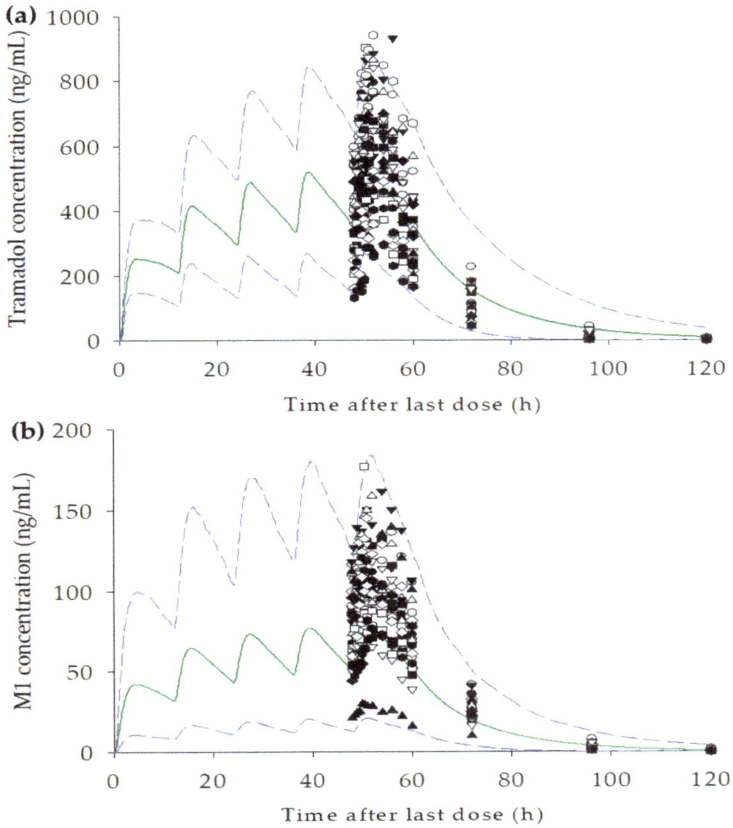

Figure 3. The observed (each symbol, n = 23) and simulated mean (solid dark green line) plasma concentration–time profiles after administration of 100 mg tramadol extended-release (ER) tablet twice daily (total five times) for (**a**) tramadol, and (**b**) *O*-desmethyltramadol (M1); blue dashed line represents 5th and 95th percentiles.

Table 4. Observed and simulated pharmacokinetic (PK) parameters for tramadol and *O*-desmethyltramadol (M1) after oral administration of 100 mg tramadol ER tablet twice daily (five times in total).

Parameters	Observed (Range)	Simulated (Range)	Ratio (90% CI)
	Tramadol		
Geometric mean $C_{max,ss}$ (ng/mL)	643.8; (294.0–942.1)	508.4; (122.1–1226)	0.79; (0.69–0.91)
Geometric mean $AUC_{last,ss}$ (ng/mL·h)	8965; (4127–16,038)	9346; (1217–42,462)	1.04; (0.85–1.28)
	M1		
Geometric mean $C_{max,ss}$ (ng/mL)	103.8; (29.8–176.7)	65.68; (1.07–368.1)	0.63; (0.51–0.79)
Geometric mean $AUC_{last,ss}$ (ng/mL·h)	1775; (445.3–2875)	1.187; (6.236–7522)	0.67; (0.54–0.84)

AUC_{last}: area under the curve from 48 h to 120 h at steady-state; CI: confidence interval; $C_{max,ss}$: maximum drug concentration in plasma at steady-state.

Table 5. Maximum simulated concentrations at steady-state for tramadol and *O*-desmethyltramadol (M1) in each organ ($C_{max,ss}$) after oral administration of 100 mg tramadol ER tablet twice daily (five times in total).

Organ	Maximum Concentration at Steady-State in Each Organ (ng/mL)	
	Tramadol	**M1**
Adipose tissue	400.6	12.89
Bone	899.8	23.88
Brain	1034	19.74
Gut	2741	88.38
Heart	763.0	94.97
Kidney	1452	78.46
Liver	3034	157.5
Lung	991.0	21.09
Muscle	2411	79.13
Pancreas	2000	56.25
Skin	1355	42.03
Spleen	2821	88.53

3.5. Prediction of Changes in Concentration–Time Profiles for Tramadol and M1 According to CYP2D6 Genotype and Dosage

To investigate the effect of CYP2D6 genotype and dosage on PK profiles, simulations were performed for the administration of 100 and 200 mg of tramadol every 12 h (total 5 times). The tramadol/M1 concentration–time profiles were captured from the pre-dose (0 h) to 120 h. The differences on PK profiles according to CYP2D6 genotypes were assessed in the general Korean population in CYP2D6 groups: PM, IM, EM, and UM. As a result, plasma concentration–time profiles for tramadol were within the therapeutic range in all groups after administration of 100 mg tramadol ER. Predicted plasma M1 concentrations were very low in the PM group (mean $C_{max,ss}$ 0.643 ng/mL) compared to the CYP2D6 IM, EM, and UM groups (mean values 40.93, 83.80, and 126.8 ng/mL, respectively).

The plasma concentration–time profiles for tramadol and M1, and changes in PK parameters, in the various CYP2D6 genotype groups following oral administration of 100 and 200 mg tramadol ER tablet twice daily (total five times) are shown in Figure 4 and Table 6 (the plasma concentration–time profiles for each CYP2D6 phenotype after administration of 100 and 200 mg of tramadol were presented in Supplementary Materials Figures S1 and S2). Following tramadol 100 mg administrations, the $C_{max,ss}$ of tramadol in CYP2D6 PMs reached to toxic range. For CYP2D6 UMs, the $C_{max,ss}$ of M1 exceeded the therapeutic margin (Supplementary Materials Figure S1). Following tramadol 200 mg administrations, the $C_{max,ss}$ of tramadol were reached to the toxic range in all CYP2D6 metabolizer groups. For M1, the $C_{max,ss}$ exceeded the therapeutic margin in the CYP2D6 IMs, EMs, and UMs (Figure S2). In Table 7, observed and predicted $C_{max,ss}$ and $AUC_{last,ss}$ values, and predicted/observed geometric mean ratios are presented. The CYP2D6 UM group was excluded from this table because UM subjects did not exist in the clinical study. In the CYP2D6 EM and IM groups, the predicted/observed geometric mean ratios for $C_{max,ss}$ and $AUC_{last,ss}$ for tramadol satisfied the acceptance criteria (0.7–1.43) however, the tramadol $AUC_{last,ss}$ ratio for the CYP2D6 PM group was overestimated at 1.95. The prediction results for M1 showed that $AUC_{last,ss}$ satisfied the acceptance criteria in the CYP2D6 EM group; however, $C_{max,ss}$ and $AUC_{last,ss}$ values were underestimated in both the CYP2D6 IM and PM groups, where the predicted values were much lower than observed values.

Table 6. Predicted geometric mean $C_{max,ss}$ and $AUC_{last,ss}$ values for tramadol and *O*-desmethyltramadol (M1) following oral administration of 100 and 200 mg tramadol ER tablet twice daily (total five times) in various CYP2D6 metabolizer groups.

Parameters	UM		EM		IM		PM	
	Tramadol	M1	Tramadol	M1	Tramadol	M1	Tramadol	M1
Tramadol 100 mg								
$C_{max,ss}$ (ng/mL)	357.2	126.8	469.6	83.80	593.8	40.93	721.3	0.6433
(range)	(72.43–927.6)	(21.39–449.0)	(122.2–1117)	(12.62–368.1)	(165.8–1379)	(5.511–240.9)	(209.5–1675)	(0.0975–5.312)
$AUC_{last,ss}$ (ng/mL·h)	5353	1881	8206	1445	12,049	813.5	16,795	2.919
(range)	(648.7–25,267)	(278.6–8560)	(1217–34,213)	(175.2–7522)	(1932–42,462)	(79.54–5234)	(2682–61,319)	(0.3351–34.42)
Tramadol 200 mg								
$C_{max,ss}$ (ng/mL)	714.3	253.5 #	939.1 *	167.6	1188 **	81.86	1443 **	1.287
(range)	(144.9–1855)	(42.77–898.0)	(244.3–2235)	(25.24–736.3)	(331.7–2758)	(11.02–481.7)	(418.9–3349)	(0.1950–10.62)
$AUC_{last,ss}$ (ng/mL·h)	10,706	3761	16,411	2890	24,097	1627	33,591	5.839
(range)	(1297–50,533)	(557.1–17,119)	(2434–68,426)	(350.3–15,044)	(3864–84,923)	(159.1–10,467)	(5365–122,637)	(0.67–68.83)

$AUC_{last,ss}$: area under the curve from 48 h to 120 h at steady-state; $C_{max,ss}$: maximum drug concentration in plasma at steady-state; EM: extensive metabolizer; IM: intermediate metabolizer; PM: poor metabolizer; UM: ultra-rapid metabolizer. * Above the therapeutic range for tramadol (>800 ng/mL); ** in toxic range for tramadol (1000–2000 ng/mL); # above maximum therapeutic range for M1 (>200 ng/mL).

Table 7. Predicted and observed geometric mean PK parameters for tramadol and M1 according to CYP2D6 genotype following oral administration of 100 mg tramadol ER tablet twice daily (total five times).

Tramadol	EM			IM			PM		
	Observed (*n* = 13)	Predicted (*n* = 1000)	Ratio (90% CI)	Observed (*n* = 8)	Predicted (*n* = 1000)	Ratio (90% CI)	Observed (*n* = 1)	Predicted (*n* = 1000)	Ratio (90% CI)
$C_{max,ss}$ (ng/mL)	551.2	469.6	0.85	828.5	593.8	0.72	751.10	721.3	0.96
(range)	(294.0–904.4)	(122.2–1117)	(0.72–1.01)	(676.6–942.1)	(165.8–1379)	(0.59–0.87)		(209.5–1675)	
$AUC_{last,ss}$ (ng/mL·h)	7116	8206	1.15	13,501	12,049	0.89	8591.72	16,795	1.95
(range)	(4127–9345)	(1217–34,213)	(0.90–1.48)	(10,527–16,038)	(1932–42,462)	(0.66–1.20)		(2682–61,319)	
M1	**EM**			**IM**			**PM**		
	Observed (*n* = 13)	Predicted (*n* = 1000)	Ratio (90% CI)	Observed (*n* = 8)	Predicted (*n* = 1000)	Ratio (90% CI)	Observed (*n* = 1)	Predicted (*n* = 1000)	Ratio (90% CI)
$C_{max,ss}$ (ng/mL)	125.0	83.80	0.67	87.79	40.93	0.47	29.8	0.6433	0.02
(range)	(81.8–176.7)	(12.62–368.1)	(0.52–0.86)	(66.0–114.1)	(5.511–240.9)	(0.32–0.69)		(0.0975–5.312)	
$AUC_{last,ss}$ (ng/mL·h)	1996	1445	0.72	1718	813.5	0.47	445.3	2.919	0.01
(range)	(1373–2875)	(175.2–7522)	(0.56–0.94)	(1223–2199)	(79.54–5234)	(0.31–0.72)		(0.3351–34.42)	

$AUC_{last,ss}$: area under the curve from 48 h to 120 h at steady-state; CI: confidence interval; $C_{max,ss}$: maximum drug concentration in plasma at steady-state; EM: extensive metabolizer; IM: intermediate metabolizer; PM: poor metabolizer; Ratio = predicted/observed. Since the observed data for the PM group are for 1 subject, the CI value cannot be obtained.

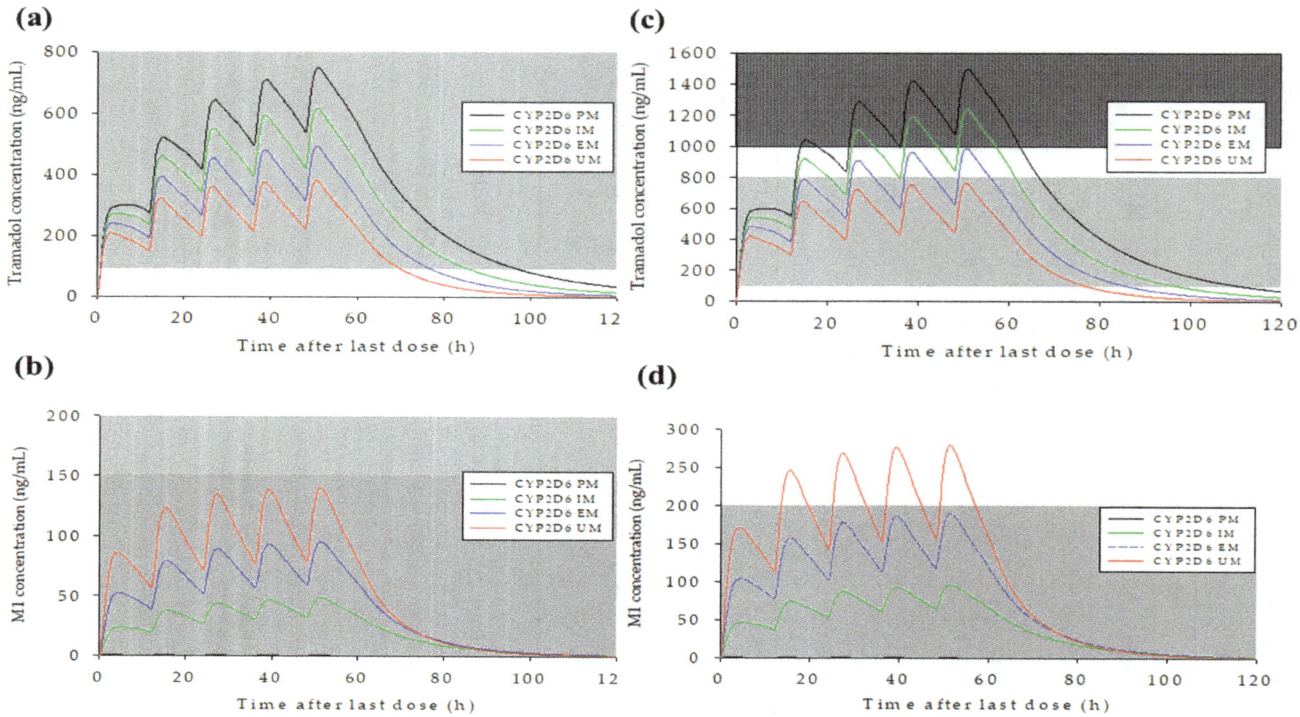

Figure 4. The predicted mean concentration–time profiles after administration of 100 mg and 200 mg tramadol ER tablet twice daily (total five times) for tramadol (**a** and **c**), and *O*-desmethyltramadol (**b** and **d**), respectively. Gray areas in (**a**) and (**c**) represent the therapeutic concentration range (100–800 ng/mL); checked gray area in (**c**) represents the toxic range (above 1000 ng/mL) for tramadol; and the gray area in (**b**) and (**d**) represents the maximum therapeutic range for M1 (up to 200 ng/mL).

4. Discussion

PBPK models for tramadol and M1 were developed. Tramadol plasma concentration–time profiles were well predicted from the proposed model. Prediction results for M1 included values in the 5th to 95th percentiles of most observed plasma concentration–time values, and the predicted mean plasma concentration was also similar to the observed concentration–time profile. However, geometric mean $C_{max,ss}$ and $AUC_{last,ss}$ ratios were under-predicted (0.63 and 0.67 for $C_{max,ss}$ and $AUC_{last,ss}$, respectively). To predict concentration-dependent toxicities, the therapeutic range (100–800 ng/mL for tramadol, and up to 200 ng/mL for M1) and the tramadol toxic range and lethal concentration (>1000 ng/mL, and >2000 ng/mL, respectively) were obtained from the literatures [34,35]. In general, the recommended dose of tramadol is up to 400 mg per day for immediate-release formulations and 300 mg per day for ER formulations [2]. Simulations were performed for 100 and 200 mg with 12-h intervals (5 times) according to CYP2D6 genotypes. After administration of 100 mg of tramadol, the predicted $C_{max,ss}$ of tramadol reached to toxic range in CYP2D6 PMs and exceeded therapeutic range in some IMs, and the predicted $C_{max,ss}$ of M1 exceeded therapeutic margin in CYP2D6 UMs. After tramadol 200 mg administrations, the predicted tramadol $C_{max,ss}$ reached to toxic ranges in all CYP2D6 metabolizer groups, even in some EMs and the predicted M1 $C_{max,ss}$ exceeded the therapeutic margin in CYP2D6 IMs, EMs, and UMs. The concentrations exceeded the therapeutic margins or reached to the toxic range might be related to potential toxicities after tramadol administrations, even though recommended doses of tramadol were administered.

PBPK modeling is useful for predicting PK profiles for rare genotypes in the population. The frequency of CYP2D6 UM in the Korean population has been reported as approximately 1.25% [36]. In the clinical study used for our PBPK model development, there was only one PM subject, and no UM subject was found. The model developed in this study could predict the plasma concentration–time profiles of tramadol and M1 for these two groups. Using the developed model, plasma tramadol/M1 concentration–time profiles for CYP2D6 UM, a very rare genotype in Koreans, were also predicted.

Tramadol inhibits reuptake of 5-HT and norepinephrine. M1 binds to μ-opioid receptors and exhibits analgesic effects. Due to these actions, the side effects of tramadol differ depending on CYP2D6 genotype. In the PM group, a high risk of side effects due to tramadol, such as serotonin syndrome, can be expected; and in the UM group, a high risk of μ-opioid receptor-related side effects, such as respiratory depression, can be expected relative to other CYP2D6 genotypes [16]. In our simulation, the plasma concentrations of tramadol and M1 exceeded the therapeutic concentration range, even after administration of recommended doses. These results suggest that the frequency of concentration-related adverse drug reactions may be reduced by optimizing the dosing regimen according to CYP2D6 genotype of the patient or population.

Tramadol and M1 distribution in each tissue were estimated using the PBPK model, and tramadol and M1 were distributed most to the liver. In cases of fatal intoxication due to tramadol, the highest concentration of tramadol was evident in the liver, after the blood and urine. These distribution characteristics are considered due to the hepatic metabolism of tramadol and its metabolites [37]. The distribution of tramadol to adipose tissue differed from that for M1. Indeed, tramadol is considered to distribute widely to lipid-rich tissues because of its higher affinity for lipids than M1 (logD for tramadol and M1: 1.13 and 0.4, respectively) [38]. Further research is needed about the distribution characteristics of tramadol and M1 to each tissue.

The predicted plasma M1 concentration–time profiles were under-predicted due to a lack of information about distribution and elimination properties. Since M1 is produced by tramadol metabolism, elimination profiles (intrinsic clearance by CYP, renal clearance and additional clearance) of tramadol were adjusted to improve the M1 model; however, there were no significant changes in M1 concentration–time profiles. This might be due to poor distribution of M1 from liver to plasma, or to exaggeration of elimination. For improvement, the M1 model was built using parameter estimation by observed plasma concentration–time profiles as distribution and elimination profiles (tissue–plasma partition coefficient, additional clearance, renal clearance, bile clearance). When estimating several parameters, the predicted plasma M1 concentration–time profiles changed significantly when values of the unbound fraction in incubated microsomes (fu_{mic}) and active hepatic scalar were changed. Thus, the plasma M1 concentration–time profile might be greatly influenced by metabolism. More detailed information and parameters for M1 metabolism are needed for more accurate predictions of plasma M1 concentration–time profiles.

Regarding limitations of our study, tramadol is metabolized not only to M1, but also to *N*-desmethyltramadol (M2) by CYP2D6, CYP2B6, and CYP3A4. In accordance with the literature, the toxicity of tramadol and M1 can be determined using M1/M2 ratio [34]. Therefore, an M2 model could improve the predictability of concentration-related adverse drug reactions after tramadol administration. Moreover, organic cation transporter 1 (OCT1) and multidrug resistance protein 1 (MDR1) influence the disposition of tramadol and M1. Significant differences in drug disposition according to OCT1 and MDR1 genotypes have been shown, even in same CYP2D6 phenotype [39–41]. Due to lack of information of transporter kinetic parameter for each organ, the transport kinetic parameters for M1 were excluded for the model. For elaborate model prediction, OCT1 and MDR1 genotypes (*OCT**1, *2, *3, *4, *5, and *MDR1* C3435T) could be incorporated.

5. Conclusions

In summary, our PBPK model for tramadol and M1 was developed and predicted concentration–time profiles after multiple administrations of a tramadol ER formulation in the Korean population. Differences in PK profiles and concentration-dependent toxicities were predicted according to CYP2D6 phenotype and dosage. Most modeling studies of tramadol used a population PK approach, and the literature using PBPK modeling focused on the PK profile of tramadol itself. However, this study developed a model with predictive power for tramadol and M1, the major active metabolite. This model could be applied to predict concentration-dependent toxicity profiles in cases of tramadol overdose or abuse and also, CYP2D6-related drug interactions.

Supplementary Materials:
Figure S1: The predicted mean tramadol and *O*-desmethyltramadol concentration-time profiles after administration of 100 mg tramadol ER tablet twice daily (five times in total) for CYP2D6 poor metabolizer, intermediate metabolizer extensive metabolizer and ultra-rapid metabolizer, respectively; Figure S2: The predicted mean tramadol and *O*-desmethyltramadol concentration-time profiles after administration of 200 mg tramadol ER tablet twice daily (five times in total) for CYP2D6 poor metabolizer, intermediate metabolizer, extensive metabolizer and ultra-rapid metabolizer, respectively.

Author Contributions: J.-W.B., S.L. and K.-H.S. conceived and designed the experiments; H.-C.J., S.H.B. and K.-H.S. performed the experiments, simulations, and analyzed the data; H.-C.J., Y.J., S.H.B., A.K. and K.-H.S reviewed the data and wrote the paper. All authors approved the final manuscript.

References

1. Shipton, E. Tramadol—Present and future. *Anaesth. Intensive Care* **2000**, *28*, 363–374. [CrossRef] [PubMed]
2. Miotto, K.; Cho, A.K.; Khalil, M.A.; Blanco, K.; Sasaki, J.D.; Rawson, R. Trends in Tramadol: Pharmacology Metabolism, and Misuse. *Anesth. Analg.* **2017**, *124*, 44–51. [CrossRef] [PubMed]
3. Lassen, D.; Damkier, P.; Brøsen, K. The Pharmacogenetics of Tramadol. *Clin. Pharmacokinet.* **2015**, *54*, 825–836 [CrossRef] [PubMed]
4. Kaye, A.D. Tramadol, pharmacology, side effects, and serotonin syndrome: A review. *Pain Physician* **2015** *18*, 395–400.
5. Leppert, W. Tramadol as an analgesic for mild to moderate cancer pain. *Pharmacol. Rep.* **2009**, *61*, 978–992 [CrossRef]
6. Lehtonen, P.; Sten, T.; Aitio, O.; Kurkela, M.; Vuorensola, K.; Finel, M.; Kostiainen, R. Glucuronidation of racemic *O*-desmethyltramadol, the active metabolite of tramadol. *Eur. J. Pharm. Sci.* **2010**, *41*, 523–530 [CrossRef]
7. Grond, S.; Sablotzki, A. Clinical pharmacology of tramadol. *Clin. Pharmacokinet.* **2004**, *43*, 879–923. [CrossRef]
8. Kostewicz, E.S.; Aarons, L.; Bergstrand, M.; Bolger, M.B.; Galetin, A.; Hatley, O.; Jamei, M.; Lloyd, R. Pepin, X.; Rostami-Hodjegan, A. PBPK models for the prediction of in vivo performance of oral dosage forms. *Eur. J. Pharm. Sci.* **2014**, *57*, 300–321. [CrossRef]
9. Zhao, P.; Zhang, L.; Grillo, J.; Liu, Q.; Bullock, J.; Moon, Y.; Song, P.; Brar, S.; Madabushi, R.; Wu, T Applications of physiologically based pharmacokinetic (PBPK) modeling and simulation during regulatory review. *Clin. Pharmacol. Ther.* **2011**, *89*, 259–267. [CrossRef]
10. Abbiati, R.A.; Manca, D. A modeling tool for the personalization of pharmacokinetic predictions *Comput. Chem. Eng.* **2016**, *91*, 28–37. [CrossRef]
11. Price, P.S.; Conolly, R.B.; Chaisson, C.F.; Gross, E.A.; Young, J.S.; Mathis, E.T.; Tedder, D.R. Modeling interindividual variation in physiological factors used in PBPK models of humans. *Crit. Rev. Toxicol.* **2003** *33*, 469–503. [CrossRef] [PubMed]
12. Marsousi, N.; Desmeules, J.A.; Rudaz, S.; Daali, Y. Usefulness of PBPK Modeling in Incorporation of Clinical Conditions in Personalized Medicine. *J. Pharm. Sci.* **2017**, *106*, 2380–2391. [CrossRef] [PubMed]
13. T'Jollyn, H.; Snoeys, J.; Colin, P.; Van Bocxlaer, J.; Annaert, P.; Cuyckens, F.; Vermeulen, A.; Van Peer, A. Allegaert, K.; Mannens, G.; et al. Physiology-Based IVIVE Predictions of Tramadol from in Vitro Metabolism Data. *Pharm. Res.* **2015**, *32*, 260–274. [CrossRef] [PubMed]
14. Salman, S.; Sy, S.K.; Ilett, K.F.; Page-Sharp, M.; Paech, M.J. Population pharmacokinetic modeling of tramadol and its *O*-desmethyl metabolite in plasma and breast milk. *Eur. J. Clin. Pharmacol.* **2011**, *67*, 899–908 [CrossRef]
15. Garrido, M.J.; Habre, W.; Rombout, F.; Trocóniz, I.F. Population Pharmacokinetic/Pharmacodynamic Modelling of the Analgesic Effects of Tramadol in Pediatrics. *Pharm. Res.* **2006**, *23*, 2014–2023. [CrossRef]
16. Faria, J.; Barbosa, J.; Moreira, R.; Queirós, O.; Carvalho, F.; Dinis-Oliveira, R. Comparative pharmacology and toxicology of tramadol and tapentadol. *Eur. J. Pain* **2018**, *22*, 827–844. [CrossRef]
17. Lee, J.; Yoo, H.D.; Bae, J.W.; Lee, S.; Shin, K.H. Population pharmacokinetic analysis of tramadol and O-desmethyltramadol with genetic polymorphism of CYP2D6. *Drug Des. Dev. Ther.* **2019**, *13*, 1751 [CrossRef]

18. Yu, H.; Hong, S.; Jeong, C.H.; Bae, J.W.; Lee, S. Development of a linear dual column HPLC–MS/MS method and clinical genetic evaluation for tramadol and its phase I and II metabolites in oral fluid. *Arch. Pharmacal Res.* **2018**, *41*, 288–298. [CrossRef]
19. Byeon, J.Y.; Kim, Y.H.; Lee, C.M.; Kim, S.H.; Chae, W.K.; Jung, E.H.; Choi, C.I.; Jang, C.G.; Lee, S.Y.; Bae, J.W. CYP2D6 allele frequencies in Korean population, comparison with East Asian, Caucasian and African populations, and the comparison of metabolic activity of CYP2D6 genotypes. *Arch. Pharmacal Res.* **2018**, *41*, 921–930. [CrossRef]
20. Byeon, J.Y.; Kim, Y.H.; Na, H.S.; Jang, J.H.; Kim, S.H.; Lee, Y.J.; Bae, J.W.; Kim, I.S.; Jang, C.G.; Chung, M.W.; et al. Effects of the CYP2D6* 10 allele on the pharmacokinetics of atomoxetine and its metabolites. *Arch. Pharmacal Res.* **2015**, *38*, 2083–2091. [CrossRef]
21. Doki, K.; Homma, M.; Kuga, K.; Kusano, K.; Watanabe, S.; Yamaguchi, I.; Kohda, Y. Effect of CYP2D6 genotype on flecainide pharmacokinetics in Japanese patients with supraventricular tachyarrhythmia. *Eur. J. Clin. Pharmacol.* **2006**, *62*, 919–926. [CrossRef] [PubMed]
22. Findling, R.L.; Nucci, G.; Piergies, A.A.; Gomeni, R.; Bartolic, E.I.; Fong, R.; Carpenter, D.J.; Leeder, J.S.; Gaedigk, A.; Danoff, T.M. Multiple dose pharmacokinetics of paroxetine in children and adolescents with major depressive disorder or obsessive–compulsive disorder. *Neuropsychopharmacology* **2006**, *31*, 1274. [CrossRef] [PubMed]
23. Yoo, H.D.; Lee, S.N.; Kang, H.A.; Cho, H.Y.; Lee, I.K.; Lee, Y.B. Influence of ABCB1 genetic polymorphisms on the pharmacokinetics of risperidone in healthy subjects with CYP2D6* 10/* 10. *Br. J. Pharmacol.* **2011**, *164*, 433–443. [CrossRef] [PubMed]
24. Chen, X.; Murawski, A.; Patel, K.; Crespi, C.L.; Balimane, P.V. A Novel Design of Artificial Membrane for Improving the PAMPA Model. *Pharm. Res.* **2008**, *25*, 1511–1520. [CrossRef]
25. Bae, S.H.; Kwon, M.J.; Park, J.B.; Kim, D.; Kim, D.H.; Kang, J.S.; Kim, C.G.; Oh, E.; Bae, S.K. Metabolic drug-drug interaction potential of macrolactin A and 7-*O*-succinyl macrolactin A assessed by evaluating cytochrome P450 inhibition and induction and UDP-glucuronosyltransferase inhibition in vitro. *Antimicrob. Agents Chemother.* **2014**, *58*, 5036–5046. [CrossRef]
26. Li, A.P. In vitro approaches to evaluate ADMET drug properties. *Curr. Top. Med. Chem.* **2004**, *4*, 701–706. [CrossRef]
27. Kanaan, M.; Daali, Y.; Dayer, P.; Desmeules, J. Uptake/Efflux Transport of Tramadol Enantiomers and O-Desmethyl-Tramadol: Focus on P-Glycoprotein. *Basic Clin. Pharmacol. Toxicol.* **2009**, *105*, 199–206. [CrossRef]
28. Saarikoski, T.; Saari, T.I.; Hagelberg, N.M.; Backman, J.T.; Neuvonen, P.J.; Scheinin, M.; Olkkola, K.T.; Laine, K. Effects of terbinafine and itraconazole on the pharmacokinetics of orally administered tramadol. *Eur. J. Clin. Pharmacol.* **2015**, *71*, 321–327. [CrossRef]
29. Mattia, C.; Coluzzi, F. Once-daily tramadol in rheumatological pain. *Expert Opin. Pharmacother.* **2006**, *7*, 1811–1823. [CrossRef]
30. T'jollyn, H.; Vermeulen, A.; Van Bocxlaer, J. PBPK and its virtual populations: The impact of physiology on pediatric pharmacokinetic predictions of tramadol. *AAPS J.* **2019**, *21*, 8. [CrossRef]
31. Pubchem. *O*-Desmethyltramadol. Available online: https://pubchem.ncbi.nlm.nih.gov/compound/9838803 (accessed on 31 January 2019).
32. Wojsławski, J.; Białk-Bielińska, A.; Stepnowski, P.; Dołżonek, J. Leaching behavior of pharmaceuticals and their metabolites in the soil environment. *Chemosphere* **2019**, *231*, 269–275. [CrossRef] [PubMed]
33. T'jollyn, H.; Snoeys, J.; Vermeulen, A.; Michelet, R.; Cuyckens, F.; Mannens, G.; Van Peer, A.; Annaert, P.; Allegaert, K.; Van Bocxlaer, J.; et al. Physiologically Based Pharmacokinetic Predictions of Tramadol Exposure Throughout Pediatric Life: An Analysis of the Different Clearance Contributors with Emphasis on CYP2D6 Maturation. *AAPS J.* **2015**, *17*, 1376–1387. [CrossRef] [PubMed]
34. Barbera, N.; Fisichella, M.; Bosco, A.; Indorato, F.; Spadaro, G.; Romano, G. A suicidal poisoning due to tramadol. A metabolic approach to death investigation. *J. Forensic Leg. Med.* **2013**, *20*, 555–558. [CrossRef] [PubMed]
35. Perdreau, E.; Iriart, X.; Mouton, J.B.; Jalal, Z.; Thambo, J.B. Cardiogenic shock due to acute tramadol intoxication. *Cardiovasc. Toxicol.* **2015**, *15*, 100–103. [CrossRef]

36. Lee, S.Y.; Sohn, K.M.; Ryu, J.Y.; Yoon, Y.R.; Shin, J.G.; Kim, J.W. Sequence-based CYP2D6 genotyping in the Korean population. *Ther. Drug Monit.* **2006**, *28*, 382–387. [CrossRef]
37. Vazzana, M.; Andreani, T.; Fangueiro, J.; Faggio, C.; Silva, C.; Santini, A.; Garcia, M.; Silva, A.; Souto, E. Tramadol hydrochloride: Pharmacokinetics, pharmacodynamics, adverse side effects, co-administration of drugs and new drug delivery systems. *Biomed. Pharmacother.* **2015**, *70*, 234–238. [CrossRef]
38. Costa, I.; Oliveira, A.; Guedes de Pinho, P.; Teixeira, H.M.; Moreira, R.; Carvalho, F.; Jorge Dinis-Oliveira, R. Postmortem Redistribution of Tramadol and *O*-Desmethyltramadol. *J. Anal. Toxicol.* **2013**, *37*, 670–675. [CrossRef]
39. Tzvetkov, M.V.; Saadatmand, A.R.; Lötsch, J.; Tegeder, I.; Stingl, J.C.; Brockmöller, J. Genetically polymorphic OCT1: Another piece in the puzzle of the variable pharmacokinetics and pharmacodynamics of the opioidergic drug tramadol. *Clin. Pharmacol. Ther.* **2011**, *90*, 143–150. [CrossRef]
40. Stamer, U.M.; Frank, M.; Stuber, F.; Brockmoller, J.; Steffens, M.; Tzvetkov, M.V. Loss-of-function polymorphisms in the organic cation transporter OCT1 are associated with reduced postoperative tramadol consumption. *Pain* **2016**, *157*, 2467–2475. [CrossRef]
41. Slanar, O.; Nobilis, M.; Kvétina, J.; Matousková, O.; Idle, J.R.; Perlík, F. Pharmacokinetics of tramadol is affected by MDR1 polymorphism C3435T. *Eur. J. Clin. Pharmacol.* **2007**, *63*, 419–421. [CrossRef]

7

Subset Analysis for Screening Drug–Drug Interaction Signal Using Pharmacovigilance Database

Yoshihiro Noguchi [1,*], Tomoya Tachi [1] and Hitomi Teramachi [1,2,*]

1 Laboratory of Clinical Pharmacy, Gifu Pharmaceutical University, 1-25-4, Daigakunishi, Gifu-shi, Gifu 501-1196, Japan; tachi@gifu-pu.ac.jp
2 Laboratory of Community Healthcare Pharmacy, Gifu Pharmaceutical University, Daigakunishi, Gifu-shi, Gifu 501-1196, Japan
* Correspondence: noguchiy@gifu-pu.ac.jp (Y.N.); teramachih@gifu-pu.ac.jp (H.T.);

Abstract: Many patients require multi-drug combinations, and adverse event profiles reflect not only the effects of individual drugs but also drug–drug interactions. Although there are several algorithms for detecting drug–drug interaction signals, a simple analysis model is required for early detection of adverse events. Recently, there have been reports of detecting signals of drug–drug interactions using subset analysis, but appropriate detection criterion may not have been used. In this study, we presented and verified an appropriate criterion. The data source used was the Japanese Adverse Drug Event Report (JADER) database; "hypothetical" true data were generated through a combination of signals detected by three detection algorithms. The accuracy of the signal detection of the analytic model under investigation was verified using indicators used in machine learning. The newly proposed subset analysis confirmed that the signal detection was improved, compared with signal detection in the previous subset analysis, on the basis of the indicators of *Accuracy* (0.584 to 0.809), *Precision (= Positive predictive value; PPV)* (0.302 to 0.596), *Specificity* (0.583 to 0.878), *Youden's index* (0.170 to 0.465), *F-measure* (0.399 to 0.592), and *Negative predictive value* (*NPV*) (0.821 to 0.874). The previous subset analysis detected many false drug–drug interaction signals. Although the newly proposed subset analysis provides slightly lower detection accuracy for drug–drug interaction signals compared to signals compared to the Ω shrinkage measure model, the criteria used in the newly subset analysis significantly reduced the amount of falsely detected signals found in the previous subset analysis.

Keywords: subset analysis; signal detection algorithms; drug-drug interaction; spontaneous reporting systems

1. Introduction

Drug-induced adverse events (AEs) caused by individual drugs and drug combinations not only hinder treatment but also cause new health hazards. To alleviate this problem, AEs caused by individual drug candidates are closely monitored and investigated during the drug development and approval process [1]. Pre-marketing randomized clinical trials are performed under certain conditions associated with age, gender, and co-morbidities, and some AEs may not be detected. In particular, in pre-marketing randomized clinical trials, patients on combination therapy are usually excluded because the focus is to establish the safety and efficacy of single drugs and not to investigate drug–drug interactions [2]. However, in the real world, many patients suffer from a variety of co-morbidities and use a number of drugs to treat them. The concomitant use of two or more drugs increases the risk of AEs due to drug–drug interactions; the proportion of such AEs is estimated to be up to 30% of unexpected AEs [3].

Therefore, in order to use drugs appropriately in the real world, it is important to understand in advance, the AEs caused by drug–drug interactions. Post-marketing analysis of AE reports could significantly contribute to the discovery of AEs caused by single drugs or drug–drug interactions that could not be detected before marketing.

For the safety surveillance of drugs, AE reports collected post-marketing are maintained by regulatory agencies as a spontaneous reporting system. There are several algorithms for detecting adverse event signals using the spontaneous reporting system [4]. Of these, the algorithms commonly used for quantitative signal detection include the proportional reporting ratio (PRR) [5], the reporting odds ratio (ROR) [6], the Bayesian confidence propagation neural network (BCPNN) [7], and the empirical Bayesian geometric mean (EBGM) [8].

Additionally, multiple statistical algorithms have been proposed for detecting drug–drug interaction signals [9,10]. However, calculation of the PRR, similar to the risk ratio, and the ROR similar to the odds ratio, is simple, but that of other algorithms (particularly the algorithm for detecting drug–drug interaction signals) is very complicated.

Therefore, in order to detect the drug–drug interaction signals between *drug* D_1 and *drug* D_2 the subset analysis that detects the signal of *drug* D_1 using the ROR, which is easy to calculate in a subset of patient groups, is often reported [11–13].

Of previous studies, several [11,12] have used animal experiments and/or pharmacological data to ensure signal reliability, but the signals obtained with this analysis model are not strictly drug–drug interaction signals; they only showed the effect of drug combinations for the following two reasons [14]

1. The subset analysis used in this study detects signals from the target AE when the patient group using *drug* D_1 takes *drug* D_2. In all patient groups, when the signal value of the target AE is large for drug D_2, the signal is detected regardless of whether the patient group is using *drug* D_1.
2. Target AE signal intensities when a patient group using *drug* D_1 takes *drug* D_2 vs. that when a patient group using *drug* D_2 takes *drug* D_1 do not necessarily match. In other words, the value to be adopted as the target AE signal value when *drug* D_1 and *drug* D_2 are used concomitantly has not been fixed (i.e., no clear detection criteria have been defined for detecting drug–drug interaction signals).

On the other hand, because the ROR, often used in subset analysis, is easy to calculate, if these shortcomings are improved and the appropriate detection criterion can be set, it might lead to early detection of AEs caused by drug–drug interactions.

In this study, we proposed a new detection criterion for the subset analysis (the newly proposed subset analysis) and verified the detection power using the spontaneous reporting system.

2. Materials and Methods

The design of this study is based on a previous paper that discussed trends in methods to detect the signals of AEs caused by individual drugs [15] or drug–drug interactions [14].

2.1. Data Sources

The validation dataset was created from the Japanese Adverse Drug Event Report database (JADER), using data from the first quarter of 2004 to the fourth quarter of 2015. The JADER consists of four comma-separated values (csv) files as data tables: DEMO.csv (patient information), DRUG.csv (medicine information), HIST.csv (patient past history), and REAC.csv (AE event information) This study used 374,327 cases registered in the verification dataset.

However, the Japanese authority, the Pharmaceuticals and Medical Devices Agency (PMDA) which owns these data, does not permit sharing the data directly. Therefore, we do not own the JADER. It can be accessed directly here: [http://www.info.pmda.go.jp/fukusayoudb/CsvDownload.jsp] (in Japanese only).

2.2. *Definitions of Adverse Drug Events*

The drugs targeted for the survey are all registered and classified as "suspect drugs" in the validation dataset. The AEs in JADER are based on the preferred terms (PTs) in the Medical Dictionary for Regulatory Activities Japanese version (MedDRA/J). The AE targeted for this study was Stevens–Johnson syndrome (SJS), which was extracted from the dataset using the PT in MedDRA/J. However, the choice of target adverse events is the same as in previous similar studies [14,15], and there was no medical or pharmacological reason for this choice.

2.3. *"Hypothetical" True Data of Adverse Events for Comparative Verification*

The signals obtained from the spontaneous reporting system including the JADER used in this study included unknown AEs that were also detected, which needs to be verified in order to confirm they were true AEs. Moreover, the information provided by the regulatory authorities, of course, does not include unknown AEs. That is, there are no "real" true data for every AE. Therefore, we set "hypothetical" true data because we cannot use "real" true data for validation in this study.

To verify the power of the subset analysis, we prepared "hypothetical" true data of AEs. To generate "hypothetical" true data, we excluded the Ω shrinkage measure model [16] that detected the most conservative signal and the combination risk ratio model [17], which would not detect a signal with a small number of reports, from the five detection algorithms. That is, this study used the combination of signals detected by three algorithms (the additive model [18], the multiplicative model [18], and the chi-square statistical model [19]) as "hypothetical" true data.

2.4. *Statistical Models and Criteria*

2.4.1. Subset Analysis

To detect the signal for the interaction between *drug* D_1 and *drug* D_2, we created subsets of the patient group using *drug* D_1 (or the patient group using *drug* D_2) (Table 1).

Table 1. The 4 × 2 contingency table for signal detection: AE: adverse event; n: the number of reports (e.g., n_{+++}: the number of all reports, n_{111}: the number of *drug* D_1- and *drug* D_2-induced target AE reports).

	Target AE	**Other AEs**	**Total**
Concomitant use of *drug* D_1 and *drug* D_2	n_{111}	n_{110}	n_{11+}
only *drug* D_1	n_{101}	n_{100}	n_{10+}
only *drug* D_2	n_{011}	n_{010}	n_{01+}
Neither *drug* D_1 or *drug* D_2	n_{001}	n_{000}	n_{00+}
Total	n_{++1}	n_{++0}	n_{+++}

The following equations (Equations (1) and (2)) were used to calculate the ROR and 95% confidence interval (95% CI) of the target AE caused by *drug* D_1 (or *drug* D_2) from the generated subset, respectively. For the signal of a patient group on *drug* D_1 that takes *drug* D_2, the number of each report can be expressed as follows: $N_{11} = n_{111}, N_{10} = n_{110}, N_{01} = n_{101}, N_{00} = n_{100}$. On the other hand, for the signal of a patient group on *drug* D_2 that takes *drug* D_1, the number of each report can be expressed as follows: $N_{11} = n_{111}, N_{10} = n_{110}, N_{01} = n_{011}, N_{00} = n_{010}$.

$$\text{ROR} = \frac{N_{11}/N_{00}}{N_{01}/N_{10}} \tag{1}$$

$$\text{ROR (95\% CI)} = e^{\ln(\text{ROR}) \pm 1.96\sqrt{\frac{1}{N_{11}} + \frac{1}{N_{10}} + \frac{1}{N_{01}} + \frac{1}{N_{00}}}} \tag{2}$$

In previous studies [11–13], if the signal for *drug* D_2 was detected in the subset of a patient group using *drug* D_1 or if the signal for *drug* D_1 was detected in the subset of a patient group using *drug* D_2, this signal was considered the drug–drug interaction signal. The criterion that a signal only needs to be detected from a subset of either patient group is ambiguous, highlighting the two shortcomings mentioned earlier. Therefore, for the newly proposed subset analysis, a case was redefined as the drug–drug interaction signal if a signal was detected in both subsets of a patient group using *drug* D_1 and a patient group using *drug* D_2.

2.4.2. Ω Shrinkage Measure Model

The Ω shrinkage measure model [16] is based on a measure calculated as the ratio of the observed reporting ratio of the AE associated with the combination of two drugs and its expected value; this model is used by the Uppsala Monitoring Center (UMC) and the World Health Organization (WHO) Collaborating Centre for International Drug Monitoring for signal analysis of drug–drug interactions (Table 1, Equations (3)–(7)).

$$\Omega = log_2 \frac{n_{111} + 0.5}{E_{111} + 0.5} \quad (3)$$

where n_{111} is the reported number of AEs caused by the combination of two drugs, and E_{111} is the expected value of AEs caused by the combination of two drugs.

$\phi(0.975)$ is 97.5% of the standard normal distribution and $\Omega_{025} > 0$ is used as a threshold to screen for signals under the combination of two drugs (Equation (4)).

$$\Omega_{025} = \Omega - \frac{\phi(0.975)}{log(2)\sqrt{n_{111}}} \quad (4)$$

To calculate E_{111}, we used the following Equations (5)–(7).

$$f_{00} = \frac{n_{001}}{n_{00+}}, f_{10} = \frac{n_{101}}{n_{10+}}, f_{01} = \frac{n_{011}}{n_{01+}}, f_{11} = \frac{n_{111}}{n_{11+}} \quad (5)$$

$$g_{11} = 1 - \frac{1}{\max\left(\frac{f_{00}}{1-f_{00}}, \frac{f_{10}}{1-f_{10}}\right) + \max\left(\frac{f_{00}}{1-f_{00}}, \frac{f_{01}}{1-f_{01}}\right) - \frac{f_{00}}{1-f_{00}} + 1} \quad (6)$$

When $f_{10} < f_{00}$ (which denotes no risk of AE caused by drug D_1), the most sensible estimator g_{11} = max (f_{00}, f_{01}) is yielded and vice versa when $f_{01} < f_{00}$.

Norén et al. re-expressed the observed and expected RRR f_{11} and g_{11} in terms of the observed number of reports n_{111} and expected numbers of reports $E_{111} = g_{11} \times n_{11+}$, respectively:

$$\frac{f_{11}}{g_{11}} = \frac{n_{111}/n_{11+}}{E_{111}/n_{11+}} = \frac{n_{111}}{E_{111}} \quad (7)$$

2.5. *Evaluation of Detection Models*

2.5.1. Using Evaluations of Classification in Machine Learning

The evaluation indicators that we set were *Accuracy* (Table 2, Equation (8)), *Precision* (*Positive predictive value; PPV*) (Table 2, Equation (9)), *Recall* (*Sensitivity*) (Table 2, Equation (10)), *Specificity* (Table 2, Equation (11)), *Youden's index* (Table 2, Equation (12)), *F*-measure (Table 2, Equation (13)), and *Negative predictive value* (*NPV*) (Table 2, Equation (14)).

$$Accuracy = \frac{TP + TN}{TP + FP + TN + FN} \quad (8)$$

$$Precision\ (Positive\ predictive\ value; PPV) = \frac{TP}{TP + FP} \quad (9)$$

$$Recall\ (Sensitivity) = \frac{TP}{TP + FN} \tag{10}$$

$$Specificity = \frac{TN}{FP + TN} \tag{11}$$

$$Youden's\ index = Sensitivity + Specificity - 1 \tag{12}$$

$$F - measure = \frac{2 \times Recall \times Precision}{Recall + Precision} \tag{13}$$

$$Negative\ predictive\ value\ (NPV) = \frac{TN}{TN + FN} \tag{14}$$

Table 2. Agreement between the criterion A and the "hypothetical" true data. AE: adverse event, *TP*: *True Positive*, *FP*: *False Positive*, *FN*: *False Negative*, *TN*: *True Negative*.

		"Hypothetical" True Data	
		AE	**non-AEs**
analysis model	signal	*TP*	*FP*
	Non-signal	*FN*	*TN*

2.5.2. Cohen's Kappa Coefficient

The commonality of the signals detected by each statistical model was evaluated using *Cohen's kappa coefficient* (κ), proportionate agreement for positive rating (P_{positive}), and proportionate agreement for negative rating (P_{negative}), as reported in a previous study [14,15]. In this study, we investigated the similarities with Ω shrinkage measure model for the previous/newly proposed subset analysis.

2.6. *Analysis Software*

The analysis software in this study used Visual Mining Studio (NTT DATA Mathematical Systems Inc., Shinjuku-ku, Tokyo, Japan) version 8.4 and Microsoft Excel 2019 (Microsoft Corp., Redmond, WA, USA).

3. Results

3.1. *Evaluations of Classification in Machine Learning*

Among all 374,327 cases analyzed, there were 3924 *drug* D_1–*drug* D_2–SJS combinations. Of these, 923 combinations were detected by all three algorithms—the additive model [18], the multiplicative model [18], and the chi-square statistics model [19]. In this study, these combinations were treated as "hypothetical" true data.

The evaluation of the analysis model is shown in Tables 3 and 4.

Table 3. The number of True positive, False positive, True negative, and False negative.

Analysis Model	*TP*	*FP*	*TN*	*FN*
Previous subset analysis	542	1251	1750	381
Newly proposed subset analysis	542	367	2634	381
Ω shrinkage measure model	538	174	2827	385

TP: True positive, FP: False positive, TN: True negative, FN: False negative.

Table 4. Evaluation of detected drug–drug interaction signals.

Analysis Model	*Accuracy*	*Precision (PPV)*	*Recall (Sensitivity)*	*Specificity*	*Youden's Index*	*F-Measure*	*NPV*
Previous subset analysis	0.584	0.302	0.587	0.583	0.170	0.399	0.821
Newly proposed subset analysis	0.809	0.596	0.587	0.878	0.465	0.592	0.874
Ω shrinkage measure model	0.858	0.756	0.583	0.942	0.525	0.658	0.880

PPV: Positive predictive value, NPV: Negative predictive value.

Table 3 shows the number of True positive (TP), False Positive (FP), True Negative (TN), and False Negative (FN).

A total of 1793 combinations were detected by the previous subset analysis (*True positive*: 542 *False positive*: 1251). On the other hand, the newly proposed subset analysis detected 909 combinations of signals (*True positive*: 542, *False positive*: 367) (Table 3).

The detection accuracy shown in Table 4 was calculated from the values shown in Table 3.

In addition, the newly proposed subset analysis confirmed that the signal detection was improved with respect to the indicators of *Accuracy* (0.584 to 0.809), *Precision (PPV)* (0.302 to 0.596), *Specificity* (0.583 to 0.878), *Youden's index* (0.170 to 0.465), *F-measure* (0.399 to 0.592), and *NPV* (0.821 to 0.874) as compared with the signal detection in the previous subset analysis (Table 3).

The values of each indicator of the Ω shrinkage measure model were *Accuracy* (0.858), *Precision* (PPV) (0.756), *Recall* (*Sensitivity*) (0.583), *Specificity* (0.942), *Youden's index* (0.525), *F-measure* (0.658), and *NPV* (0.880) (Table 4).

3.2. Cohen's Kappa Coefficient

The similarity between the detection results of the Ω shrinkage measure model and that of the newly proposed subset analysis was κ (95% CI): 0.375 (0.355–0.395), P_{positive}: 0.502, and P_{negative}: 0.870 The similarity was κ (95% CI): 0.355 (0.327–0.384), P_{positive}: 0.678, and P_{negative}: 0.674 when targeting three or more reports (Table 5).

Table 5. The similarity between the Ω shrinkage measure model and subset analysis.

Analysis Model	All Case			$n_{111} \geq 3$		
	κ (95% CI)	P_{positive}	P_{negative}	κ (95% CI)	P_{positive}	P_{negative}
Previous subset analysis	0.088 (0.071–0.105)	0.325	0.684	−0.120 (−0.151–0.088)	0.556	0.296
Newly proposed subset analysis	0.375 (0.355–0.395)	0.502	0.870	0.355 (0.327–0.384)	0.678	0.674

n_{111}: targeting three or more reports, κ: *Cohen's kappa coefficient*, P_{positive}: proportionate agreement for positive rating, P_{negative}: proportionate agreement for negative rating.

4. Discussions

In this study, we evaluated the accuracy of drug–drug interaction signals for the newly proposed subset analysis that modified two shortcomings of the previous subset analysis on the basis of data from the spontaneous reporting system.

There were 3924 pairs of *drug* D_1–*drug* D_2–SJS in the spontaneous reporting system, JADER. There are several known combinations of drugs that onset SJS by drug–drug interactions [20]. On the other hand, there are some combinations that have not yet been reported. Recently, we used the Ω shrinkage measure model to report potential drug combinations for the onset of SJS in concomitant use with antiepileptic drugs [21]. Not all AEs have been identified and there are still many unknown AEs Unfortunately, unknown AE data do not exist anywhere in the world; there were no "real" true data for AEs. Therefore, to verify the accuracy of the subset analysis, we needed to prepare "hypothetical" true data of AEs. A previous comparative study [14] of five algorithms for detecting drug–drug interaction signals revealed that the Ω shrinkage measure model [16] detected the most conservative signal, while the combination risk ratio model [17] did not detect any interaction signal in less than three reports due to the detection criterion. Therefore, of the five algorithms, we used the combination of signals detected by the three algorithms (the additive model, the multiplicative model, and the chi-square statistical model) as "hypothetical" true data.

Among the previous subset analysis, the newly proposed subset analysis, and the Ω shrinkage measure model, most signals were detected by the previous subset analysis with 1793 pairs (45.7% of the total combinations, *Accuracy*: 0.584, *Precision* (*PPV*): 0.302, *Recall* (*Sensitivity*): 0.587, *Specificity*: 0.583, *Youden's index*: 0.170, *F-measure*: 0.399, and *NPV*: 0.821), followed by the newly proposed subset analysis with 909 pairs (23.2% of the total combinations, *Accuracy*: 0.809, *Precision* (*PPV*): 0.596, *Recall* (*Sensitivity*): 0.587, *Specificity*: 0.878, *Youden's index*: 0.465, *F-measure*: 0.592, and *NPV*: 0.874). In contrast, the Ω shrinkage measure model detected the fewest signals with 712 pairs (18.1% of the total combinations, *Accuracy*: 0.858, *Precision* (*PPV*): 0.756, *Recall* (*Sensitivity*): 0.583, *Specificity*: 0.942, *Youden's index*: 0.525, *F-measure*: 0.658, and *NPV*: 0.880) (Table 2, Table 4).

This result indicates that the accuracy of signal detection has been greatly improved in the newly proposed subset analysis with a simple modification of the previous subset analysis. However, the newly proposed subset analysis exhibited slightly lower power and accuracy for detecting the drug–drug interaction signals compared to the Ω shrinkage measure model.

Verification by the number of reports showed that when the number of reports (N_{11}; n_{111}) < 2, the accuracy (*Youden's index*, *F-measure*) of signal detection was higher in the newly proposed subset analysis than in the Ω shrinkage measure model (*Youden's index*: the newly proposed subset analysis (0.337) vs. the Ω shrinkage measure model (0.174), *F-measure*: the newly proposed subset analysis (0.448) vs. the Ω shrinkage measure model (0.298)).

However, as the number of reports increased, the Ω shrinkage measure model became more accurate (*Youden's index*: the newly proposed subset analysis (0.465) vs. the Ω shrinkage measure model (0.525), *F-measure*: the newly proposed subset analysis (0.592) vs. the Ω shrinkage measure model (0.658)) (Table 4).

Additionally, the *True positive* values for the previous subset analysis and the newly proposed subset analysis were the same (Table 3). Since all signals obtained by the newly proposed subset analysis were included in the previous subset analysis, this result indicates that the detection criterion of the previous subset analysis was loose and that the data contained false positives.

The similarity between the newly proposed subset analysis and the Ω shrinkage measure model was κ (95% CI): 0.375 (0.355–0.395), $P_{positive}$: 0.502, and $P_{negative}$: 0.870. On the other hand, the similarity between the previously subset analysis and the Ω shrinkage measure model was κ (95% CI): 0.088 (0.071–0.105), $P_{positive}$: 0.325, and $P_{negative}$: 0.684. Thus, the newly proposed subset analysis w more similar to the Ω shrinkage measure model than the previously subset analysis. However, the similarity of the newly proposed subset analysis and the Ω shrinkage measure model is not very high. Additionally, when the number of reports (N_{11}; n_{111}) was ≥3, no significant change was observed in the similarity between the Ω shrinkage measure model and the newly proposed subset analysis. Despite not being similar to the Ω shrinkage model, the newly subset analysis showed a high degree of accuracy. This result suggests that the newly subset analysis may be detecting signals that the Ω shrinkage model has failed to detect.

This study has the following three limitations. First, unfortunately, unknown AE data do not exist anywhere in the world [14]. Therefore, there were no "real" true data for AEs. Thus, for the purpose of verification, it was necessary to set "hypothetical" true data for AEs instead of "real" true data. Therefore, of the five algorithms for detecting drug–drug interaction signals, we used the combination of signals detected by the three algorithms (the additive model, the multiplicative model, and the chi-square statistical model) as "hypothetical" true data in this study. In other words, the hypothetical true data consisted of statistically based *drug* D_1–*drug* D_2–AE combinations, not pharmacologically based combinations.

Second, usually it is important to compare detection trends using all AEs recorded in the validation dataset created on the basis of a spontaneous reporting system; however, it takes an extremely long time to calculate signal values for all combinations of drug–drug interactions. Such a study design is not realistic. Therefore, this study targeted SJS, the same AE used in previous comparative studies [14,15]; if different reference sets were used, the possibility of obtaining different performance characteristics might not be ruled out. There are fewer enrolled cases than in the global dataset because JADER is limited to cases in Japan. However, the signal detection is based on a comparison between the ratio of reported cases (N) to expected values (E). Therefore, differences in the number of cases enrolled in the spontaneous reporting system had only a very small statistical impact in this study. Recently, validation of the number of cases enrolled in the spontaneous reporting system has also been reported by Caster et al. [22]. Moreover, differences in the way regulatory authorities think may result in a different tendency to register AEs to the spontaneous reporting system. For example, the Food and Drug Administration Adverse Events Reporting System (FAERS) in the United States has also registered reports from non-medical professionals, but JADER has not registered reports from patients until recently. It is unknown how the differences in registration tendencies affect the results of this study.

Finally, neither the general algorithms for detecting drug–drug interaction signals nor the proposed subset analysis in this study were antagonistic; only signals of synergistic interactions were detected [10].

5. Conclusions

In recent years, the need for safety signal screening has been demanded, not only for single drugs but also for drug–drug interactions. Although several methods for detecting signals of drug interaction have been reported, it is difficult to say that these methods are used because many of them are complicated in calculation. Therefore, there were several cases [11–13] where subset analysis using the algorithm for detecting signals of single drugs (e.g., ROR [6]) was used for signal detection of drug–drug interactions before its validity was verified.

This study showed that there were many false positives in the existing subset analysis, albeit under limited conditions. Additionally, very simple modifications of the detection criteria were made to solve two problems associated with the previous subset analysis for exploring recently reported drug–drug interaction signals. This modification helped to reduce falsely detected signals found in the previous subset analysis.

Moreover, the newly proposed subset analysis is more similar to the Ω shrinkage measure model than the previous subset analysis, but the similarity with the Ω shrinkage measure model is not as high. However, the newly proposed subset analysis showed that although the detection accuracy of the drug–drug interaction signal was slightly lower than that of the Ω shrinkage measure model, the detection accuracy was sufficient. This result may also indicate the possibility of detecting signals that cannot be detected by the Ω shrinkage measure model.

Author Contributions: Conceptualization, Y.N.; funding acquisition, Y.N.; investigation, Y.N.; methodology, Y.N. and T.T.; project administration, Y.N. and H.T.; supervision, Y.N.; validation, Y.N. and T.T.; visualization, Y.N.; writing—original draft, Y.N.; writing—review and editing, Y.N., T.T., and H.T. All authors have read and agreed to the published version of the manuscript.

References

1. Berlin, J.A.; Glasser, S.C.; Ellenberg, S.S. Adverse event detection in drug development: Recommendations and obligations beyond phase 3. *Am. J. Public Health* **2008**, *98*, 1366–1371. [CrossRef] [PubMed]
2. Noguchi, Y.; Ueno, A.; Otsubo, M.; Katsuno, H.; Sugita, I.; Kanematsu, Y.; Yoshida, A.; Esaki, H.; Tachi, T.; Teramachi, H. A New Search Method Using Association Rule Mining for Drug-Drug Interaction Based on Spontaneous Report System. *Front. Pharmacol.* **2018**, *9*, 197. [CrossRef] [PubMed]
3. Iyer, S.V.; Harpaz, R.; LePendu, P.; Bauer-Mehren, A.; Shah, N.H. Mining clinical text for signals of adverse drug-drug interactions. *J. Am. Med. Inf. Assoc.* **2013**, *21*, 353–362. [CrossRef] [PubMed]

4. Suling, M.; Pigeot, I. Signal Detection and Monitoring Based on Longitudinal Healthcare Data. *Pharmaceutics* **2012**, *4*, 607–640. [CrossRef] [PubMed]
5. Evans, S.J.; Waller, P.C.; Davis, S. Use of proportional reporting ratios (PRRs) for signal generation from spontaneous adverse drug reaction reports. *Pharmacoepidemiol. Drug Saf.* **2001**, *10*, 483–486. [CrossRef] [PubMed]
6. Rothman, K.J.; Lanes, S.; Sacks, S.T. The reporting odds ratio and its advantages over the proportional reporting ratio. *Pharmacoepidemiol. Drug Saf.* **2004**, *13*, 519–523. [CrossRef]
7. Bate, A.; Lindquist, M.; Edwards, I.R.; Olsson, S.; Orre, R.; Lansner, A.; De Freitas, R.M. A Bayesian neural network method for adverse drug reaction signal generation. *Eur. J. Clin. Pharmacol.* **1998**, *54*, 315–321. [CrossRef]
8. DuMouchel, W. Bayesian Data Mining in Large Frequency Tables, with an Application to the FDA Spontaneous Reporting System. *Am. Stat.* **1999**, *53*, 177–190. [CrossRef]
9. Vilar, S.; Friedman, C.; Hripcsak, G. Detection of drug-drug interactions through data mining studies using clinical sources, scientific literature and social media. *Brief. Bioinform.* **2018**, *19*, 863–877. [CrossRef]
10. Noguchi, Y.; Tachi, T.; Teramachi, H. Review of Statistical Methodologies for Detecting Drug-Drug Interactions Using Spontaneous Reporting Systems. *Front. Pharmacol.* **2019**, *10*, 1319. [CrossRef]
11. Nagashima, T.; Shirakawa, H.; Nakagawa, T.; Kaneko, S. Prevention of antipsychotic-induced hyperglycaemia by vitamin D: A data mining prediction followed by experimental exploration of the molecular mechanism. *Sci. Rep.* **2016**, *6*, 26375. [CrossRef] [PubMed]
12. Uno, T.; Wada, K.; Hosomi, K.; Matsuda, S.; Ikura, M.M.; Takenaka, H.; Terakawa, N.; Oita, A.; Yokoyama, S.; Kawase, A.; et al. Drug interactions between tacrolimus and clotrimazole troche: A data mining approach followed by a pharmacokinetic study. *Eur. J. Clin. Pharmacol.* **2020**, *76*, 117–125. [CrossRef] [PubMed]
13. Sanagawa, A.; Hotta, Y.; Kondo, M.; Nishikawa, R.; Tohkin, M.; Kimura, K. Tumor lysis syndrome associated with bortezomib: A post-hoc analysis after signal detection using the US Food and Drug Administration Adverse Event Reporting System. *Anti-Cancer Drugs* **2020**, *31*, 183–189. [CrossRef] [PubMed]
14. Noguchi, Y.; Tachi, T.; Teramachi, H. Comparison of signal detection algorithms based on frequency statistical model for drug-drug interaction using spontaneous reporting systems. *Pharm. Res.* **2020**, *37*, 86. [CrossRef]
15. Kubota, K.; Koide, D.; Hirai, T. Comparison of data mining methodologies using Japanese spontaneous reports. *Pharmacoepidemiol. Drug Saf.* **2004**, *13*, 387–394. [CrossRef]
16. Norén, G.N.; Sundberg, R.; Bate, A.; Edwards, I.R. A statistical methodology for drug-drug interaction surveillance. *Stat. Med.* **2008**, *27*, 3057–3070. [CrossRef]
17. Susuta, Y.; Takahashi, Y. Safety risk evaluation methodology in detecting the medicine concomitant use risk which might cause critical drug rash. *Jpn. J. Pharmacoepidemiol.* **2014**, *19*, 39–49. [CrossRef]
18. Thakrar, B.T.; Grundschober, S.B.; Doessegger, L. Detecting signals of drug-drug interactions in a spontaneous reports database. *Br. J. Clin. Pharmacol.* **2007**, *64*, 489–495. [CrossRef]
19. Gosho, M.; Maruo, K.; Tada, K.; Hirakawa, A. Utilization of chi-square statistics for screening adverse drug-drug interactions in spontaneous reporting systems. *Eur. J. Clin. Pharmacol.* **2017**, 73779–73786. [CrossRef]
20. Cheng, F.J.; Syu, F.K.; Lee, K.H.; Chen, F.C.; Wu, C.H.; Chen, C.C. Correlation between drug-drug interaction-induced Stevens-Johnson syndrome and related deaths in Taiwan. *J. Food Drug Anal.* **2016**, *24*, 427–432. [CrossRef]
21. Noguchi, Y.; Takaoka, M.; Hayashi, T.; Tachi, T.; Teramachi, H. Antiepileptic combination therapy with Stevens-Johnson syndrome and toxic epidermal necrolysis: Analysis of a Japanese pharmacovigilance database. *Epilepsia* **2020**. [CrossRef] [PubMed]
22. Caster, O.; Aoki, Y.; Gattepaille, L.M.; Grundmark, B. Disproportionality Analysis for Pharmacovigilance Signal Detection in Small Databases or Subsets: Recommendations for Limiting False-Positive Associations. *Drug Saf.* **2020**, *43*, 479–487. [CrossRef] [PubMed]

8

Mechanisms of CYP450 Inhibition: Understanding Drug-Drug Interactions due to Mechanism-Based Inhibition in Clinical Practice

Malavika Deodhar [1], Sweilem B Al Rihani [1], Meghan J. Arwood [1], Lucy Darakjian [1], Pamela Dow [1], Jacques Turgeon [1,2] and Veronique Michaud [1,2,*]

[1] Tabula Rasa HealthCare Precision Pharmacotherapy Research and Development Institute, Orlando, FL 32827, USA; mdeodhar@trhc.com (M.D.); srihani@trhc.com (S.B.A.R.); marwood@trhc.com (M.J.A.); ldarakjian@trhc.com (L.D.); pdow@trhc.com (P.D.); jturgeon@trhc.com (J.T.)

[2] Faculty of Pharmacy, Université de Montréal, Montreal, QC H3C 3J7, Canada

[*] Correspondence: vmichaud@trhc.com

Abstract: In an ageing society, polypharmacy has become a major public health and economic issue. Overuse of medications, especially in patients with chronic diseases, carries major health risks. One common consequence of polypharmacy is the increased emergence of adverse drug events, mainly from drug–drug interactions. The majority of currently available drugs are metabolized by CYP450 enzymes. Interactions due to shared CYP450-mediated metabolic pathways for two or more drugs are frequent, especially through reversible or irreversible CYP450 inhibition. The magnitude of these interactions depends on several factors, including varying affinity and concentration of substrates, time delay between the administration of the drugs, and mechanisms of CYP450 inhibition. Various types of CYP450 inhibition (competitive, non-competitive, mechanism-based) have been observed clinically, and interactions of these types require a distinct clinical management strategy. This review focuses on mechanism-based inhibition, which occurs when a substrate forms a reactive intermediate, creating a stable enzyme–intermediate complex that irreversibly reduces enzyme activity. This type of inhibition can cause interactions with drugs such as omeprazole, paroxetine, macrolide antibiotics, or mirabegron. A good understanding of mechanism-based inhibition and proper clinical management is needed by clinicians when such drugs are prescribed. It is important to recognize mechanism-based inhibition since it cannot be prevented by separating the time of administration of the interacting drugs. Here, we provide a comprehensive overview of the different types of mechanism-based inhibition, along with illustrative examples of how mechanism-based inhibition might affect prescribing and clinical behaviors.

Keywords: drug–drug interactions; mechanism-based inhibition; competitive inhibition, non-competitive inhibition; substrate; inhibitor; cytochromes P450

1. Introduction

In clinical practice, the need for the use of multiple drugs is common, as patients often present with numerous chronic diseases. To improve commodity and drug adherence, several medications are often administered concomitantly. Although this may represent a preferred clinical strategy, the administration of two or more drugs at overlapping times increases the likelihood of drug–drug interactions [1,2]. As the risk of drug–drug interactions increases, the risk of debilitating, even fatal, adverse drug events also increases [3]. From a pharmacokinetics standpoint, drug–drug interactions occur when one drug—the perpetrator drug—alters the disposition of another co-administered drug—the victim drug.

Inhibition of cytochrome P450 (CYP450) enzymes is the most common mechanism leading to drug–drug interactions [4]. CYP450 inhibition can be categorized as reversible (including competitive and non-competitive inhibition) or irreversible (or quasi-irreversible), such as mechanism-based inhibition. Each type of interaction involves a distinct clinical management strategy. This is why a comprehensive understanding of mechanisms of CYP450-mediated metabolism inhibition is needed to prevent or mitigate these harmful drug interactions. This review will focus on the CYP450 enzymatic system with a special look at one specific type of CYP450 inhibition, namely mechanism-based inhibition; clinical cases involving mechanism-based inhibitors will be discussed in this context.

2. Basic Concepts of Enzyme, Substrate, and Inhibitor

For clarity, as we address the various types of drug metabolism inhibition, the concepts of active (orthosteric) and allosteric sites, substrates, and inhibitors need to first be reviewed.

2.1. Active Site or Orthosteric Site of the Enzyme

The active or orthosteric site is a physical space or pocket within the protein structure of an enzyme where a molecule can bind and from where a catalytic reaction takes place to convert the molecule into a metabolite (addition of a hydroxyl moiety, removal of alkyl moieties, etc.). (Figure 1) For CYP450 isoforms, binding to the active site is independent of the NADPH-P450 oxidase reactions; however, the chemical reaction leading to the formation of the metabolite will employ electrons originated from NADPH.

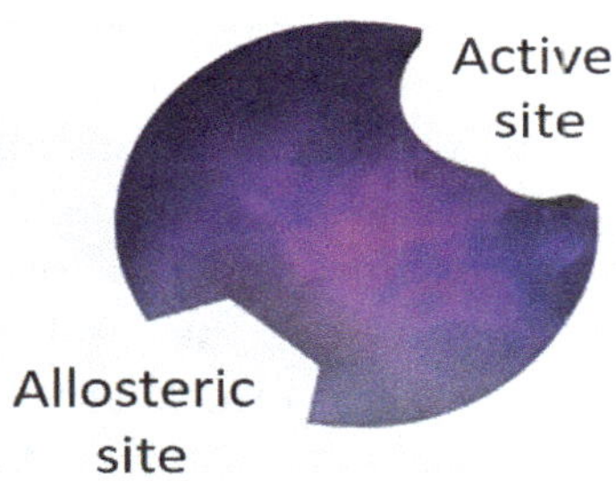

Figure 1. Illustration of an enzyme with its active binding site for drug transformation and allosteric binding site (or regulatory site).

2.2. Allosteric Site

The allosteric site is a physical space or pocket within the protein structure of an enzyme spatially separated from the active site. (Figure 1) The allosteric site allows molecules to modulate enzyme activity. These molecules can be allosteric activators or allosteric inhibitors, depending on how they influence enzyme activity. Drugs can bind to this site and change the three-dimensional structure of the enzyme (conformational change). Allosteric inhibitors may render the active site no longer accessible for substrate binding or make the site unable to catalyze reactions. It is widely known that almost all cases of non-competitive inhibition are caused by allosteric regulation (see discussion in Section 3).

2.3. Substrates

Substrates are drugs that bind to the active site of an enzyme and are transformed into metabolites while being present in this active site. The biotransformation process of a drug may involve multiple enzymes leading to various metabolites; each metabolic route relies on specific characteristics.

The strength of attraction between an enzyme and a substrate is measured as the "binding affinity". A substrate can exhibit varying binding affinity for an active site depending on their chemical structure and physical properties. Based on their binding affinity for a specific enzyme, substrates can be classified into weak, intermediate, and strong affinity substrates. Advanced clinical decision support systems (such as MedWise™) depict the various degrees of affinity by different colors: light yellow (weak), dark yellow (intermediate), and orange (strong affinity).

2.4. Binding Affinity

Binding affinity to an enzyme is measured by the K_m, i.e., the concentration at which 50% of the maximum metabolic reaction (V_{max}) occurs; the lower the K_m, the greater the affinity. The intrinsic clearance measures the ability of an organ to clear unbound drug when there are no limitations to blood flow and binding considerations. The intrinsic clearance (CL_{int}) of a substrate is defined by:

$$CL_{int} = \frac{Vmax}{(Km + [S])}$$

where $[S]$ is the substrate concentration. In most clinical situations, liver enzymes are rarely saturated so that, generally, the substrate concentration is much smaller than the K_m and the equation can be simplified to:

$$CL\ int \approx \frac{Vmax}{Km}$$

The binding affinity of a substrate can be modified by the presence of other molecules (in many drug–drug interaction situations, the K_m is increased for the victim drug such that its CL_{int} is decreased).

2.5. Inhibitors

Drugs defined as inhibitors bind either to the active site or to an allosteric site of the enzyme. However, they can also bind to both; in these cases, the process is called "mixed inhibition" and can often be more potent than simple competitive or non-competitive inhibition. Inhibitors can be either substrates or non-substrates of the enzyme. As mentioned previously, non-substrate inhibitors typically bind to an allosteric site of the enzyme. If the inhibitor is a substrate transformed by the enzyme, the substrate itself or its metabolites could contribute to the inhibition mechanism. For example, studies on the inhibitory potency of gemfibrozil indicated that gemfibrozil is a potent inhibitor of CYP2C9 in vitro, but that it is a more potent inhibitor of CYP2C8 than CYP2C9 in vivo [5–7]. This observation is substantiated by several clinical reports of interactions between gemfibrozil and CYP2C8 substrates including cerivastatin, repaglinide, and glitazones [8–11]. The mechanism of this clinical interaction is explained by the formation of the major metabolite of gemfibrozil, gemfibrozil 1-O-β-glucuronide, which was found to potently inhibit CYP2C8 [10,12].

3. Mechanism of CYP450 Inhibition

Drug interactions due to drug metabolism inhibition are frequent since (1) CYP450-mediated metabolism is the major route of elimination for a large number of drugs, and (2) multiple drugs can compete for the same CYP450 active site. Mechanisms of CYP450 inhibition can be categorized as reversible (including competitive or non-competitive) or irreversible/quasi-irreversible (mechanism-based inhibition).

3.1. Reversible CYP450 Inhibition

Reversible inhibition is a result of rapid association and dissociation between the substrate drugs and the enzyme and can be categorized as competitive or non-competitive. A third category, uncompetitive inhibitor, also considered as a reversible inhibition type, is a very rare phenomenon and will not be considered in this current review; this type of inhibitor binds only the enzyme–substrate complex, leading to a dead-end complex.

3.1.1. Competitive Inhibition

The ability of a single CYP450 isoform to metabolize multiple substrates is responsible for several drug interactions associated with reversible competitive inhibition. Competitive inhibition occurs when two substrates compete for the same active site—such as the prosthetic heme iron or substrate-binding region—of CYP450s. The competition is a function of the respective affinities of the two substrates for the binding site and their concentrations in the proximity of the enzyme. First, the most clinically relevant situation will be discussed.

Two Substrates with Different Affinities Administered Concomitantly

This situation is often encountered in clinical practice. Under a competitive inhibition condition, a substrate with strong affinity (acting as a perpetrator) can displace a weaker substrate (behaving as a victim) from the active site (Figure 2), thus increasing the K_m of the victim drug (decreased affinity) and reducing the extent of its breakdown (decrease in its CL_{int}) over a period of time.

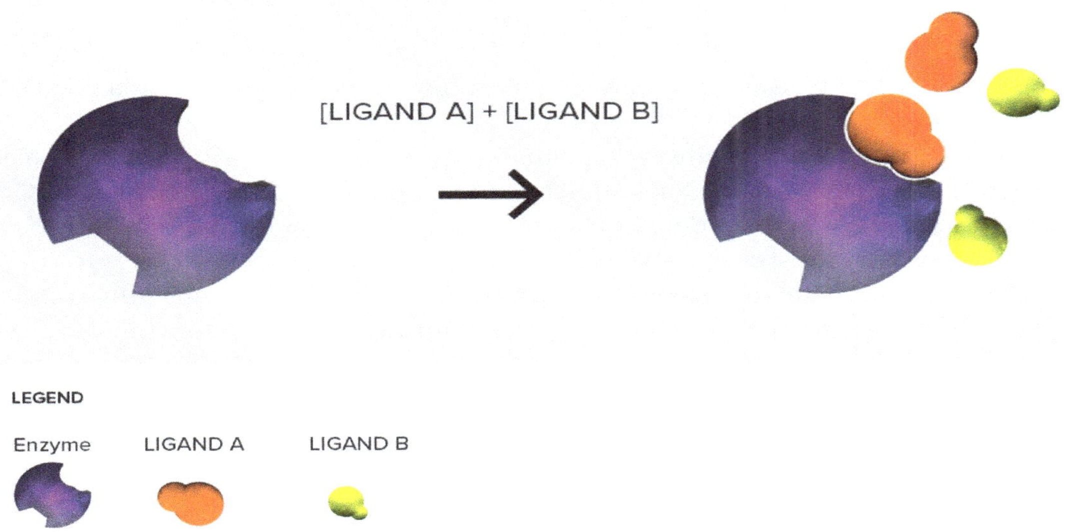

Figure 2. Illustration of reversible competitive inhibition where ligand A (**orange**) is a substrate with strong affinity and ligand B (**yellow**) is a substrate with a weaker affinity for a specific enzyme (**purple**). As long as the concentrations of the two substrates are comparable, the stronger affinity substrate with higher binding affinity will be preferred at the active site of the enzyme resulting in an accumulation of ligand B.

For an active drug, the decrease in the CL_{int} of one of its metabolic pathways can lead to a decrease in the total clearance of the drug (capacity for eliminating the drug) and can result in increased plasma concentrations, potentially precipitating adverse effects. However, for prodrugs, this interaction can instead result in a decrease in the formation of the active metabolite, reducing drug efficacy. The magnitude of changes observed in the overall disposition of the victim drug (increase in its plasma levels) will be a function of the relative contribution of the inhibited metabolic pathway to the clearance of this drug. For example, if 15% of a drug is excreted unchanged in urine—35% by enzyme 1 and 50% by enzyme 2—a 50% decrease in the total CL of the victim drug is expected if enzyme 2 is inhibited:

$$CL = CL_{renal} + CL_{metabolic} = 0.15 + 0.85$$

and,

$$CL_{metabolic} = CL_{enzyme\ 1} + CL_{enzyme\ 2}$$

or,

$$0.85 = 0.35 + 0.5$$

under conditions of enzyme 2 inhibition (whether it is reversible or irreversible),

$$CL_{metabolic} = CL_{enzyme\ 1} + CL_{enzyme\ 2}$$

or,

$$0.35 = 0.35 + 0.0$$

and,

$$CL = CL_{renal} + CL_{metabolic} = 0.15 + 0.35 = 0.5$$

Since,

$$CL = Dose/AUC_{0\text{-}\infty}$$

Under steady-state conditions, the area under the drug concentration curve (AUC) measured over a dosing interval (τ) is equal to $AUC_{0-\infty}$. Since the average concentration over a dosing interval (C_{av}) at steady state can be estimated by $AUC_{0\text{-}\tau}/\tau$, the equation could be rearranged in a simpler manner to yield:

$$CL = Dose/(C_{av} \times \tau)$$

A 50% decrease in CL will be associated with a doubling in the average plasma concentrations of the victim drug.

According to a competitive inhibition mechanism, every substrate of an enzyme is a potential perpetrator drug (inhibitor) towards another substrate metabolized by the same enzyme. Competitive inhibition is almost immediate and the degree of inhibition of the enzyme does not change with time if the concentration of the two substrates remains the same.

In an example illustrating this scenario, theophylline (weak CYP1A2 substrate) is largely metabolized by CYP1A2 by binding to its active site. (Figure 3) If that active site is occupied by a stronger substrate like duloxetine (moderate CYP1A2 affinity substrate), breakdown of theophylline will be reduced ($\downarrow CL_{int}$), leading to increased plasma levels of theophylline and possibly side effects (e.g., headache, nausea, vomiting). To minimize competitive inhibition, two competing substrates should be administered with as much time apart as possible.

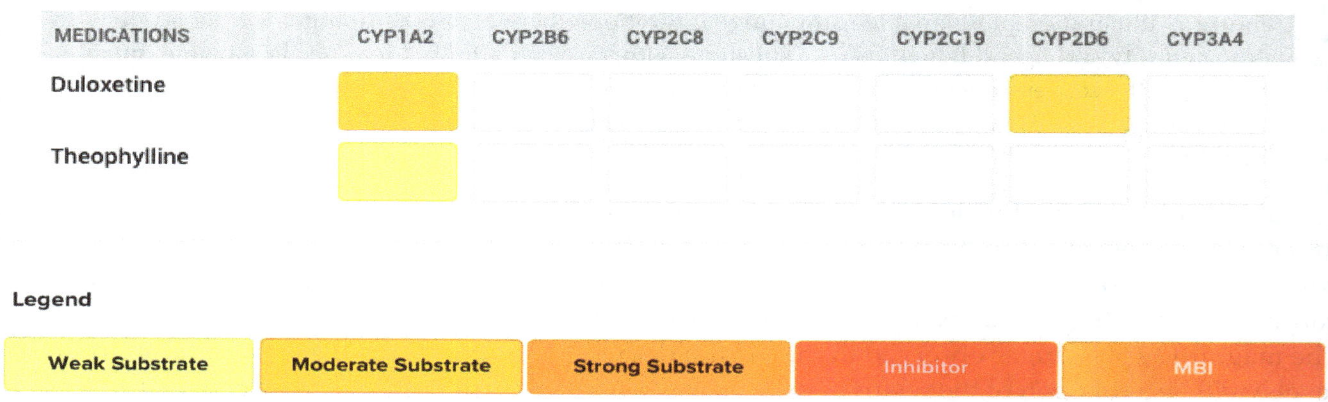

Figure 3. CYP450 metabolic pathways involved in the metabolism of duloxetine and theophylline and their respective affinities are depicted. Competitive inhibition between duloxetine and theophylline will be expected at CYP1A2. Duloxetine acts as the perpetrator drug over theophylline, the victim drug.

Two Substrates with Largely Different Concentrations

As mentioned previously, the competitive inhibition process is sensitive to substrate concentrations. If concentrations of the weaker affinity substrate are much higher than concentrations of the stronger affinity substrate, the weaker affinity substrate can displace the stronger affinity substrate and overcome the enzyme inhibition, which is why this type of inhibition is deemed reversible. (Figure 4) The greater the difference there is between the affinity of the weaker affinity substrate and the stronger affinity substrate, the more the concentration of the weaker affinity substrate needs to be increased to displace the stronger affinity substrate. This situation can be observed clinically when very high concentrations of a weak affinity substrate are present in the intestine or liver (high micromolar concentrations), following its oral administration, while concentrations of another higher affinity substrate have long been absorbed and distributed to various tissues leading to plasma concentrations in the low nanomolar range. In this case, the extent of victim drug inhibition would be minimal. A direct application of this principle is to alleviate the degree of inhibition by separating the time of administration of the two competing drugs.

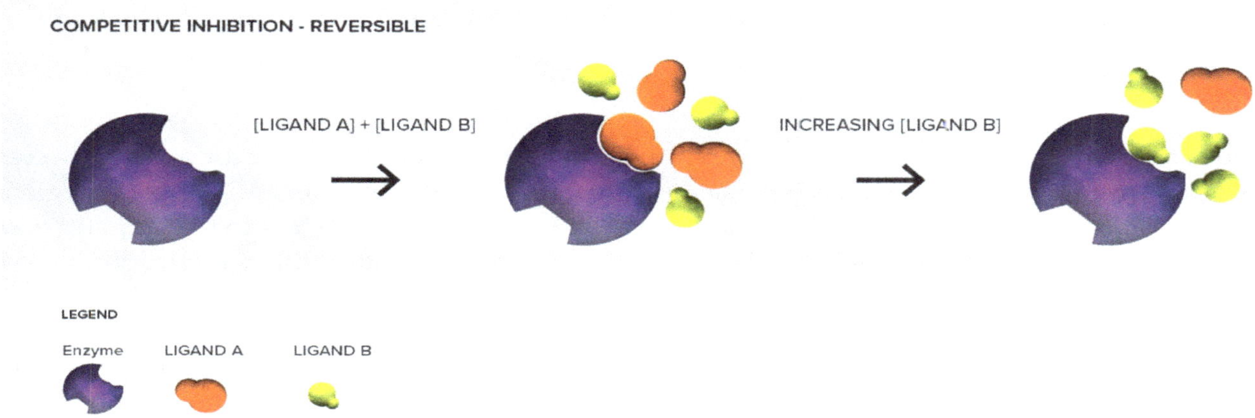

Figure 4. Illustration of reversible competitive inhibition where ligand A (**orange**) is a substrate with strong affinity and ligand B (**yellow**) is a substrate with weaker affinity for a specific enzyme (**purple**). When the concentrations of the weaker affinity substrate are sufficiently high, it can outcompete the stronger affinity substrate for the active site of the enzyme.

3.1.2. Non-Competitive Inhibition

The non-competitive inhibitor does not generally have any structural resemblance to the substrate as it binds to an allosteric site. The non-competitive inhibitor will cause a conformational change in the structure of the active site such that the active site loses its affinity for the substrate. (Figure 5) Thus, there is no direct competition between the inhibitor and the substrate at the active site. This type of inhibition is often long lasting and cannot be overcome by increasing substrate concentrations. Under these conditions, a decrease in the CL_{int} of the substrate due to a decrease in its V_{max} is observed. Similar to competitive inhibitors, non-competitive inhibitors also have an almost immediate effect. As long as the concentration of the inhibitor is not changed, the amount of inhibition will not increase over time. This type of inhibition does not require the involvement of NADPH as a cofactor, i.e., the inhibitor is not metabolized by the enzyme, but merely sits in an allosteric site. Other non-competitive inhibition conditions may involve CYPb5 and/or CYP450 oxidoreductase as these factors have been shown to modulate CYP450 activities, at least in in vitro systems [13,14]. Separating the time of dosing will not alleviate non-competitive inhibition. Fluvoxamine (CYP2C19) and terbinafine (CYP2D6) are some common examples of non-competitive inhibitors at other CYP isoforms [15–17].

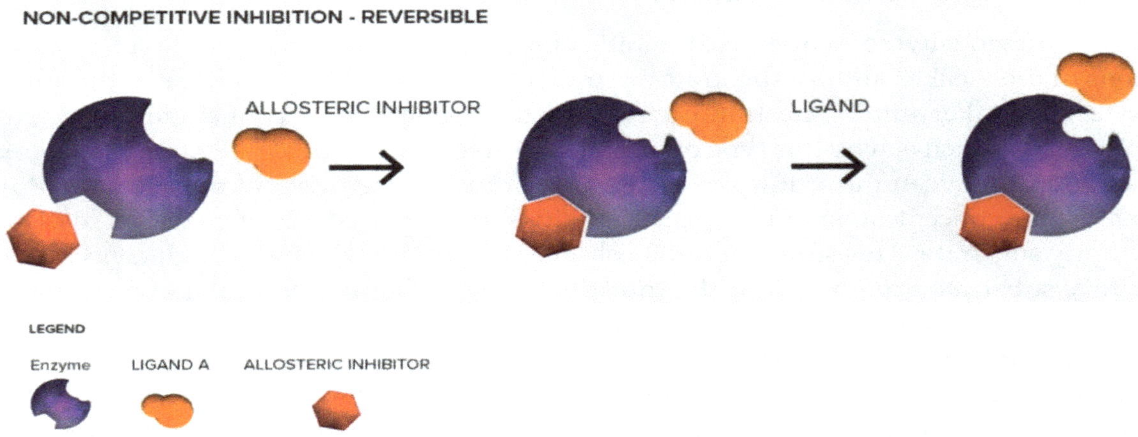

Figure 5. Illustration of reversible non-competitive inhibition. An inhibitor (**red**) binds to an allosteric site on the enzyme and causes conformational changes that prevent a substrate (**orange**) from binding to the active site. Over time, as the inhibitor is flushed out, the conformation of the enzyme can return to normal and substrate (**orange**) can bind to the active site again.

3.1.3. Mixed inhibition

In the case of mixed inhibition, both competitive and non-competitive inhibition occur. Mixed inhibitors can simultaneously bind to both the heme iron atom (at the active site) and lipophilic regions of the protein (allosteric site). Mixed inhibitors are usually more potent inhibitors than competitive or non-competitive inhibitors. Ketoconazole and fluconazole, both imidazole antifungals, exhibit potent mixed reversible inhibition of CYP3As. However, fluconazole is a weaker mixed reversible inhibitor compared to ketoconazole, mainly due to its lower lipophilicity (less binding to an allosteric site).

For a CYP3A substrate like midazolam, concomitant use of non-competitive or mixed CYP3A inhibitors will reduce its transformation to α-hydroxy midazolam, increasing midazolam plasma levels and augmenting the risk of adverse drug events [18].

3.2. Irreversible CYP450 Inhibition

Several clinically important pharmacokinetic drug interactions result from a decrease in the metabolic clearance of a substrate due to CYP450 irreversible inhibition. Mechanism-based inhibition is a condition often encountered with irreversible CYP450 inhibitors.

3.2.1. Mechanism-Based Inhibition

Mechanism-based inhibition can be irreversible or quasi-irreversible. It generally derives from the activation of a substrate drug by a CYP450 isoform into a reactive metabolite, which binds to the enzyme heme prosthetic site (part of the active site), resulting in irreversible long-lasting loss of enzyme activity (decrease in V_{max}). (Figure 6) Several drugs undergo metabolic activation by a specific CYP450 isoform to produce inhibitory intermediate metabolites, which can form stable intermediate complexes. As a result, the CYP450 isoform is sequestered in an inactive state. Even though the reactive intermediate metabolite plays a key role in the mechanism-based inactivation of the CYP450 isoform, in many instances, the exact reactive metabolite involved in this phenomenon is unknown.

In the case of quasi-irreversible inhibition, the metabolites form very stable complexes with the heme prosthetic site (metabolite–intermediate complex), so that the enzyme is sequestered in a functionally inactive state. This phenomenon is called quasi-irreversible since, in theory, this complex can be disrupted. In the case of irreversible inhibition, the metabolites covalently bind to the heme prosthetic site or the protein part of the CYP450, leading to irreversible inactivation [19,20].

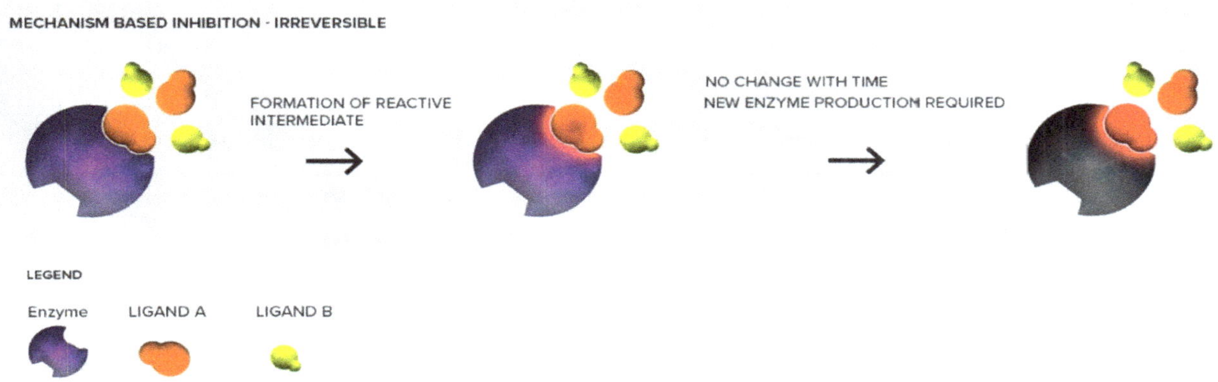
MECHANISM BASED INHIBITION - IRREVERSIBLE
FORMATION OF REACTIVE INTERMEDIATE
NO CHANGE WITH TIME
NEW ENZYME PRODUCTION REQUIRED
LEGEND
Enzyme
LIGAND A
LIGAND B

Figure 6. Illustration of mechanism-based inhibition. The mechanism-based inhibitor (**orange**) binds to the active site as a substrate. During the normal process of metabolism, it forms either stable intermediate–enzyme complexes or reactive electrophilic species that can lock up or destroy the enzyme, and new enzyme synthesis is required to restore the enzymatic activity.

Hence, mechanism-based inhibition is active site mediated, and the allosteric site is not involved. In contrast to reversible inhibition mechanisms, mechanism-based inhibition is time dependent and NADPH dependent. This means that the enzyme has to start breaking down the substrate in order for inhibition to proceed. As more drug molecules are metabolized, more complexes are stably formed in the active sites, increasing inhibition over time before it reaches a plateau. Mechanism-based inhibition is therefore also saturable. New enzyme formation is necessary to restore activity: the relationship between the amount of intermediate complex formed and the speed of new enzyme synthesis dictate the equilibrium and extent of enzyme inhibition.

Mechanism-based inhibitors can be classified into two categories: metabolic–intermediate complex formation inhibitors and protein and/or heme alkylation inhibitors.

Metabolic–Intermediate Complex Formation (or Alternate Substrate Inhibition)

Such a condition occurs when a stable intermediate metabolite formed during the normal metabolic cycle forms covalent bonds at the active site. This stable intermediate–enzyme complex is not easily broken by increasing substrate concentration. Since the enzyme structure remains otherwise unchanged, theoretically this reaction is reversible with time. However, in in vivo conditions, with this metabolic intermediate complex being excessively stable, the metabolic intermediate cannot be displaced and the enzyme remains inaccessible for metabolism so the reaction seems irreversible.

An example of alternate substrate inhibition is observed with paroxetine as its methoxy diene carbon moiety was found to be responsible for the formation of covalent bonds at the active site of CYP2D6 [21,22]. Another example of this type of inhibition was observed with clarithromycin when the nitrosoalkene intermediate generated by N-demethylation forms covalent bonds with the active site of CYP3A4 [23].

Protein and/or Heme Alkylation (or Suicide Inhibition)

This situation takes place when a latent highly reactive (generally electrophilic) intermediate is formed in the catalysis process. The reactive intermediate forms covalent bonds (strong irreversible bonds) with the enzyme in a step that is not part of the normal metabolic pathway. This process can change the conformational structure of the enzyme significantly—it can even destroy the enzyme in some cases—making it functionally unviable. For example, inhibition of CYP2C19 by esomeprazole was found to be mediated by crosslinking the heme and apoprotein moieties in the enzyme, changing its conformational structure [24].

It is important to note that since mechanism-based inhibitors are substrates of the enzyme, they can also cause acute competitive inhibition when co-administered with other sensitive substrates.

The difference between competitive inhibition and mechanism-based inhibition is that as the time period of exposure to mechanism-based inhibitors increases, the degree of inhibition also increases (Table 1)

Table 1. Summary of major pharmacokinetic characteristics of various drug inhibition models.

Characteristics	Inhibitor Type		
	Competitive	Non-Competitive Non-Mechanism Based	Mechanism-Based
Metabolism required	No	No	Yes
Active site mediated	Yes	No	Yes
Time dependent	No	No	Yes
Substrate concentration dependent	Yes	No	Yes
K_m (victim drug)	↑	↔	↔
V_{max} (victim drug)	↔	↓	↓
CL_{int} (victim drug)	↓	↓	↓

4. Clinical Cases

4.1. The Case of Omeprazole and Clopidogrel

Proton pump inhibitors (PPIs) are commonly prescribed along with antiplatelet drugs like clopidogrel to reduce the incidence of gastric bleeding during treatment with antiplatelet therapy [25,26]. Omeprazole has long been one of the most widely used PPIs [27]. Omeprazole is a known strong affinity substrate of CYP2C19, leading to the formation of its hydroxy and desmethyl metabolites. The antiplatelet drug clopidogrel is sequentially activated by CYP450 isoforms, including CYP2C19, into its active metabolite (H4) [28]. When omeprazole is co-administered with clopidogrel, omeprazole acts as a strong affinity substrate of CYP2C19 (perpetrator), whereas clopidogrel is a weaker sensitive substrate (victim). (Figure 7) Multiple in vitro studies have reported a potential pharmacokinetic interaction between omeprazole and clopidogrel [29–32]. A clinical study conducted by Angiolillo et al. demonstrated that plasma levels of clopidogrel's active metabolite H4, and consequently the platelet aggregation induced by adenosine diphosphate, were decreased when omeprazole and clopidogrel were administered concomitantly [30]. Various other clinical studies have demonstrated that co-administration of omeprazole and clopidogrel diminishes the antiplatelet activity of clopidogrel [31,32].

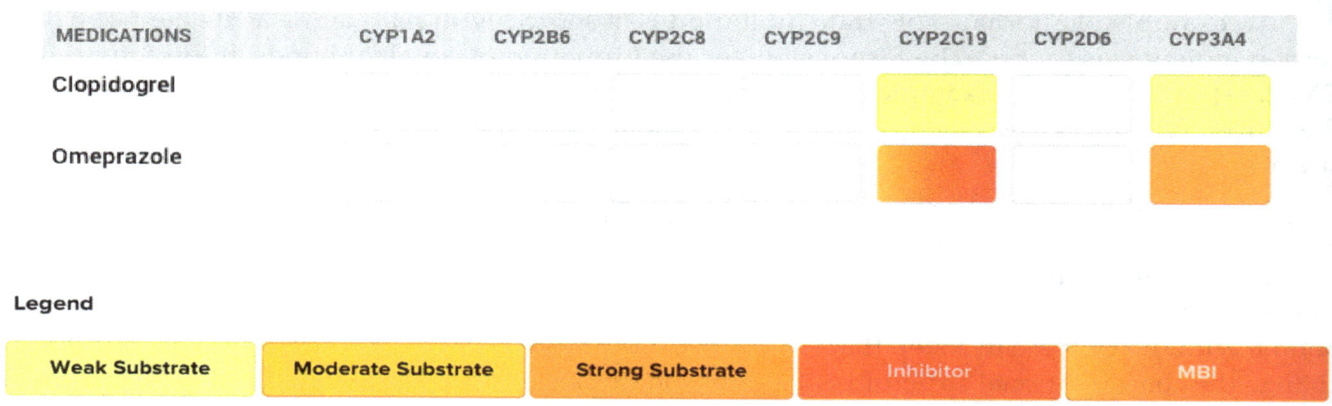

Figure 7. CYP450 metabolic pathways involved in the metabolism of clopidogrel and omeprazole, and their respective affinities are depicted. Competitive inhibition will be expected at CYP3A4 and mechanism-based inhibition at the CYP2C19 enzymatic level. Clopidogrel is the victim drug and omeprazole acts as the perpetrator drug.

Since omeprazole is a strong affinity substrate for CYP2C19, an "immediate" competitive inhibition is expected between these two drugs. Since competitive inhibition was expected, separating time of administration was considered a logical mitigation strategy to avoid or alleviate the extent of the drug interaction [29]. Others have suggested that increasing the dose of clopidogrel might compensate for the diminished formation of the active metabolite [29]. These recommendations to separate the time of administration of the two drugs or to increase the dose of the victim drug (clopidogrel) come from a sound rationale and have been proven to be efficacious in mitigating drug interactions associated with competitive inhibition. However, it has been shown that following chronic administration, separating the time of administration does not alleviate the reduction in clopidogrel active metabolite (H4) caused by omeprazole [30,33]. This is due to the fact that omeprazole is not only a competitive inhibitor, but also a mechanism-based inhibitor of CYP2C19, which results in a gradual increase in irreversible inhibition of the CYP2C19 enzyme, to a point where clopidogrel activation and its clinical efficacy are significantly impaired. From these observations, the FDA warns that separating the time of administration between these two substrates will not alleviate this interaction [34].

Multiple studies have been conducted to determine the clinical impact of the potential reduced antiplatelet efficacy resulting from this interaction. In two retrospective studies looking at interactions between clopidogrel and PPIs and the effects on clinical outcomes, it was reported either that PPIs were associated with increased cardiac adverse events in acute coronary syndrome patients, or that cardiac adverse events were less common in PPI non-users [35,36]. Short-term mortality odds ratios also favored PPI non-users, but no significant differences were observed in long-term mortality [35]. Though a wide range of PPIs were reviewed, omeprazole and esomeprazole remained the most widely prescribed when all studies were combined. A similar study was conducted by Mahabaleshwarkar et al., which found that PPIs were slightly, but significantly, associated with all-cause mortality [37]. The odds ratio of adverse cardiac events and all-cause mortality for omeprazole in particular was 1.23. In another retrospective cohort study, clopidogrel use post discharge for acute coronary syndrome hospitalizations was studied [38]. Concurrent clopidogrel and PPI use was associated with an increased risk of death or rehospitalization; among patients prescribed a PPI, 60% were on omeprazole [38]. PPI plus clopidogrel use also remained significantly associated with recurrent acute coronary syndrome and revascularization procedures [38]. Another study evaluated the association between various PPIs (all PPIs combined) and individual PPI agents with clopidogrel use and increased risk of hospitalization [39]. There was no significant association between any PPI and increased risk of rehospitalization with clopidogrel, but this association was significant with omeprazole [39].

Several studies also report no change in the frequency of cardiovascular adverse events with omeprazole administration during clopidogrel treatment [26,40–42]. Dosing regimens in these studies suggest that the extent of interaction between clopidogrel (75 mg vs. 600 mg) and omeprazole (20 mg vs. 80 mg) may be dose dependent. If an alternative PPI has to be considered, in vitro studies using human liver microsomes have confirmed that PPIs like rabeprazole, lansoprazole, dexlansoprazole, and pantoprazole do not show evidence of mechanism-based inhibition [29]. Clinical studies have also reported that effects of lansoprazole and pantoprazole on clopidogrel antiplatelet activity are not as potent as omeprazole [43–45]. When clopidogrel and PPI coadministration is necessary, switching to a PPI other than omeprazole or esomeprazole may be considered, in light of the evidence presented herein.

4.2. The Case of Paroxetine

The antidepressant paroxetine is a known substrate of CYP2D6, but also a potent mechanism-based inhibitor of this enzyme. As such, paroxetine is expected to inhibit its own metabolism over time. This has been illustrated in two clinical studies, where the C_{max} and AUC of paroxetine were increased 5.2- and 7-fold after 2 weeks of paroxetine administration, respectively [46,47]. In the second study, Laine et al. revealed that ultra-rapid metabolizers of CYP2D6 were converted to extensive or poor metabolizers with chronic paroxetine use [47]. The FDA-approved label states that paroxetine takes nearly 10 days to achieve steady-state concentrations even though the drug has a reported elimination half-life of 21 h; so, within 4–5 days, steady-state levels should be reached under normal circumstances. The label also states that saturation of CYP2D6 contributes to the non-linear pharmacokinetics of paroxetine. Thus, it may be assumed that inhibition of its own mechanism contributes to achieving later than expected steady-state levels and clinical efficacy [48].

As paroxetine is a strong CYP2D6 affinity substrate, it can exhibit acute competitive inhibition when co-administered with sensitive substrates like nortriptyline. (Figure 8) Though separating the time of administration may seem appropriate initially, the effects of mechanism-based inhibition over time should be factored into medication risk management; dosage adjustment or substitution of the victim substrate may be necessary. The extent of this interaction also depends on when paroxetine and the victim drug are added to the regimen. If paroxetine is newly added to a victim drug that has already reached steady-state plasma levels, the extent of inhibition and plasma concentrations of the victim drug will increase over time until reaching a new steady state. However, if steady-state levels of paroxetine are already achieved before adding another sensitive substrate, the extent of inhibition will be maximum at initiation and will remain stable, since saturation of enzyme inhibition is already established.

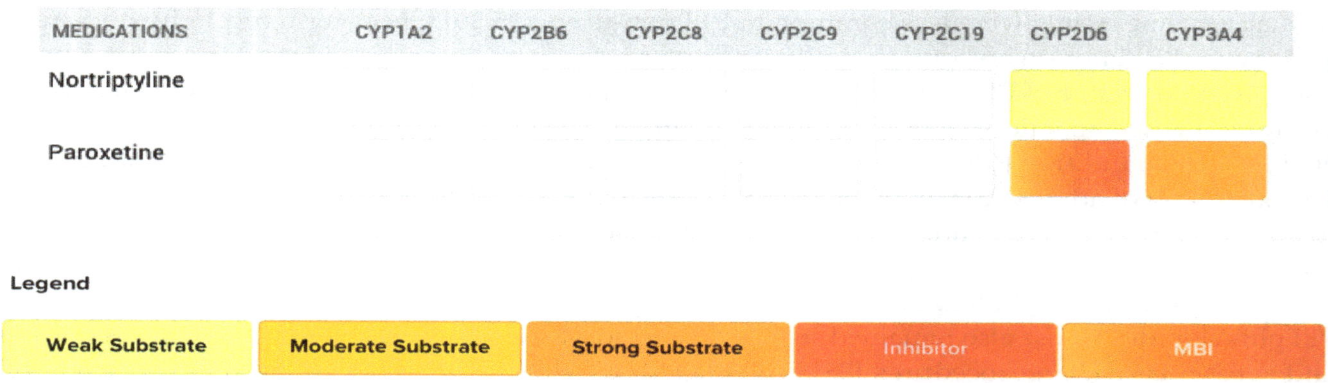

Figure 8. CYP450 metabolic pathways involved in the metabolism of nortriptyline and paroxetine and their respective affinities for the isoform are depicted. Mechanism-based inhibition at CYP2D6 enzymatic level will be expected. Nortriptyline is the victim drug and paroxetine acts as the perpetrator drug for the CYP2D6 elimination pathway.

4.3. The Case of Erythromycin

Another example that illustrates the concept of saturability in mechanism-based inhibition is observed with the commonly used macrolide antibiotics erythromycin (Figure 9) or clarithromycin. These drugs are known to cause mechanism-based inhibition of CYP3A4. Clinical studies have demonstrated saturability (i.e., degree of inhibition reaches a maximum value) of enzyme inhibition using CYP3A4-sensitive substrates like alfentanil or midazolam with or without erythromycin pretreatment (treatment or control, respectively). In a study with healthy males after single or multiple oral dose(s) of erythromycin 500 mg, the effects on alfentanil pharmacokinetics were measured [49]. A 25% increase of alfentanil half-life was observed following a single erythromycin dose compared to control. After a 7-day pretreatment with erythromycin, the half-life of alfentanil was further increased by 25% (up to 56% compared to control), suggesting an increase in inhibition with time [49]. Similar effects were seen on clearance. Although a direct association of this potential drug interaction on clinical outcomes has not been systematically reported, two case reports suggest that erythromycin pretreatment may cause prolonged respiratory depression when alfentanil is administered compared to patients who did not receive erythromycin [50,51].

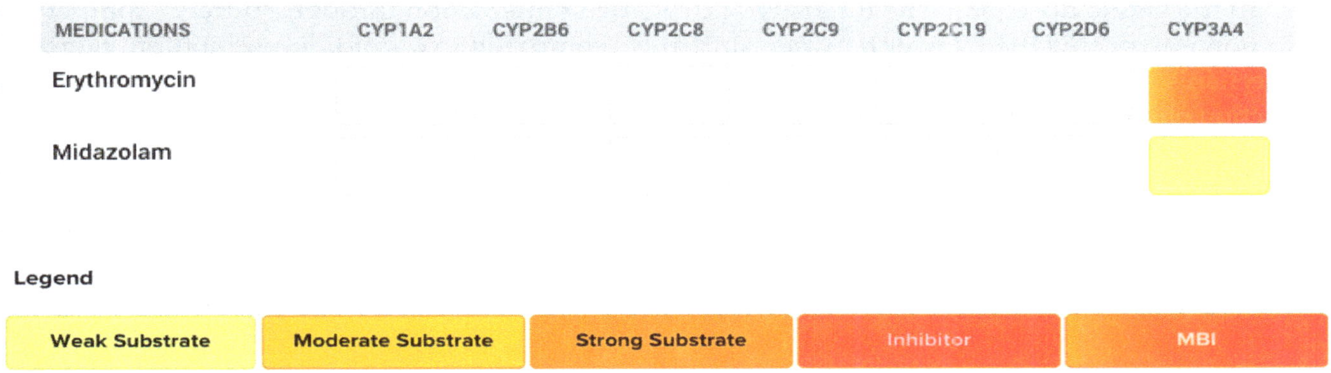

Figure 9. CYP450 metabolic pathways involved in the metabolism of erythromycin and midazolam and their respective affinities for the isoform are depicted. Mechanism-based inhibition at the CYP3A4 enzymatic level will be expected. Midazolam is the victim drug and erythromycin acts as the perpetrator drug.

In another study with 12 healthy volunteers, the effects of erythromycin on midazolam metabolism were studied [52]. It was observed that the *AUC* of midazolam increased 2.3-fold after 2 days of erythromycin pretreatment, compared to control. Following 4 days of pretreatment, midazolam's *AUC* increase was 3.38-fold. After a 7-day pretreatment, a similar increase (3.38-fold) was observed, indicating an increase in inhibition with repeated administration of erythromycin and that a plateau effect had been reached after 4 days of exposure [52].

4.4. The Case of Mirabegron

A widely prescribed drug in the treatment of overactive bladder, mirabegron, also displays characteristics of mechanism-based inhibition for CYP2D6. (Figure 10) The difference in the degree of metabolism inhibition between a competitive inhibitor and a mechanism-based inhibitor is perceived when they are compared using the same victim drug. One study investigated the victim drug desipramine, with the potential competitive inhibitor duloxetine and the mechanism-based inhibitor mirabegron. In this study, duloxetine (moderate CYP2D6 affinity substrate) 30 mg twice a day was administered for 10 days, after which desipramine (weak CYP2D6 affinity substrate) 50 mg was administered as a single dose. Here, duloxetine would act as a competitive inhibitor and desipramine as a victim drug. Accordingly, a 1.2-fold increase in *AUC* and 0.6-fold increase in C_{max} of desipramine was observed [53]. In a similar study design, desipramine was administered with or without mirabegron pretreatment. First, desipramine was administered alone and, after a washout period, mirabegron (100 mg) was administered for 13 days. On the fourteenth day, mirabegron 100 mg and desipramine 50 mg were co-administered. A 3.41-fold increase in the desipramine *AUC* was observed with mirabegron pretreatment compared to control [54]. This increase in the *AUC* of desipramine was much larger than the increase observed with duloxetine, a "purely" potential competitive inhibitor. It is important to note that in the short term, mechanism-based inhibitors can act as competitive inhibitors if the other drug has lower affinity for the metabolizing enzyme. Duloxetine and mirabegron are both substrates of CYP2D6 with moderate affinity, exhibiting potential competitive inhibition over desipramine; therefore, following a single dose of each drug, a similar level of CYP2D6 inhibition is expected towards the CYP2D6 victim drug. (Figure 10) The higher inhibition observed with multiple doses of mirabegron versus single dose of duloxetine is explained by the mechanism-based inhibition observed over time. Similar effects of chronic mirabegron administration on metoprolol (a weak CYP2D6 substrate) pharmacokinetics are also reported [54]. A 3.3-fold increase in the metoprolol AUC was observed following a pretreatment of 5 days with mirabegron in CYP2D6 normal (i.e., previously called "extensive") metabolizer subjects [55]. The coadministration of quinidine (a potent

CYP2D6 inhibitor) with metoprolol was associated with a similar magnitude of increase in metoprolol's AUC after a single dose [56]. The intensity of drug–drug interaction through "purely" competitive inhibition is expected to be lower between substrates compared to quinidine's inhibition; therefore the mechanism-based inhibition property of mirabegron can explain why the magnitude of drug–drug interaction observed between mirabegron and metoprolol is similar to that observed between quinidine and metoprolol.

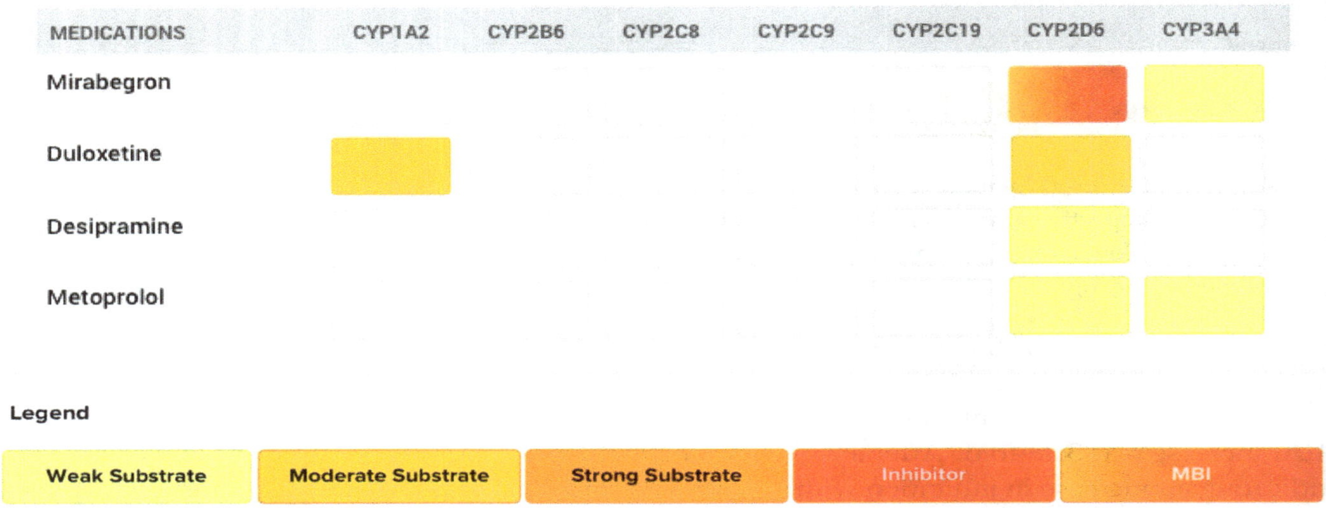

Figure 10. CYP450 metabolic pathways involved in the metabolism of desipramine, duloxetine, metoprolol, mirabegron, and their respective affinities for the isoform are depicted. Competitive inhibition will be expected at CYP2D6 between duloxetine (perpetrator; CYP2D6 substrate with higher affinity) and either desipramine or metoprolol (victim drugs; both CYP2D6 substrates with weaker affinity). Mechanism-based inhibition at CYP2D6 will be expected between mirabegron and desipramine, metoprolol, or duloxetine.

In addition to the case examples discussed above, Figure 11 provides a list of CYP450 mechanism-based inhibitors, along with the enzyme inhibited and relevant CYP450 pathways involved in their metabolism. This list is not exhaustive, but provides a quick reference for commonly used medications.

In addition to drug–drug interactions, high variability in terms of CYP450 expression and/or activities can be explained by genetic polymorphisms in genes encoding specific isoforms (such as *CYP2C9*, *CYP2C19*, and *CYP2D6*). This variability on CYP450 expression/activities translates into intersubject variability in drug disposition and drug response. Often, the impact of genetic polymorphisms and drug–drug interactions on CYP450s have been studied separately. However, an interaction exists between these factors. Genetic polymorphisms could also contribute to variability observed in the magnitude of drug–drug interactions observed between two drugs. So, genetic polymorphisms in drug-metabolizing enzymes can affect the occurrence of phenoconversion induced by drug inhibitors. As reported by Storelli et al., differences in CYP2D6 inhibition observed in vitro with paroxetine (mechanism-based inhibitor) or duloxetine (competitive inhibitor) across *CYP2D6* genotypes were not related to their inhibition parameters but likely due to a differential level of functional enzymes as a function of the *CYP2D6* genotype [57,58].

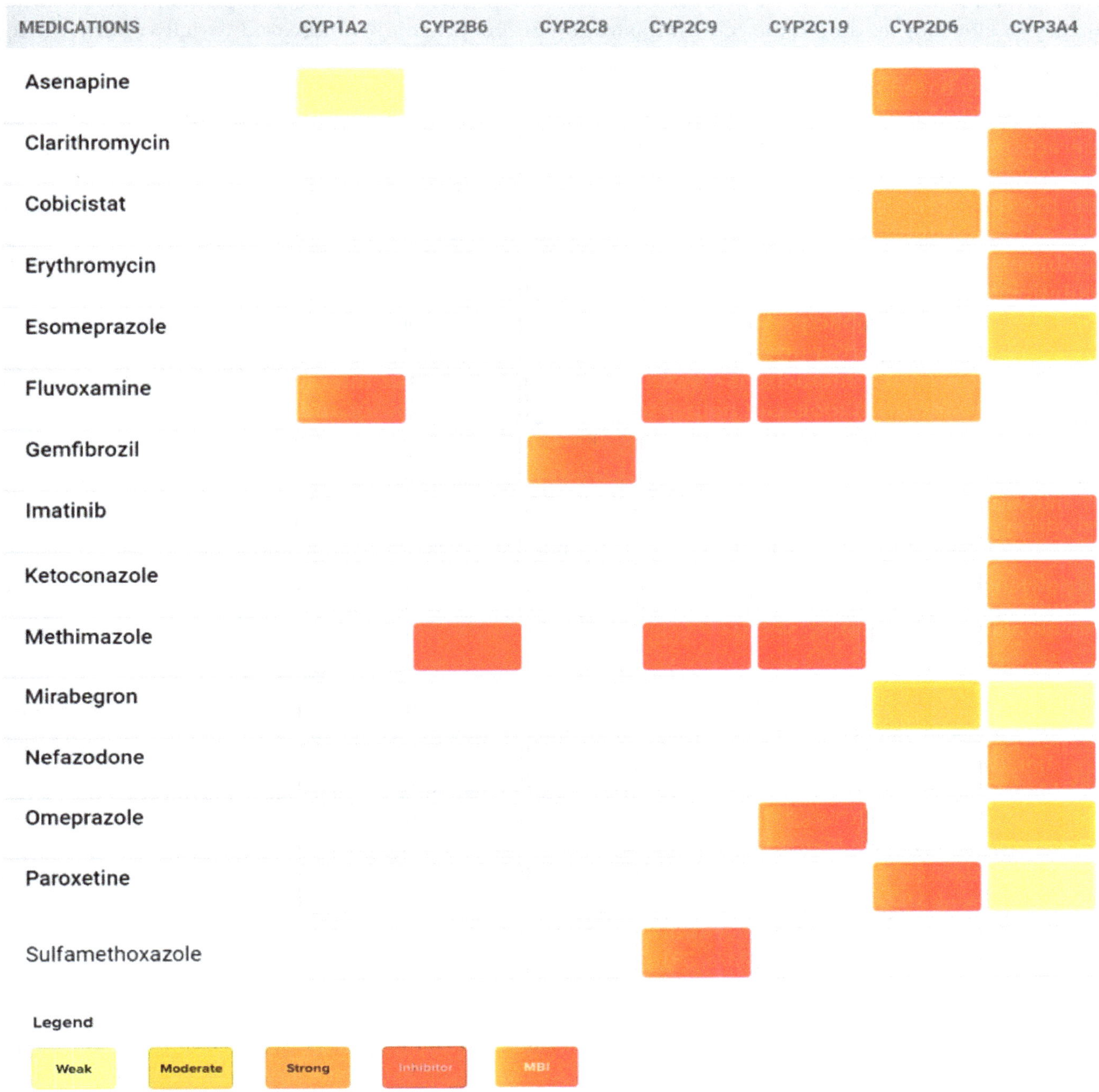

Figure 11. List of commonly prescribed medications producing mechanism-based inhibition.

5. Conclusions

Polypharmacy in many cases is deemed to be required and elderly patients are particularly prone to this phenomenon. Aging is associated with the presence of multiple independent chronic diseases and is almost always accompanied by multiple drug regimens. Polypharmacy has been associated with many adverse clinical outcomes, such as drug–drug interactions, leading to adverse drug events. Among these, mechanism-based inhibitor–victim drug combinations like clopidogrel and omeprazole are commonly prescribed. Drugs for overactive bladder like mirabegron and tricyclic antidepressants like paroxetine are also commonly prescribed in elderly populations. Polypharmacy is not necessarily synonymous with inappropriate treatment, but in several situations, it can lead to significant drug–drug interactions especially in the presence of mechanism-based inhibitor drugs, as described in the current review. In these cases, polypharmacy might cause problems like blunted efficacy of clopidogrel due to the co-administration of omeprazole, or increased toxicity of other drugs co-administered with paroxetine or mirabegron. Clinicians must be able to recognize and intervene appropriately based on the mechanism of these interactions.

As highlighted in this current review, mechanism-based inhibition can cause severe clinical interactions. The magnitude of these interactions and their impacts depend on the duration of the mechanism-based inhibitor exposure and the exact time-point when the victim drug is introduced into the drug regimen. Without a comprehensive understanding of this mechanism, healthcare professionals might find it difficult to diagnose and mitigate these interactions. Separating the time of administration of interacting drugs cannot mitigate an interaction caused by mechanism-based inhibition. A careful titration of dose, monitoring of clinical effects, or switching to an alternate drug with a different metabolic pathway may become necessary to avoid such interactions. Advanced clinical decision support systems that consider and distinguish competitive versus mechanism-based inhibition drug–drug interactions would help identify potential interactions mediated by enzyme inhibition. Using such tools can help pharmacists quickly identify and mitigate drug interactions, thus helping reduce preventable drug interactions.

Author Contributions: Conceptualization, M.D. and V.M.; methodology, M.D., J.T., and V.M.; resources, M.D., P.D., J.T., and V.M.; writing—original draft preparation, M.D., S.B.A.R., M.J.A., L.D., P.D., J.T., and V.M.; writing—review and editing, M.D., P.D., J.T., and V.M.; visualization, M.D.; supervision, J.T. and V.M.; project administration, P.D., J.T., and V.M. All authors have read and agreed to the published version of the manuscript.

Acknowledgments: The authors recognize the contribution of Ernesto Lucio for his design of the included figures. The authors would like to thank Dana Filippoli for her comprehensive review and comments pertaining to the contents of this manuscript.

References

1. Doan, J.; Zakrzewski-Jakubiak, H.; Roy, J.; Turgeon, J.; Tannenbaum, C. Prevalence and risk of potential cytochrome P450-mediated drug-drug interactions in older hospitalized patients with polypharmacy. *Ann. Pharmacother.* **2013**, *47*, 324–332. [CrossRef] [PubMed]
2. Mallet, L.; Spinewine, A.; Huang, A. The challenge of managing drug interactions in elderly people. *Lancet* **2007**, *370*, 185–191. [CrossRef]
3. Bankes, D.L.; Jin, H.; Finnel, S.; Michaud, V.; Knowlton, C.H.; Turgeon, J.; Stein, A. Association of a Novel Medication Risk Score with Adverse Drug Events and Other Pertinent Outcomes Among Participants of the Programs of All-Inclusive Care for the Elderly. *Pharmacy* **2020**, *8*, 87. [CrossRef] [PubMed]
4. Lynch, T.; Price, A. The effect of cytochrome P450 metabolism on drug response, interactions, and adverse effects. *Am. Fam. Physician* **2007**, *76*, 391–396. [PubMed]
5. Wen, X.; Wang, J.S.; Backman, J.T.; Kivistö, K.T.; Neuvonen, P.J. Gemfibrozil is a potent inhibitor of human cytochrome P450 2C9. *Drug Metab. Dispos.* **2001**, *29*, 1359–1361.
6. Shitara, Y.; Hirano, M.; Sato, H.; Sugiyama, Y. Gemfibrozil and its glucuronide inhibit the organic anion transporting polypeptide 2 (OATP2/OATP1B1:SLC21A6)-mediated hepatic uptake and CYP2C8-mediated metabolism of cerivastatin: Analysis of the mechanism of the clinically relevant drug-drug interaction between cerivastatin and gemfibrozil. *J. Pharmacol. Exp. Ther.* **2004**, *311*, 228–236.
7. Lilja, J.J.; Backman, J.T.; Neuvonen, P.J. Effect of gemfibrozil on the pharmacokinetics and pharmacodynamics of racemic warfarin in healthy subjects. *Br. J. Clin. Pharmacol.* **2005**, *59*, 433–439. [CrossRef]
8. Backman, J.T.; Kyrklund, C.; Neuvonen, M.; Neuvonen, P.J. Gemfibrozil greatly increases plasma concentrations of cerivastatin. *Clin. Pharmacol. Ther.* **2002**, *72*, 685–691. [CrossRef]
9. Varma, M.V.S.; Lin, J.; Bi, Y.-A.; Kimoto, E.; Rodrigues, A.D. Quantitative Rationalization of Gemfibrozil Drug Interactions: Consideration of Transporters-Enzyme Interplay and the Role of Circulating Metabolite Gemfibrozil 1-O-β-Glucuronide. *Drug Metab. Dispos.* **2015**, *43*, 1108–1118. [CrossRef]
10. Niemi, M.; Backman, J.T.; Neuvonen, M.; Neuvonen, P.J. Effects of gemfibrozil, itraconazole, and their combination on the pharmacokinetics and pharmacodynamics of repaglinide: Potentially hazardous interaction between gemfibrozil and repaglinide. *Diabetologia* **2003**, *46*, 347–351. [CrossRef]
11. Jaakkola, T.; Backman, J.T.; Neuvonen, M.; Neuvonen, P.J. Effects of gemfibrozil, itraconazole, and their combination on the pharmacokinetics of pioglitazone. *Clin. Pharmacol. Ther.* **2005**, *77*, 404–414. [CrossRef] [PubMed]

12. Ogilvie, B.W.; Zhang, D.; Li, W.; Rodrigues, A.D.; Gipson, A.E.; Holsapple, J.; Toren, P.; Parkinson, A. Glucuronidation converts gemfibrozil to a potent, metabolism-dependent inhibitor of CYP2C8: Implications for drug-drug interactions. *Drug Metab. Dispos.* **2006**, *34*, 191–197. [CrossRef] [PubMed]
13. Zhang, H.; Gao, N.; Liu, T.; Fang, Y.; Qi, B.; Wen, Q.; Zhou, J.; Jia, L.; Qiao, H. Effect of Cytochrome b5 Content on the Activity of Polymorphic CYP1A2, 2B6, and 2E1 in Human Liver Microsomes. *PLoS ONE* **2015**, *10*, e0128547. [CrossRef] [PubMed]
14. Bart, A.G.; Scott, E.E. Structural and functional effects of cytochrome b(5) interactions with human cytochrome P450 enzymes. *J. Biol. Chem.* **2017**, *292*, 20818–20833. [CrossRef] [PubMed]
15. Abdel-Rahman, S.M.; Gotschall, R.R.; Kauffman, R.E.; Leeder, J.S.; Kearns, G.L. Investigation of terbinafine as a CYP2D6 inhibitor in vivo. *Clin. Pharmacol. Ther.* **1999**, *65*, 465–472. [CrossRef]
16. Vickers, A.E.M.; Sinclair, J.R.; Zollinger, M.; Heitz, F.; Glänzel, U.; Johanson, L.; Fischer, V. Multiple Cytochrome P-450s Involved in the Metabolism of Terbinafine Suggest a Limited Potential for Drug-Drug Interactions. *Drug Metab. Dispos.* **1999**, *27*, 1029–1038. [PubMed]
17. Rasmussen, B.B.; Nielsen, T.L.; Brøsen, K. Fluvoxamine inhibits the CYP2C19-catalysed metabolism of proguanil in vitro. *Eur. J. Clin. Pharmacol.* **1998**, *54*, 735–740. [CrossRef] [PubMed]
18. Lam, Y.W.; Alfaro, C.L.; Ereshefsky, L.; Miller, M. Pharmacokinetic and pharmacodynamic interactions of oral midazolam with ketoconazole, fluoxetine, fluvoxamine, and nefazodone. *J. Clin. Pharmacol.* **2003**, *43*, 1274–1282. [CrossRef]
19. Drolet, B.; Khalifa, M.; Daleau, P.; Hamelin, B.A.; Turgeon, J. Block of the rapid component of the delayed rectifier potassium current by the prokinetic agent cisapride underlies drug-related lengthening of the QT interval. *Circulation* **1998**, *97*, 204–210. [CrossRef]
20. Naritomi, Y.; Teramura, Y.; Terashita, S.; Kagayama, A. Utility of microtiter plate assays for human cytochrome P450 inhibition studies in drug discovery: Application of simple method for detecting quasi-irreversible and irreversible inhibitors. *Drug Metab. Pharmacokinet.* **2004**, *19*, 55–61. [CrossRef]
21. Uttamsingh, V.; Gallegos, R.; Liu, J.F.; Harbeson, S.L.; Bridson, G.W.; Cheng, C.; Wells, D.S.; Graham, P.B.; Zelle, R.; Tung, R. Altering Metabolic Profiles of Drugs by Precision Deuteration: Reducing Mechanism-Based Inhibition of CYP2D6 by Paroxetine. *J. Pharmacol. Exp. Ther.* **2015**, *354*, 43–54. [CrossRef] [PubMed]
22. Bertelsen, K.M.; Venkatakrishnan, K.; Von Moltke, L.L.; Obach, R.S.; Greenblatt, D.J. Apparent mechanism-based inhibition of human CYP2D6 in vitro by paroxetine: Comparison with fluoxetine and quinidine. *Drug Metab. Dispos.* **2003**, *31*, 289–293. [CrossRef] [PubMed]
23. Kouladjian, L.; Chen, T.F.; Gnjidic, D.; Hilmer, S.N. Education and Assessment of Pharmacists on the Use of the Drug Burden Index in Older Adults Using a Continuing Professional Development Education Method. *Am. J. Pharm. Educ.* **2016**, *80*, 63. [CrossRef] [PubMed]
24. Ogilvie, B.W. An In Vitro Investigation into the Mechanism of the Clinically Relevant Drug-Drug Interaction between Omeprazole or Esomeprazole and Clopidogrel. Ph.D. Thesis, University of Kansas, Lawrence, KS, USA, 23 April 2015.
25. Ray, W.A.; Murray, K.T.; Griffin, M.R.; Chung, C.P.; Smalley, W.E.; Hall, K.; Daugherty, J.R.; Kaltenbach, L.A.; Stein, C.M. Outcomes with concurrent use of clopidogrel and proton-pump inhibitors: A cohort study. *Ann. Int. Med.* **2010**, *152*, 337–345. [CrossRef]
26. Bhatt, D.L.; Cryer, B.L.; Contant, C.F.; Cohen, M.; Lanas, A.; Schnitzer, T.J.; Shook, T.L.; Lapuerta, P.; Goldsmith, M.A.; Laine, L.; et al. Clopidogrel with or without omeprazole in coronary artery disease. *N. Engl. J. Med.* **2010**, *363*, 1909–1917. [CrossRef]
27. Sidney, M.; Wolfe, M.D. *Proton Pump Inhibitors: Dangerous and Habit-Forming Heartburn Drugs*; Citizen, P., Ed.; The Citizen: Washington, DC, USA, 2011; Volume 27, p. 9.
28. Karaźniewicz-Łada, M.; Danielak, D.; Burchardt, P.; Kruszyna, L.; Komosa, A.; Lesiak, M.; Główka, F. Clinical pharmacokinetics of clopidogrel and its metabolites in patients with cardiovascular diseases. *Clin. Pharmacokinet.* **2014**, *53*, 155–164. [CrossRef]
29. Zvyaga, T.; Chang, S.-Y.; Chen, C.; Yang, Z.; Vuppugalla, R.; Hurley, J.; Thorndike, D.; Wagner, A.; Chimalakonda, A.; Rodrigues, A.D. Evaluation of Six Proton Pump Inhibitors As Inhibitors of Various Human Cytochromes P450: Focus on Cytochrome P450 2C19. *Drug Metab. Dispos.* **2012**, *40*, 1698–1711. [CrossRef]

30. Angiolillo, D.J.; Gibson, C.M.; Cheng, S.; Ollier, C.; Nicolas, O.; Bergougnan, L.; Perrin, L.; LaCreta, F.P. Hurbin, F.; Dubar, M. Differential Effects of Omeprazole and Pantoprazole on the Pharmacodynamics and Pharmacokinetics of Clopidogrel in Healthy Subjects: Randomized, Placebo-Controlled, Crossover Comparison Studies. *Clin. Pharmacol. Ther.* **2011**, *89*, 65–74. [CrossRef]
31. Furtado, R.H.M.; Giugliano, R.P.; Strunz, C.M.C.; Filho, C.C.; Ramires, J.A.F.; Filho, R.K.; Neto, P.A.L. Pereira, A.C.; Rocha, T.R.; Freire, B.T.; et al. Drug Interaction Between Clopidogrel and Ranitidine or Omeprazole in Stable Coronary Artery Disease: A Double-Blind, Double Dummy, Randomized Study. *Am. J Cardiovasc. Drugs* **2016**, *16*, 275–284. [CrossRef]
32. Gilard, M.; Arnaud, B.; Cornily, J.-C.; Le Gal, G.; Lacut, K.; Le Calvez, G.; Mansourati, J.; Mottier, D. Abgrall, J.-F.; Boschat, J. Influence of Omeprazole on the Antiplatelet Action of Clopidogrel Associated With Aspirin: The Randomized, Double-Blind OCLA (Omeprazole CLopidogrel Aspirin) Study. *J. Am. Coll Cardiol.* **2008**, *51*, 256–260. [CrossRef]
33. Frelinger, A.L., III; Lee, R.D.; Mulford, D.J.; Wu, J.; Nudurupati, S.; Nigam, A.; Brooks, J.K.; Bhatt, D.L. Michelson, A.D. A randomized, 2-period, crossover design study to assess the effects of dexlansoprazole, lansoprazole, esomeprazole, and omeprazole on the steady-state pharmacokinetics and pharmacodynamics of clopidogrel in healthy volunteers. *J. Am. Coll. Cardiol.* **2012**, *59*, 1304–1311. [CrossRef] [PubMed]
34. U.S. Food and Drug Administration. Information for Healthcare Professionals: Update to the Labeling of Clopidogrel Bisulfate (Marketed as Plavix) to Alert Healthcare Professionals about a Drug Interaction with Omeprazole (Marketed as Prilosec and Prilosec OTC). Available online http://www.fda.gov/Drugs/DrugSafety/PostmarketDrugSafetyInformationforPatientsandProviders/DrugSafetyInformationforHeathcareProfessionals/ucm190787 (accessed on 25 July 2020).
35. Bundhun, P.K.; Teeluck, A.R.; Bhurtu, A.; Huang, W.-Q. Is the concomitant use of clopidogrel and Proton Pump Inhibitors still associated with increased adverse cardiovascular outcomes following coronary angioplasty? A systematic review and meta-analysis of recently published studies (2012–2016). *BMC Cardiovasc. Disord* **2017**, *17*, 3. [CrossRef] [PubMed]
36. Bhurke, S.M.; Martin, B.C.; Li, C.; Franks, A.M.; Bursac, Z.; Said, Q. Effect of the clopidogrel-proton pump inhibitor drug interaction on adverse cardiovascular events in patients with acute coronary syndrome *Pharmacotherapy* **2012**, *32*, 809–818. [CrossRef] [PubMed]
37. Mahabaleshwarkar, R.K.; Yang, Y.; Datar, M.V.; Bentley, J.P.; Strum, M.W.; Banahan, B.F.; Null, K.D. Risk of adverse cardiovascular outcomes and all-cause mortality associated with concomitant use of clopidogrel and proton pump inhibitors in elderly patients. *Curr. Med. Res. Opin.* **2013**, *29*, 315–323. [CrossRef] [PubMed]
38. Ho, P.M.; Maddox, T.M.; Wang, L.; Fihn, S.D.; Jesse, R.L.; Peterson, E.D.; Rumsfeld, J.S. Risk of Adverse Outcomes Associated With Concomitant Use of Clopidogrel and Proton Pump Inhibitors Following Acute Coronary Syndrome. *JAMA* **2009**, *301*, 937–944. [CrossRef] [PubMed]
39. Lin, C.F.; Shen, L.J.; Wu, F.L.; Bai, C.H.; Gau, C.S. Cardiovascular outcomes associated with concomitant use of clopidogrel and proton pump inhibitors in patients with acute coronary syndrome in Taiwan. *Br. J. Clin. Pharmacol.* **2012**, *74*, 824–834. [CrossRef] [PubMed]
40. Vaduganathan, M.; Cannon, C.P.; Cryer, B.L.; Liu, Y.; Hsieh, W.H.; Doros, G.; Cohen, M.; Lanas, A. Schnitzer, T.J.; Shook, T.L.; et al. Efficacy and Safety of Proton-Pump Inhibitors in High-Risk Cardiovascular Subsets of the COGENT Trial. *Am. J. Med.* **2016**, *129*, 1002–1005. [CrossRef]
41. Sherwood, M.W.; Melloni, C.; Jones, W.S.; Washam, J.B.; Hasselblad, V.; Dolor, R.J. Individual Proton Pump Inhibitors and Outcomes in Patients with Coronary Artery Disease on Dual Antiplatelet Therapy: A Systematic Review. *J. Am. Heart Assoc.* **2015**, *4*, e002245. [CrossRef]
42. Yano, H.; Tsukahara, K.; Morita, S.; Endo, T.; Sugano, T.; Hibi, K.; Himeno, H.; Fukui, K.; Umemura, S. Kimura, K. Influence of omeprazole and famotidine on the antiplatelet effects of clopidogrel in addition to aspirin in patients with acute coronary syndromes: A prospective, randomized, multicenter study. *Circ. J.* **2012**, *76*, 2673–2680. [CrossRef]
43. Lau, W.C.; Gurbel, P.A. The drug–drug interaction between proton pump inhibitors and clopidogrel. *Can. Med. Assoc. J.* **2009**, *180*, 699–700. [CrossRef]
44. Juurlink, D.N.; Gomes, T.; Ko, D.T.; Szmitko, P.E.; Austin, P.C.; Tu, J.V.; Henry, D.A.; Kopp, A.; Mamdani, M.M A population-based study of the drug interaction between proton pump inhibitors and clopidogrel. *Can. Med. Assoc. J.* **2009**, *180*, 713–718. [CrossRef] [PubMed]

45. Zhang, J.R.; Wang, D.Q.; Du, J.; Qu, G.S.; Du, J.L.; Deng, S.B.; Liu, Y.J.; Cai, J.X.; She, Q. Efficacy of Clopidogrel and Clinical Outcome When Clopidogrel Is Coadministered With Atorvastatin and Lansoprazole: A Prospective, Randomized, Controlled Trial. *Medicine* **2015**, *94*, e2262. [CrossRef] [PubMed]
46. Chen, R.; Shen, K.; Hu, P. Single- and multiple-dose pharmacokinetics and tolerability of a paroxetine controlled-release tablet in healthy Chinese subjects. *Int. J. Clin. Pharmacol. Ther.* **2017**, *55*, 231–236. [CrossRef] [PubMed]
47. Laine, K.; Tybring, G.; Härtter, S.; Andersson, R.N.K.; Svensson, J.-O.; Widén, J.; Bertilsson, L. Inhibition of cytochrome P4502D6 activity with paroxetine normalizes the ultrarapid metabolizer phenotype as measured by nortriptyline pharmacokinetics and the debrisoquin test. *Clin. Pharmacol. Ther.* **2001**, *70*, 327–335. [CrossRef]
48. U.S. Food and Drug Administration. Paxil [Drug Label]. Available online: https://www.accessdata.fda.gov/drugsatfda_docs/label/2008/020031s060,020936s037,020710s024lbl.pdf (accessed on 31 July 2020).
49. Bartkowski, R.R.; Goldberg, M.E.; Larijani, G.E.; Boerner, T. Inhibition of alfentanil metabolism by erythromycin. *Clin. Pharmacol. Ther.* **1989**, *46*, 99–102. [CrossRef]
50. Bartkowski, R.R.; McDonnell, T.E. Prolonged Alfentanil Effect Following Erythromycin Administration. *Anesthesiology* **1990**, *73*, 566–567. [CrossRef]
51. Yate, P.M.; Short, S.M.; Sebel, P.S.; Thomas, D.; Morton, J. Comparison of infusions of alfentanil or pethidine for sedation of ventilated patients on THE ITU. *Br. J. Anaesth.* **1986**, *58*, 1091–1099. [CrossRef]
52. Okudaira, T.; Kotegawa, T.; Imai, H.; Tsutsumi, K.; Nakano, S.; Ohashi, K. Effect of the Treatment Period With Erythromycin on Cytochrome P450 3A Activity in Humans. *J. Clin. Pharmacol.* **2007**, *47*, 871–876. [CrossRef]
53. Patroneva, A.; Connolly, S.M.; Fatato, P.; Pedersen, R.; Jiang, Q.; Paul, J.; Guico-Pabia, C.; Isler, J.A.; Burczynski, M.E.; Nichols, A.I. An assessment of drug-drug interactions: The effect of desvenlafaxine and duloxetine on the pharmacokinetics of the CYP2D6 probe desipramine in healthy subjects. *Drug Metab. Dispos.* **2008**, *36*, 2484–2491. [CrossRef]
54. U.S. Food and Drug Administration. Consultation for NDA 202611. In *Clinical Pharmacology and Biopharmaceutics Review(s), Center for Drug Evaluation and Research Division of Cardiovascular and Renal Products*; U.S. Food and Drug Administration: Pharr, TX, USA, 2012; p. 218.
55. Krauwinkel, W.; Dickinson, J.; Schaddelee, M.; Meijer, J.; Tretter, R.; van de Wetering, J.; Strabach, G.; van Gelderen, M. The effect of mirabegron, a potent and selective β3-adrenoceptor agonist, on the pharmacokinetics of CYP2D6 substrates desipramine and metoprolol. *Eur. J. Drug Metab. Pharmacokinet.* **2014**, *39*, 43–52. [CrossRef]
56. Bramer, S.L.; Suri, A. Inhibition of CYP2D6 by Quinidine and its Effects on the Metabolism of Cilostazol. *Clin. Pharmacokinet.* **1999**, *37*, 41–51. [CrossRef] [PubMed]
57. Storelli, F.; Matthey, A.; Lenglet, S.; Thomas, A.; Desmeules, J.; Daali, Y. Impact of CYP2D6 Functional Allelic Variations on Phenoconversion and Drug-Drug Interactions. *Clin. Pharmacol. Ther.* **2018**, *104*, 148–157. [CrossRef] [PubMed]
58. Storelli, F.; Desmeules, J.; Daali, Y. Genotype-sensitive reversible and time-dependent CYP2D6 inhibition in human liver microsomes. *Basic Clin. Pharmacol. Toxicol.* **2019**, *124*, 170–180. [CrossRef] [PubMed]

9

Interpretation of Drug Interaction Using Systemic and Local Tissue Exposure Changes

Young Hee Choi

College of Pharmacy and Integrated Research Institute for Drug Development, Dongguk University_Seoul, 32 Dongguk-lo, Ilsandong-gu, Goyang-si 10326, Gyeonggi-do, Korea; choiyh@dongguk.edu;

Abstract: Systemic exposure of a drug is generally associated with its pharmacodynamic (PD) effect (e.g., efficacy and toxicity). In this regard, the change in area under the plasma concentration-time curve (AUC) of a drug, representing its systemic exposure, has been mainly considered in evaluation of drug-drug interactions (DDIs). Besides the systemic exposure, the drug concentration in the tissues has emerged as a factor to alter the PD effects. In this review, the status of systemic exposure, and/or tissue exposure changes in DDIs, were discussed based on the recent reports dealing with transporters and/or metabolic enzymes mediating DDIs. Particularly, the tissue concentration in the intestine, liver and kidney were referred to as important factors of PK-based DDIs.

Keywords: drug interaction; pharmacokinetics; tissue-specific; systemic exposure

1. Introduction

Drug-drug interactions (DDIs) are described as the pharmacokinetic (PK) or pharmacodynamic (PD) influence of a perpetrator drug on a victim drug, resulting in an unexpected effect. In practice, DDIs have gained much attention due to their changes of pharmacologic effects (i.e., the loss of efficacy or unintentional toxicity) [1]. The importance of DDIs is well-recognized by the fact that mismanaged DDIs constitute one of the major causes of drug withdrawal from the market (e.g., mibefradil, terfenadine, and cisapride) [2–4]. Numerous drug withdrawal cases, as well as serious side-effects caused by DDIs, including PK-based interactions, can be the result of accompanying clinically relevant PD interactions [1–4]. The DDIs that can change PK profiles involve: (1) Gastrointestinal absorption, (2) protein binding in plasma and/or tissue, (3) carrier-mediated transport across plasma membranes (e.g., hepatic or renal uptake and biliary or urinary secretion), and (4) metabolism. PD interactions, such as acting an agonist or antagonist at the receptor may also increase or decrease the effects of a drug [5].

Since the drug concentration at the target site drives its efficacy and toxicity [6], accurate measurement or prediction of drug concentrations at the target sites is necessary to evaluate DDIs [7–11]. Generally, it is assumed that the plasma drug concentration reflects its concentration in tissue, and drug concentrations in plasma and tissue are mostly thought to be similar. The direct measurement of drug concentration in tissue is practically limited, and the plasma drug concentration has been used as a surrogate for drug concentrations in tissue for PK-PD investigations [11–13]. Among possibly changed PK profiles in DDIs, transporter- and/or metabolic enzyme-mediated alteration of plasma concentration of a victim drug by a perpetrator drug is a major proportion to be considered in PK-based DDI evaluations [12,13]. Of course, plasma drug concentrations do not always reflect tissue concentrations [6,14–17], and moreover, a closer correlation of tissue concentration, not plasma concentration, with PD effects of drugs has emerged (e.g., an increased hepatic concentration of metformin is closely associated with improving its glucose-lowering effect [18,19]; a decreased hepatic concentration of pravastatin is closely associated with a reduction of its lipid-lowering effect [20,21]).

Owing to the accumulation of scientific knowledge for understanding PK-related mechanisms of DDIs and awareness of DDIs, it has become a key issue when assessing DDIs to determine how a victim drug concentration changes at the target (pharmacological action) sites or in the whole body [22–24]. Regulatory agencies, such as the United States Food and Drug Administration (FDA) and European Medicines Agency (EMA) have published guidance for drug interaction studies, and they recommend that evaluation of PK-based DDIs be conducted for drugs under development and on the market [22,23]. As a result, detailed information about DDIs via metabolic enzymes and transporters have become available at the time of market approval. Nevertheless, the clinically relevant DDIs, leading to the loss of efficacy or advent of toxicity, have been increasing because polypharmacotherapy is becoming progressively more common. In addition, the underlying mechanisms of DDIs have been variously interpreted, which makes it difficult to explain a correlation of PK and PD changes in DDIs, as well as to predict their clinical relevance [25–29]. In other words, if the alteration of a PD effect is negligible even through a PK change of a victim drug was observed later, the DDI would be ignored at the time. In some cases, if the PK and PD changes of a victim drug are not related, it is likely that the critical underlying mechanism, that triggers a PK change of a victim drug, is mainly associated with a PD effect has not been investigated [25].

Considering that drug concentrations in plasma and tissue are important parameters to investigate DDIs in aspects of PK, as well as PD, we summarized how transporters or metabolic enzymes are involved in the changes of systemic exposure (represented by an area under the plasma concentration versus time curve (AUC)) and/or local tissue concentration of a victim drug in PK-based DDIs.

2. Transporter and/or Metabolic Enzymes as Main Determinant Factors in PK-Based DDIs

The individual chemical properties of a victim drug or a perpetrator drug (i.e., molecular size, lipophilicity, ionization, and binding affinity, etc.) can determine its own PK characteristics and affect the PK change of counterpart individual drugs in DDIs [30–32]. In addition to the physicochemical properties of drugs, other factors determine the drug concentrations in plasma and tissue, like regulation of inward or outward flow of a drug into blood vessels or tissues by passive diffusion and/or transporters, metabolism by phase I and phase II metabolic enzymes, and/or transporter-mediated excretion (e.g., renal or biliary excretion) [25,33,34]. First of all, a perpetrator drug can affect transporter-mediated uptake and/or efflux of a victim drug across cell membranes of tissues, as well as its excretion from the tissue (e.g., to the blood or outside of the body). Also, a perpetrator drug is able to induce or inhibit metabolic enzymes and consequently change the enzyme-mediated elimination of a victim drug [25,35–37]. A transporter-mediated metabolite and/or parent form of a victim drug excretion can be altered by a perpetrator drug as well in DDIs. In other words, the interplay of transporters and metabolic enzymes in enterocytes, hepatocytes, and renal proximal tubules is shown in Figure 1, and their effects on systemic exposure and/or tissue concentration of a victim drug have been increasingly reported [25,33,34,38].

The functions of transporters are to uptake drugs into cells and to export drugs or drug metabolites from the cells. Each transporter has specific expression pattern in individual tissues. In particular, transporters expressed in the small intestine, liver, and kidneys are important for drug disposition and DDIs [39–42]. We summarized the possible transporters in the human intestine, liver, and kidneys that are able to cause clinically relevant DDIs in Table 1. Considering the absorption, distribution, metabolism and excretion (ADME) process of a drug, efflux transporters such as P-glycoprotein (P-gp; gene symbol ABCB1), the multidrug resistance protein 2 (MRP2; gene symbol ABCC2), and the breast cancer resistance protein (BCRP; gene symbol ABCG2) are localized to the apical membrane of enterocytes (Figure 1A), thereby regulating the bioavailability of orally administered substrate drugs. The concomitantly administered perpetrator drugs inhibited these efflux transporters, resulting in an increase in the bioavailability of the victim drug. In contrast, the bioavailability of the drug was reduced when these efflux transporters were induced by perpetrator drugs. After the absorbed drugs pass through the portal vein and reach the basolateral (i.e., sinusoidal) membrane of hepatocytes (Figure 1B), uptake transporters in the basolateral membrane of hepatocytes mediate the drugs into hepatocytes as the most important site of drug metabolism. For example, organic anion-transporting polypeptides (OATPs) such as OATP1B1 (gene symbol SLCO1B1) and organic cation transporters (OCTs), such as OCT1 (gene symbol SLC22A1), mediate the transport of organic anions and organic cations, respectively After which efflux transporters localized in the canalicular membrane of hepatocytes [(e.g., P-gp, BCRP multidrug and toxin extrusion protein 1 (MATE1, gene symbol SLC47A1), multidrug resistance protein 2 (MRP2), and bile salt export pump (BSEP, gene symbol ABCB11)] mediate drug transport into the bile [34,43]. In hepatocytes, the drugs can be metabolized by phase I or phase II metabolic enzymes and some of them are transported into bile [34,43]. Sometimes, for a small proportion, the efflux of the drug or metabolites across the basolateral membrane into can occur [34].

Drug transporters also play a major role in drug secretion from the renal proximal tubular cells into the urine (Figure 1C). Transporter-mediated uptake across the basolateral membrane of the proximal tubular cells and efflux across the luminal membrane mainly coordinate the renal secretion of a drug which affects the drug concentration in the blood and kidneys. For the secretion of organic cation drugs, OCT2 (gene symbol SLC22A2), localized in the basolateral membrane uptakes the drug and subsequently, MATE1 and MATE2-K (gene symbol SLC47A2), localized in the luminal membrane, efflux the drug in the proximal tubular cells. Similarly, the uptake and efflux transporters for organic anions are also expressed in the kidney. Alternation of these processes by a concomitantly administered drug leads to reduced or increased renal clearance of the victim drug [43].

After uptake of a victim drug into the tissue, metabolic pathways are involved in PK-based DDIs as an elimination pathway. Cytochrome P450s (CYPs) and UDP-glucuronosyltransferases (UGTs) are the primary metabolic enzymes in phase I and phase II metabolism, as shown in Figure 1 [44,45] CYP enzymes play a major role in drug elimination through oxidation, reduction, and hydroxylation They are mainly present on the smooth endoplasmic reticulum and mitochondria of the hepatocytes and small intestinal epithelia, and to a lesser extent in the proximal tubules of the kidneys [46] Their by-products of metabolism known as metabolites can be either, pharmacologically active or inactive [47]. Among the CYP enzymes in the human liver, CYP3A4 is the most abundant, followed by CYP2E1 and CYP2C9, representing approximately 22.1%, 15.3%, and 14.6% of the total CYP450s (based on protein content), respectively [48], among which the highly expressed CYP isoforms show high potential to cause metabolic DDIs. In addition, drugs or metabolites formed from phase I metabolism are conjugated with a hydrophilic compound with the help of transferase enzymes during the process of phase II metabolism. The most common phase II drug-metabolizing enzymes are UGTs, sulfotransferases (SULTs), *N*-acetyltransferases (NATs), glutathione *S*-transferases (GSTs), thiopurine *S*-methyltransferase (TPMT), and catechol *O*-methyltransferase (COMT), and glucuronidation by UGTs have been reported as major phase II enzyme-mediated DDIs [5,49]. Glucuronide conjugated products are mostly hydrophilic and are readily excreted from the body, mainly through efflux transporters in the liver, intestines, and kidneys (e.g., biliary excretion and renal excretion) [5,49,50]. UGTs are normally highly expressed in the liver and intestine, and their substrates are relatively more overlapping with each other compared to substrate for CYPs. Especially, UGT1A1, 1A3, 1A9, 2A1, or 2B7-mediated DDIs have commonly occurred. These pathways, including interplay of metabolic enzymes and transporters during the ADME of drugs, and any alterations of them may result in changes in the PK and PD of a victim drug [5,45].

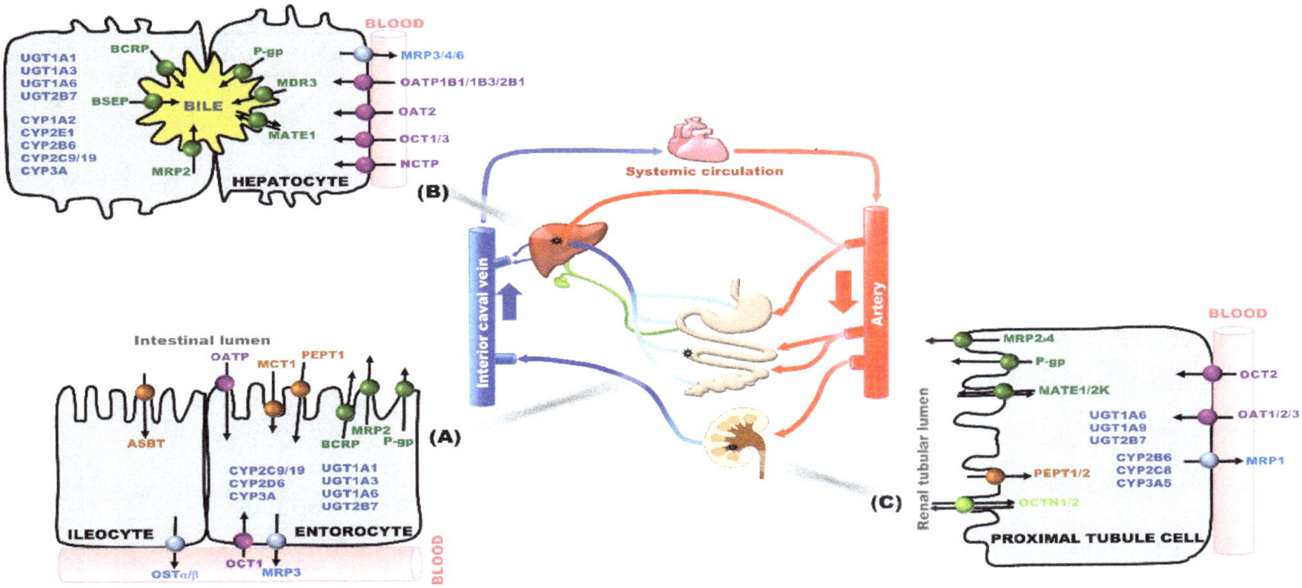

Figure 1. Representative transporters and metabolic enzymes in enterocytes (**A**), hepatocytes (**B**) and renal proximal renal tubules (**C**), which are possibly involved in DDIs.

Table 1. Characteristics of transporters mediating the occurrence of clinically relevant DDIs.

Protein	Location	Direction	Ref.
P-gp (MDR1)	Apical membrane in enterocyte	efflux	[43,51]
	Canalicular membrane in hepatocyte	efflux	
	[1] Luminal membrane in renal proximal tubule cell	efflux	
MDR3	Canalicular membrane in hepatocyte	efflux	[43]
BSEP	Canalicular membrane in hepatocyte	efflux	[43]
BCRP	Apical membrane in enterocyte	efflux	[43]
	Canalicular membrane in hepatocyte	efflux	
	[1] Luminal membrane in renal proximal tubule cell	efflux	
MRP1	Basolateral membrane in renal proximal tubule cell	efflux	[6,43]
MRP2	Apical membrane in enterocyte	efflux	
	Canalicular membrane in hepatocyte	efflux	
	[1] Luminal membrane in renal proximal tubule cell	efflux	
MRP3	Basolateral membrane in enterocyte	uptake	
	Basolateral membrane in hepatocyte	efflux	
	Basolateral membrane in renal proximal tubule cell	efflux	
MRP4	Basolateral membrane in hepatocyte	efflux	[38,43]
	[1] Luminal membrane in renal proximal tubule cell	efflux	
MRP5,6	Basolateral membrane in hepatocyte	efflux	[43]
OATP1B1	Basolateral membrane in enterocyte	uptake	[43,52]
	Basolateral membrane in hepatocyte	uptake	
OATP1B3	Basolateral membrane in enterocyte	uptake	
	Basolateral membrane in hepatocyte	uptake	

Table 1. *Cont.*

Protein	Location	Direction	Ref.
OATP2B1	Basolateral membrane in enterocyte	uptake	[43,53]
	Basolateral membrane in hepatocyte	uptake	
OAT1	Basolateral membrane in renal proximal tubule cell	uptake	[43]
OAT2	Basolateral membrane in hepatocyte	uptake	[38,43]
	Basolateral membrane in renal proximal tubule cell	uptake	
OAT3	Basolateral membrane in renal proximal tubule cell	uptake	[43]
OAT4	[1] Luminal membrane in renal proximal tubule cell	efflux/uptake [2]	
OCT1	Basolateral membrane in enterocyte	uptake	[43,54–56]
	Basolateral membrane in hepatocyte	uptake	
OCT2	Basolateral membrane in renal proximal tubule cell	uptake	
OCT3	Basolateral membrane in enterocyte	uptake	
	Canalicular membrane in hepatocyte	efflux/uptake	
	Basolateral membrane in renal proximal tubule cell	uptake	
MATE1	Canalicular membrane in hepatocyte	efflux/uptake	[43,51]
	[1] Luminal membrane in renal proximal tubule cell	efflux/uptake [2]	
MATE2-K	[1] Luminal membrane in renal proximal tubule cell	efflux/uptake [2]	
PEPT1	Apical membrane in enterocyte	uptake	[43,57]
	[1] Luminal membrane in renal proximal tubule cell	uptake [2]	
PEPT2	[1] Luminal membrane in renal proximal tubule cell	uptake [2]	

[1] Luminal membrane means apical membrane. [2] Uptake in apical membrane in kidneys represents a reabsorption pathway.

3. Effects of Transporter- or Metabolic Enzyme Mediated Changes of Systemic Exposure and/or Local Tissue Concentration on PD Effects

Regarding the effects of PK profile changes on DDIs, it is important to consider which PK parameters (or concepts) are primarily or closely associated with PD effects in DDIs [1]. The accurate measurement or prediction of the unbound (free) drug concentration at the target site is essential for evaluating DDIs [6,8–11]. When considering the protein binding of a drug, it is assumed that only free drugs, not bound to proteins and lipids in the blood and tissues, are metabolized and distributed to target sites where the free drugs exert their pharmacological effects [9,10,58,59]. Protein binding is possibly able to impact PK and PD, driven by the changes of free drug concentrations [58,59]. However, it has been generally accepted that the protein binding change of a victim drug shows little clinical significance in the majority of DDIs cases [58,60].

In the following section, we describe the effects of transporter- and/or metabolic enzymes-mediated DDIs, resulting in changes in systemic exposure or local tissue concentration of a victim drug, which affect PD effects. In particular, since transporters and metabolic enzymes are determinant factors causing DDIs, they are differently expressed and variously interplay together in individual tissues. Therefore, it is difficult to generally explain the systemic exposure and tissue concentration changes with PD effects in accordance with the change (e.g., inhibition or induction) of transporters or metabolic enzymes. Thus, we focused on the change of systemic exposure or tissue concentration in the liver and kidneys of a victim drug along with how their changes affect the PD effects. Several examples are presented in Table 2.

As a major site of drug absorption, the changes in transporters in the apical and basolateral membranes, as well as the metabolic enzymes of enterocytes determine the final amount of drug absorbed into systemic circulation [54,57]. An increase of drug absorption happens due to a drug influx from the intestinal lumen into enterocytes, by an increase of influx transporter or a decrease of efflux transport in the apical membrane, a decrease of drug metabolism in enterocytes, or an increase of drug efflux from enterocytes to blood by an increase of transporter in the basolateral membrane [37,54,57]. Recently, drug catalysis by gut microbiota has emerged as one pathway to regulate drug absorption [61]. A change in drug absorption affects the systemic exposure and intestinal concentration of a drug, and they are generally similar in most cases. In particular, the changed intestinal concentration of a drug can drive the alterations of efficacy and toxicity that occur in the intestine [61,62].

In the liver, the changed final hepatic clearance of a victim drug affects its systemic and local tissue exposure depending on the contribution of the transporter and metabolic enzyme-mediated pathways (i.e., uptake or efflux of a victim drug across the basolateral membrane of hepatocyte, hepatic metabolism, and biliary excretion). There are two major cases. One is that the metabolic plus biliary efflux clearance is a determinant step in drug elimination, so the basolateral uptake becomes the rate-determining step in the hepatic clearance of the drug. In other words, the hepatic clearance is driven mainly by uptake clearance. The inhibition of uptake transporter in the basolateral membrane will increase plasma drug concentrations and systemic exposure of a victim drug, but will not significantly impact the liver AUC of a drug. This may be due to the victim drug being mainly eliminated by the liver [6], and the alteration of basolateral uptake into hepatocytes is the main factor behind the change in the plasma concentration of a victim drug.

The second is that the inhibition of metabolic enzymes or biliary efflux transporters can increase the liver AUC of a victim drug while minimally impacting its plasma AUC [63,64], which may be due to the elimination pathway after uptake into hepatocytes being a determinant factor for final hepatic clearance. In these examples, the changes of plasma and liver concentrations of the drug are not symmetric directions. This asymmetry may lead to misinterpretations of the plasma concentration and/or tissue concentration (e.g., the liver) of a victim drug in DDIs, and in particular, this issue is important to explain the association of PK and PD changes in DDIs [6].

In the kidneys, the alteration of systemic exposure (or plasma concentrations) of victim drugs in renal transporter-mediated DDIs is comparatively moderate compared with those in intestinal or hepatic-transporter mediated DDIs. However, a change in renal clearance of drugs that are mainly eliminated via renal routes can substantially affect the systemic levels of victim drugs, and sometimes these changes are related to efficacy and/or toxicity changes [38,54,65]. Moreover, if the kidneys are the pharmacological target site, a drug concentration change of a victim drug in the kidneys is a critical factor regulating the drug efficacy [66–69]. From here, we have divided the next section into three subsections as follows: (1) Systemic exposure change of a victim drug having a major PD effect; (2) tissue concentration changes of a victim drug having a major PD effect; and (3) additional factors affecting PD effects along with changes in systemic exposure or tissue concentration of a victim drug.

Table 2. Examples of transporter- or metabolic enzyme-mediated DDIs.

Victim Drug	Perpetrator Drug	Underlying Mechanism [1]	PK Change of a Victim Drug	PD Change of a Victim Drug	Ref.
Apixaban	Ketoconazole	(−) P-gp in enterocyte	AUC↑	ADR↑ (bleeding risk)	[70]
Dabigatran	Rifampin	(+) P-gp in enterocyte	AUC↓	TR↔, safety↔	[71]
Digoxin	Rifampin	(+) P-gp in enterocyte	AUC↓	TR↓	[72]
Loperamide	Quinidine	(−) P-gp in enterocyte or brain	AUC↑	ADR↑(respiratory depression) by P-gp inhibition in brain (not enterocyte)	[73]
Rosuvastatin	Eltrombopag, Fostamatinib	(−) BCRP in enterocyte	AUC↑	ADR↑ (myopathy), TR↑	[43,74,75]
Clopidogrel	Aspirin	(+) P-gp in enterocyte (+) CYP2C9 in hepatocyte	AUC↓, F↓, H4 (active metabolite)↑	Platelet inhibition effect↔	[29]
Digoxin	Clarithromycin	(−) P-gp in enterocyte (−) CYP2D6 or 3A4 inhibition in hepatocyte	AUC↑, CL↓, CL_R↓ (by non-glomerular renal clearance)	ADR↑ (digoxin toxicity)	[76]
Atorvastatin	**Cyclosporine**	(−) OATP1B1, 1B3, 2B1 in hepatocyte (−) CYP3A in hepatocyte	AUC↑, hepatic uptake↔	Muscle-related toxicity↑	[1,43,77,78]
	Itraconazole	(−) CYP3A in hepatocyte	AUC↑, hepatic uptake↔	-	[62,79,80]
Bosentan	Clarithromycin	(−) OATP1B1, 1B3 in hepatocyte	AUC↑	ADR↑ (cholestatic liver injury)	[81,82]
Pitavastatin	Cyclosporine, rifampin	(−) OATP1B1, 1B3, 2B1 in hepatocyte	AUC↑	ADR↑	[83,84]
Atrovastatin, simvastatin	Itraconazole, mibefradil, verapamil	(−) CYP3A4 in hepatocyte	AUC↑, C_{max}↑	ADR↑ (myopathy, fatal rhadomyolysis)	[85]
Atrovastatin, pravastatin, simvastatin	Clarithromycin	(−) OATP1B1, 1B3, 2B1 in hepatocyte (−) CYP3A4 in hepatocyte	AUC↑, C_{max}↑	ADR↑ (myopathy, fatal rhadomyolysis)	[85]

Table 2. *Cont.*

Victim Drug	Perpetrator Drug	Underlying Mechanism [1]	PK Change of a Victim Drug	PD Change of a Victim Drug	Ref.
Rosuvastatin	Cyclosporine	(−) OATP1B1, 1B3, 2B1 in hepatocyte	AUC↑, hepatic cons [2] $\boxed{\leftrightarrow}$	ADR↑	[86,87]
	Gemfibrozil	(−) OATP2B1 in hepatocyte	AUC↑, hepatic cons [2] $\boxed{\leftrightarrow}$	ADR↑	[87,88]
Simvastatin	Cyclosporine	(−) OATP1B1 in hepatocyte (−) CYP3A4 in hepatocyte	AUC↑	ADR↑ (myopathy)	[43]
Adefovir	Probenecid	(−) OAT1 in proximal tubule cell	AUC↑, CL_R↓	ADR↑ (nephrotoxicity)	[43,89]
Benzylpenicillin	Probenecid	(−) OAT3 in proximal tubule cell	AUC↑, CL_R↓	ADR↑	[89]
Digoxin	Quinidine	(−) CYP2D6 or 3A4 inhibition in hepatocyte (−) P-gp in proximal tubule cell	AUC↑, CL↓, CL_{NR}↓, CL_R↓	ADR↑ (digoxin toxicity)	[83,90]
Lamivudine	Trimethoprim /sulfamethoxazole	(−) OCT2, MATE1, MATE2-K in proximal tubule cell	AUC↑, CL_R↓	ADR↑ (hepatotoxicity)	[91,92]
Metformin	Trimethoprim	(−) OCT2, MATE1 in proximal tubule cell	C_{max}↑, AUC↑, CL/F↓, CL_R↓	ADR↑ (plasma lactate↑, lactic acidosis especially in renal dysfunction patients)	[93]
		(−) OCT2, MATE1, MATE2-K in proximal tubule cell	C_{max}↑, AUC↑, CL_R↓	ADR↑ (plasma lactate↑, lactic acidosis)	[94]
	Dolutegravir	(−) OCT2 in proximal tubule cell	C_{max}↑, AUC↑	ADR↑ (plasma lactate↑, lactic acidosis)	[95]
Pravastatin	**Paroxetine**	(−) Mrp2 in enterocyte; (−) Oatp2 in enterocyte/hepatocyte	Intestinal absorption↑, AUC↑, hepatic uptake↓, hepatic cons↓	Lipid-lowing effect ↓	[20,21,96]
Atorvastatin	Rifampin	(−) OATPs in hepatocyte	AUC↑, hepatic uptake↓	Lipid-lowing effect↓	[52,53,79, 97]
Atorvastatin	**Metformin**	(−) MRP2 in hepatocyte	Biliary excretion↓, hepatic cons [2]↑	Lipid-lowing effect↑	[98]
Metformin	**Rifampin**	(+) mRNA of OCT1 in blood cells	AUC↑ (probable hepatic cons [2]↑)	Glucose-lowering effect↑	[19]
Metformin	*Lonicera japonica* extract	(−) MATE1 in hepatocyte	AUC$\boxed{\leftrightarrow}$, hepatic cons [2]↑	Glucose tolerance effect↑	[67]

Table 2. *Cont.*

Victim Drug	Perpetrator Drug	Underlying Mechanism [1]	PK Change of a Victim Drug	PD Change of a Victim Drug	Ref.
Metformin	Nuciferine	(−) OCT1 and MATE1 in hepatocyte	Hepatic cons [2]↓	Glucose-lowering effect↓	[99]
Rosuvastatin	**Rifampin**	(−) OATP1B1, 1B3, 2B1 in hepatocyte	AUC↑, hepatic cons [2]↓, renal cons [2]↓, hepatic biliary excretion↔	ADR↑	[87]
Metformin	*Houttuynia cordata* extract	(−) MATE1 in hepatocyte (−) OCT2 in proximal tubule cell	AUC↑, CL_R↓, hepatic cons [2]↑	Glucose tolerance effect↑	[66]
Metformin	**Cimetidine**	(−) MATE1 in hepatocyte; (−) MATE1, MATE2-K in proximal tubule cell	AUC↑, hepatic cons [2]↑, (biliary excretion↓), renal cons [2]↑, CL_R↓	Glucose-lowering effect↑	[51,55,56, 100,101]
Metformin	Pyrimethamine	(−) MATE1 in hepatocyte; (−) MATE1 in proximal renal tubule	AUC↑, C_{max}↑, CL_R↓, CL_{CR}↓, S_{CR} [3]↑, hepatic cons [2]↑	Glucose lowering effect↑	[101–103]

The DDI cases mentioned in the main text is marked by bold style. [1] (−) and (+) present inhibition and induction, respectively. [2] Cons refers to concentration. [3] S_{CR} refers to a serum creatinine level.

3.1. *Changed Systemic Exposure of a Victim Drug Affecting the PD Effect*

First of all, it is necessary to clarify the relevance of plasma drug concentration and plasma AUC when assessing DDIs. A plasma AUC alteration implies that the systemic exposure of a victim drug is changed by a perpetrator drug in DDIs, which does not consider the exact time point. Since the AUC is an integrated value from the plasma drug concentration-time curve, the AUC change is not identical to plasma drug concentration changes at all sampling points. If the plasma drug concentration at the specific time points affect PD effects, the plasma drug concentration with the sampling time point or periods should be mentioned to prevent confusion of plasma drug concentrations for plasma AUC. For example, C_{max}, the highest plasma drug concentration that is generally related to toxicity, has been used to evaluate or predict a risk of toxicity change in DDIs [24]. Assuming that plasma drug concentrations reflect the efficacy or toxicity of a drug, the systemic exposure based on plasma AUC from time zero to last sampling time (or time infinity) is used as a proper parameter in the evaluation of DDIs by numerous investigators and regulatory regencies (e.g., FDA and EMA) [22–24]. The systemic exposure change based on plasma AUC is considered to trigger the drug efficacy or toxicity, and especially, the systemic exposure reflects the duration of drug efficacy: The higher plasma AUC results in a stronger efficacy and/or toxicity [24,25,38]. Of course, there may be an exception, such as onset time or duration time in drug efficacy not being reflected by systemic exposure of a drug (e.g., decreased plasma AUC of clopidogrel is not related to a reduction in anti-coagulant activity; [29]), which is described later in detail.

According to the guidelines for DDI studies suggested by FDA and EMA, the AUC ratio for a victim drug in the presence and absence of a perpetrator drug ($AUC_{in\ the\ presence\ of\ a\ perpetrator}/AUC_{in\ the\ absence\ of\ a\ perpetrator}$) > 5 is determined as a strong PK-based DDI occurrence, because a perpetrator drug may inhibit transporter- or metabolic enzyme-mediated clearance of a victim drug. The AUC ratio for a victim drug in the presence and absence of a perpetrator drug <0.5 is also considered, because a perpetrator drug acts as a strong inducer for transporter- or metabolic enzyme-mediated elimination. Both these strong DDI cases are recommended to be labelled as a victim drug [4,24]. Moreover, the plasma AUC represents systemic exposure of a victim drug, and is used as a critical parameter to adjust dosage regimens to clinical levels. Since the contribution of transporters and metabolic enzymes in the occurrence and/or severity of DDIs is different depending on the individual drug combinations, and because there is a pronounced inter-individual variability in the magnitude of the perpetrator effect, it is hard to predict the DDIs and it is necessary to evaluate them case-by-case.

There are several examples where the systemic exposure of a victim drug affects its pharmacological activity. For example, atorvastatin, a permeable drug (log $D_{7.4}$ = 1.53), is a substrate of the OATP transporter (e.g., OATP1B1, 1B3, and 2B1) and is eliminated primarily by hepatic CYP3A metabolism [52,77,78,97]. In a case of atorvastatin co-administered with cyclosporine as a strong OATP inhibitor and moderate CYP3A inhibitor, a 5- to 16-fold increase of plasma AUC of atorvastatin occurs, and a reduction of the atorvastatin dose is clinically recommended, due to an increased rate of muscle-related toxicity, such as myopathy and rhabdomyolysis [1,43,77,78]. Additional DDI studies of atorvastatin are useful for understanding the underlying mechanism of the AUC change of atorvastatin along with the occurrence of toxicity. Co-administered rifampin, an OATP inhibitor, leads to an increase of plasma AUC of atorvastatin, but co-administered itraconazole, a CYP3A inhibitor, does not cause any change of the plasma AUC of atorvastatin. This result suggests that hepatic uptake of atorvastatin via OATPs is the rate-determining step for the hepatic clearance of atorvastatin [62,79,80], and that the plasma concentration of atorvastatin does not reflect its liver concentration [53]. Although the relationship between an increase of atorvastatin AUC in plasma and its pharmacological activity (e.g., cholesterol lowering activity or toxicity) was not mentioned in this example, it is a good example of the contribution of transporter and metabolic enzymes to changes in plasma profiles of a victim drug that do not affect its tissue concentration (e.g., liver) in DDIs.

Co-administration of cimetidine, a MATE1 and OCT2 inhibitor [51,55,56,100,101], with metformin increases systemic exposure of metformin due to the reduction of renal clearance of metformin via inhibited tubular secretion. The effect of cimetidine on the renal excretion of metformin is time-dependent. In other words, cimetidine inhibited metformin renal secretion up to 6 h after cimetidine co-administration, accompanied by an increased blood lactate/pyruvate ratio from 4 h after cimetidine co-administration and reduced creatinine clearance as a dose and concentration-dependent adverse effect of metformin [100]. This is an example of the increased systemic exposure reflecting a toxicity risk of a victim drug in DDIs.

3.2. Changed Local Tissue Concentration of a Victim Drug Affecting the PD Effect

In contrast to the numerous DDIs evaluated by the changes of systemic exposure (i.e., plasma drug concentrations), there are also DDIs that show pharmacological action changes caused by the tissue concentration of a victim drug [53,62,98]. In vivo drug concentration at a target site triggering a PD effect is compared to in vitro efficient concentration, which has been used to explain PK-PD correlations of a victim drug in DDIs [66,98]. In vivo tissue concentration/in vitro half-maximal inhibitory concentration for inhibiting transporter or metabolic enzymes ($[I]/IC_{50}$) or in vivo tissue concentration/in vitro inhibition constant for transporter-or metabolic enzyme ($[I]/K_i$) of a perpetrator drug are used to investigate whether the tissue concentration of a perpetrator drug is sufficient to inhibit transporter-or metabolic enzyme-mediated interactions with a victim drug. When the ratio of IC_{50}/K_i is over 2, the inhibitory interaction of a perpetrator drug to a victim drug can sufficiently happen in vivo in tissue [104,105]. Especially, if there is a tissue lag time relative to peak plasma concentration, the duration of drug efficacy or toxicity should also be considered [6,106,107].

After a drug is absorbed into blood and delivered to the tissue, the drug concentration in the tissue is the sum of the net membrane permeation by influx and efflux across the membrane and the intrinsic clearance by metabolism and/or excretion (e.g., biliary excretion in the liver and renal excretion in the kidneys) [33,34,108,109]. Although membrane permeation and intrinsic clearance are variable in individual tissues, drug influx consists of transporter-mediated uptake and passive diffusion from blood to tissue, as well as transporter-mediated active efflux. After the sum of membrane permeation, a drug is exposed to metabolic enzymes and/or excretion pathways within the localized tissue, which determines the drug concentration in the tissue, as well as the plasma drug concentration as systemic exposure of a drug.

When specific tissues are the pharmacological target sites to show drug efficacy and/or toxicity, drug concentration changes in these tissues strongly affect the PD changes in DDIs. The tissue concentration of a victim drug does not necessarily change in parallel to plasma AUC of a victim drug Thus, it is necessary to choose a tissue to evaluate DDIs based on the pharmacological mechanism and major organ regulating drug disposition. The liver and/or kidneys are frequently involved in drug disposition pathways, but the pharmacological target organs absolutely depend on the individual drugs used. Time-dependent changes of drug concentrations in tissues also need to be considered, especially when onset or duration time is an important factor for drug efficacy [38].

There are several cases showing no change of AUC of a victim drug, even though there is a change of tissue drug concentration, which has been named a silent interaction [63,98]. In the case of atorvastatin with metformin co-administration as a silent interaction, co-administered metformin reduces the biliary excretion of atorvastatin by MRP2 inhibition, increasing the atorvastatin concentration in the liver without changes in total clearance or systemic exposure of atorvastatin [98]. Shin et al. [98] concluded that the increased atorvastatin concentration in the liver might consequently improve the lipid-lowering effect of atorvastatin as in similar DDI studies of statins and metformin [110,111].

In the case of rosuvastatin, the inhibition of OATP uptake by rifampin leads to an increase of blood AUC of rosuvastatin without any significant change to the hepatic AUC of rosuvastatin in rats [87] Similarly, PBPK analysis of rosuvastatin in humans illustrated that the predicted liver concentrations of rosuvastatin are not significantly impacted. Moreover, the OATP1B1 polymorphism affects the plasma concentrations of rosuvastatin without affecting its PD response [112]. These cases demonstrate that the plasma exposure changes do not reflect liver exposure changes without any relevant PD effects. This is because the rate-determining step in the hepatic clearance of rosuvastatin is uptake clearance via OATPs, even though rosuvastatin is also excreted into bile via MRP2/BCRP [74,75,86–88,112].

The case of metformin, an anti-diabetic agent, is an interesting example. Due to metformin's high pKa (most portions are positively charged at pH 7.4) and its negative logP value, the passive diffusion of metformin through cellular membranes is minor. Therefore, transporters are pivotal for metformin permeation through cellular membranes. In the intestine, apical OCT3 and basolateral OCT1 primarily mediate metformin absorption. In the liver, basolateral OCT1 and OCT3 uptake metformin from the sinusoidal blood into hepatocytes, whereas apical MATE1 is thought to efflux metformin into the bile. In renal proximal tubule cells, OCT2, MATE1, and MATE2-K are essential for the renal tubular secretory system of metformin [56]. The pharmacological action site of metformin is the liver, but renal excretion as an unchanged form, is the main elimination route of metformin, which primarily contributes to determining the systemic exposure of metformin along with intestinal absorption. Metformin disposition changes, such as in plasma and tissue concentration with relevant pharmacological effect alterations is determined by OCT and MATE mediated metformin transport. This has been proven based on studies conducted of metformin administration to patients with OCTs and MATEs genetic polymorphisms, as well as OCTs and MATEs knock-out mice [101,113–115]. With regards to DDIs of metformin, Cho et al. [19] reported that rifampin significantly enhanced the glucose-lowering action of metformin (54.5% of $AUC_{glucose}$ with $P = 0.020$) due to the increased mRNA level of OCT1 by rifampin probably enhancing hepatic uptake of metformin. Conversely, co-administration of an OCT1 inhibitor, verapamil, with metformin decreased the glucose-lowering effect of metformin without increases of systemic exposure of metformin in healthy participants [18]. In mice, co-infusion of cimetidine increases metformin concentrations in the liver and kidneys, due to the inhibition of mMate1-mediated metformin export to biliary excretion and renal excretion, respectively [51,55,56], suggesting that cimetidine exerts MATE1 inhibition-mediated interaction with metformin. In another mouse study, co-administration of metformin with pyrimethamine, a MATE inhibitor, also resulted in a ~2.5-fold increase in liver AUC of metformin compared with controls (i.e., metformin alone administration [101,102,114,115]). These examples indicate that the inhibition or induction of transporters primarily mediating drug disposition to pharmacological target tissue has a strong potential to alter the efficacy of the drug, regardless of the systemic exposure, such as plasma concentration.

Although we focused on DDIs in this review, similar phenomena have been observed in herb-drug interactions. Han et al. [67] reported that the glucose tolerance activity of metformin was enhanced without a change of metformin plasma concentration, because the metformin concentration in the liver increased as a result of a reduction of mate1-mediated biliary excretion of metformin in rats simultaneously treated with metformin and *Lonicera japonica* extract. Considering that renal clearance is the main route of metformin's elimination, only hepatic transporter-mediated interactions of metformin will impact its hepatic concentration, and therefore, affect the PD effect without the alteration of its plasma concentration.

Interestingly, there were several cases where the systemic exposure and tissue exposure of a drug changed in the opposite direction (e.g., increase of systemic exposure and decrease of hepatic exposure). For example, when paroxetine is co-administered with pravastatin in rats, paroxetine increased the systemic exposure and decreased the liver exposure of pravastatin by the combined effects of an increase in intestinal absorption and a decrease in hepatic uptake of pravastatin via Oatp2 inhibition as well as increased biliary excretion via Mrp2 inhibition [96]. The reduced hepatic exposure of pravastatin had a trend to weaken the lipid-lowing effect of pravastatin in diabetic rats [20,21] in spite of the increased systemic exposure of pravastatin. In a case of herb-drug interactions, You et al. [66] reported that the AUC of metformin was increased due to the decrease of oct2-mediated renal excretion of metformin, and thus, the metformin concentration in the kidneys increased due to the increase in oct1-mediated renal uptake of metformin along with the enhancement of its glucose-lowering effect in rats with 28-day co-treatment of metformin and *Houttuynia cordata* (*H. Cordata*) extract. Considering that metformin's pharmacological action site is the liver, the enhanced glucose-lowering effect is probably due to increased hepatic uptake of metformin by the *H. Cordata* extract. In spite of an increase of metformin's systemic exposure, any toxicity of metformin identified as renal dysfunction and lactic acidosis were not observed. Thus, the metformin-*H. Cordata* extract combination case can be included as an example of a local tissue concentration change more strongly affecting the PD effect.

3.3. Additional Factors Affecting PD Effects with Changes of Systemic Exposure or Local Tissue Concentration of a Victim Drug

Additional underlying mechanisms can also cause PD alterations in DDIs. The first case represents how a PK change of an active metabolite can affect the PD effect in DDIs. In the case of clopidogrel with co-administration of aspirin, the systemic exposure of clopidogrel is reduced due to the intestinal P-gp induction lowering the bioavailability of clopidogrel, but the relative platelet inhibition effect of clopidogrel is not changed [29]. Since co-administered aspirin increases clopidogrel metabolism via CYP2C19 and the AUC of the active thiol metabolite, H4, of clopidogrel is consequently increased, the reduced platelet inhibition effect due to the reduced AUC of clopidogrel might be compensated for by an increase of H4's AUC [29]. This example indicates that the systemic exposure of a parent drug is not always able to explain the alteration of PD effect, and the systemic exposure of active metabolites can also cause PD changes. Thus, the systemic exposure of a parent drug, as well as active metabolites need to be considered together, especially when predicting pharmacological effects.

The second case is that the co-administration interval between a victim drug and a perpetrator drug can determine the PD effect. Co-administration of nuciferine, as a potential inhibitor of OCT1 and MATE, time-dependently reduced the glucose-lowering effect of metformin and the hepatic metformin concentration. The hepatic metformin concentration was increased until 1 h after nuciferine administration, which subsequently enhanced the glucose-lowering effect of metformin only during the 2.5-4 h after nuciferine co-administration [99]. If the metformin concentration in the liver is measured at longer time intervals after nuciferine co-administration, the increased hepatic metformin concentration, due to the increased OCT1 and reduced MATE1 transport activity for metformin movement by nuciferine would not be detected, and the alteration of the glucose-lowering effect would also be in the same direction. This example indicates that the onset and duration time of pharmacological action is one factor to be considered to evaluate the PK and PD changes in DDIs.

4. Challenging Experimental Approaches for Exploring the Transporter- or Metabolic Enzyme-Mediated Ddis

It is necessary to explore the expression or activity changes of transporters- or metabolic enzymes responsible for DDI occurrences. Even though the guidance from regulatory agents (e.g., EMA and FDA), labeling recommendations, and the reported references have informed the DDI potential, general in vitro and in vivo methods, as well as clinically designed approaches have been applied in DDI evaluations [22–25,37] and elsewhere, the inconsistency between the clinical relevance and the accumulated information (or experimental results) is still present [66,67,79,98] and elsewhere. Besides the conventional tools (e.g., western blot analysis, q-PCR analysis, permeability test, etc.) to measure the protein and mRNA expression or activity of transporters or metabolic enzymes in tissues, require a guess as to the target causing PK alteration. Therefore, the proteomic quantification methods with "total protein approach" (TPA) for transporters and metabolic enzymes in liver or intestines have been attempted [116]. The TPA-based quantification of transporters and enzymes in human liver tissue samples using liquid chromatography-tandem mass spectrometry can detect their protein expression levels, which could correlate with the results from the targeted proteomic quantitation. This challenging TPA-based quantification can identify as many proteins as possible in a small volume of the same sample and does not require standards [116,117]. In addition, unexpected interplay of transporters or metabolic enzymes in DDI events can be detected by TPA-based quantification approach.

As an experimental approach to investigate the tissue exposure, microdialysis technique in tissue distribution studies has recently been introduced, making it possible to measure the drug concentration at multiple time points in one living animal [118,119]. Animals are sacrificed at each sampling point using the classical experimental approaches to measure drug concentration in tissues, and at least four sampling time points are recommended to explain the tissue distribution pattern changes in DDIs, considering C_{max} and terminal half-life [90,120]. Additionally, (1) composition of a victim drug and a perpetrator drug, and (2) the dosage regimen are suggested to be considered in designing in vivo conventional PK experiments. A perpetrator drug can be chosen as an index substrate, inhibitor or inducer of the transporter or metabolic enzyme responsible for the PK of a victim drug, or as a highly recommended drug in clinical combination therapies [3,25,28]. The dosage regimens, including doses, treatment period (i.e., single or multiple treatments), and drug-dosing schedule of a victim drug and a perpetrator drug, can result in different DDI events [6,22–25,66,67,121].

5. Concluding Remarks

Evaluations of DDIs are a crucial issue for drug efficacy and safety. Although methodologies to evaluate DDIs and information about mechanisms of PK-based DDIs have greatly advanced, the incidences and severity of DDIs still remain high in clinical cases. Moreover, previously unknown DDIs have been revealed and their mechanisms have been suggested in clinical DDI studies, but most of them have then been confirmed by, for example, in vitro studies through a reverse translation process. Since clinical DDI studies may not cover the numerous combinations and various factors that cause these outcomes, it is necessary to interpret the PK and PD data to provide a comprehensive understanding of DDIs with clinical relevance. Although there is currently no optimal way to study DDIs, its evaluation needs to be based on interpretation of the available data about PK-based DDIs, which can ensure the safety and maximal usefulness of DDI studies.

References

1. Wiggins, B.S.; Saseen, J.J.; Page, R.L., II; Reed, B.N.; Sneed, K.; Kostis, J.B.; Lanfear, D.; Virani, S.; Morris, P.B. Recommendations for management of clinically significant drug-drug interactions with statins and select agents used in patients with cardiovascular disease. *Circulations* **2016**, *134*, e468–e495.
2. Dechanont, S.; Maphanta, S.; Butthum, B.; Kongkaew, C. Hospital admissions/visits associated with drug-drug interactions: A systemic review and meta-analysis. *Pharmacoepidemiol. Drug Saf.* **2014**, *23*, 489–497. [CrossRef] [PubMed]
3. Huang, S.M.; Strong, J.M.; Zhang, L.; Reynolds, K.S.; Nallani, S.; Temple, R.; Abraham, S.; Habet, S.A.; Baweja, R.K.; Burchart, G.J.; et al. New era in drug interaction evaluations: US Food and Drug Administration update on CYP enzymes, transporters, and guideline process. *J. Clin. Pharmacol.* **2008**, *48*, 662–670. [CrossRef] [PubMed]
4. Yu, J.; Zhou, Z.; Tay-Sontheimer, J.; Levy, R.H.; Ragueneau-Majlessi, I. Risk of clinically relevant pharmacokinetic-based drug-drug interactions with drugs approved by the U.S. Food and Drug Administration between 2013 and 2016. *Drug Metab. Dispos.* **2018**, *46*, 835–845. [CrossRef]
5. Ito, K.; Iwatsubo, T.; Kanamitsu, S.; Ueda, K.; Suzuki, H.; Sugiyama, Y. Prediction of pharmacokinetic alterations caused by drug-drug interactions: Metabolic interaction in the liver. *Pharmacol. Rev.* **1998**, *50*, 387–411.
6. Zhang, D.; Hop, C.E.; Patilea-Vrana, G.; Gampa, G.; Seneviratne, H.K.; Unadkat, J.D.; Kenny, J.R.; Nagapudi, K.; Di, L.; Zhou, L.; et al. Drug concentration asymmetry in tissues and plasma for small molecule–related therapeutic modalities. *Drug Metab. Dispos.* **2019**, *47*, 1122–1135. [CrossRef]
7. Mager, D.E.; Jusko, W.J. General pharmacokinetic model for drugs exhibiting target-mediated drug disposition. *J. Pharmacokinet. Pharmacodyn.* **2001**, *28*, 507–532. [CrossRef]
8. Rankovic, Z. CNS drug design: Balancing physicochemical properties for optimal brain exposure. *J. Med. Chem.* **2015**, *58*, 2584–2608. [CrossRef]

9. Smith, D.A.; Di, L.; Kerns, E.H. The effect of plasma protein binding on in vivo efficacy: Misconceptions in drug discovery. *Nat. Rev. Drug Discov.* **2010**, *9*, 929–939. [CrossRef]
10. Di, L.; Umland, J.P.; Trapa, P.E.; Maurer, T.S. Impact of recovery on fraction unbound using equilibrium dialysis. *J. Pharm. Sci.* **2012**, *101*, 1327–1335. [CrossRef]
11. Di, L.; Breen, C.; Chambers, R.; Eckley, S.T.; Fricke, R.; Ghosh, A.; Harradine, P.; Kalvass, J.C.; Ho, S.; Lee, C.A. et al. Industry perspective on contemporary protein-binding methodologies: Considerations for regulatory drug-drug interaction and related guidelines on highly bound drugs. *J. Pharm. Sci.* **2017**, *106*, 3442–3452 [CrossRef]
12. Gabrielsson, J.; Peletier, I.A. Pharmacokinetic steady-states highlight interesting target-mediated disposition properties. *AAPS J.* **2017**, *19*, 772–786. [CrossRef] [PubMed]
13. Van Waterschoot, R.A.; Parrott, N.J.; Olivares-Moralres, A.; Lave, T.; Rowland, M.; Smith, D.A. Impact of target interactions on small-molecule drug disposition: An overlooked area. *Nat. Rev. Drug Discov.* **2018**, *17* 299–301. [CrossRef]
14. Li, R.; Kimoto, E.; Niosi, M.; Tess, D.A.; Lin, J.; Tremaine, L.M.; Di, L. A study on pharmacokinetics of bosentan with systems modeling, part 2: Prospectively predicting systemic and liver exposure in healthy subjects. *Drug Metab. Dispos.* **2018**, *46*, 357–366. [CrossRef] [PubMed]
15. Li, R.; Niosi, M.; Johnson, N.; Tess, D.A.; Kimoto, E.; Lin, J.; Yang, X.; Riccardi, K.A.; Ryu, S.; El-Kattan, A.F. et al. A study on pharmacokinetics of bosentan with systems modeling, part 1: Translating systemic plasma concentration to liver exposure in healthy subjects. *Drug Metab. Dispos.* **2018**, *46*, 346–356. [CrossRef]
16. Tsamandouras, N.; Dickinson, G.; Guo, Y.; Hall, S.; Rostami-Hodjegan, A.; Galetin, A.; Aarons, L. Development and application of a mechanistic pharmacokinetic model for simvastatin and its active metabolite simvastatin acid using an integrated population PBPK approach. *Pharm. Res.* **2015**, *32*, 1864–1883. [CrossRef] [PubMed]
17. Watanabe, T.; Kusuhara, H.; Maeda, K.; Shitara, Y.; Sugiyama, Y. Physiologically based pharmacokinetic modeling to predict transporter-mediated clearance and distribution of pravastatin in humans. *J. Pharmacol. Exp. Ther.* **2009**, *328*, 652–662. [CrossRef]
18. Cho, S.K.; Kim, C.O.; Park, E.S.; Chung, J.Y. Verapamil decreases the glucose-lowering effect of metformin in healthy volunteers. *Br. J. Clin. Pharmacol.* **2014**, *78*, 1426–1432. [CrossRef]
19. Cho, S.K.; Yoo, J.S.; Lee, M.G.; Lee, D.H.; Lim, L.A.; Park, K.; Park, M.S.; Chung, J.Y. Rifampin enhances the glucose-lowering effect of metformin and increases OCT1 mRNA levels in healthy participants *Clin. Pharmacol. Ther.* **2011**, *89*, 416–421. [CrossRef]
20. Li, F.; Zhang, M.; Xu, D.; Liu, C.; Zhong, Z.Y.; Jia, L.L.; Hu, M.Y.; Yang, Y.; Liu, L.; Liu, X.D. Co-administration of paroxetine and pravastatin causes deregulation of glucose homeostasis in diabetic rats via enhanced paroxetine exposure. *Acta. Pharmacol. Sin.* **2014**, *35*, 792–805. [CrossRef]
21. Hasegawa, Y.; Kishimoto, S.; Shibatani, N.; Inotsume, N.; Takeuchi, Y.; Fukushima, S. The disposition of pravastatin in a rat model of streptozotocin-induced diabetes and organic anion transporting polypeptide 2 and multidrug resistance associated protein 2 expression in the liver. *Biol. Pharm. Bull.* **2010**, *33*, 153–156 [CrossRef] [PubMed]
22. European Medicines Agency. Guideline on the Investigation of Drug Interactions. 2012. Available online: https://www.ema.europa.eu/documents/scientific-guideline/guideline-investigation-drug-interactions-en/pdf (accessed on 15 February 2019).
23. US Food and Drug Administration, Center for Drug Evaluation and Research. Clinical Drug Interaction Studies-Study Design, Data Analysis, and Clinical Implications Guideline for Industry. 2017. Available online: https://www.fda.gov/downloads/drugs/guidances/ucm292362.pdf (accessed on 27 February 2020).
24. Yu, J.; Petrie, I.D.; Levy, R.H.; Ragueneau-Majlessi, I. Mechanisms and clinical significance of pharmacokinetic-based drug-drug interactions with drug approved by the U.S. Food and Drug Administration in 2017. *Drug Metab. Dispos.* **2019**, *47*, 135–144. [CrossRef]
25. Tornio, A.; Filppula, A.M.; Niemi, M.; Backman, J.T. Clinical studies on drug-drug interactions involving metabolism and transport: Methodology, pitfalls, and interpretation. *Clin. Pharmacol. Ther.* **2019**, *105*, 1345–1361. [CrossRef] [PubMed]
26. Chen, X.P.; Tan, Z.R.; Huang, Z.; Ou-Yang, D.S.; Zhou, H.H. Isozyme-specific induction of low-dose aspirin on cytochrome P450 in healthy subjects. *Clin. Pharmacol. Ther.* **2003**, *73*, 264–271. [CrossRef] [PubMed]
27. Li, M.-P.; Tang, J.; Zhang, Z.-L.; Chen, X.-P. Induction of both P-glycoprotein and specific cytochrome P450 by aspirin eventually does not alter the antithrombotic effect of clopidogrel. *Clin. Pharmacol. Ther.* **2015**, *97*, 324. [CrossRef] [PubMed]

28. Morgan, P.; Brown, D.G.; Lennard, S.; Anderton, M.J.; Barrett, J.C.; Eriksson, U.; Fidock, M.; Hamren, B.; Johnson, A.; March, R.E.; et al. Impact of a five-dimensional framework on R&D productivity at AstraZeneca. *Nat. Rev. Drug Dispos.* **2018**, *17*, 167–181.
29. Oh, J.; Shin, D.; Lim, K.S.; Lee, S.; Jung, K.-H.; Chu, K.; Hong, K.S.; Shin, K.-H.; Cho, J.-Y.; Yoon, S.H.; et al. Aspirin decreases systemic exposure to clopidogrel through modulation of P-glycoprotein but does not alter its antithrombotic activity. *Clin. Pharmacol. Ther.* **2014**, *95*, 608–616. [CrossRef]
30. Poulin, P. A paradigm shift in pharmacokinetic-pharmacodynamic (PKPD) modeling: Rule of thumb for estimating free drug level in tissue compared with plasma to guide drug design. *J. Pharm. Sci.* **2015**, *104*, 2359–2368. [CrossRef]
31. Poulin, P.; Haddad, S. Advancing prediction of tissue distribution and volume of distribution of highly lipophilic compounds from simplified tissue composition-based models as a mechanistic animal alternative model. *J. Pharm. Sci.* **2012**, *101*, 2250–2261. [CrossRef]
32. Rurak, C.D.; Hack, C.E.; Robinson, P.J.; Mahle, D.A.; Gearheart, M. Predicting passive and active tissue:plasma partition coefficient: Interindividual and interspecies variability. *J. Pharm. Sci.* **2014**, *103*, 2189–2198. [CrossRef]
33. Shirata, Y.; Hoire, T.; Sigiyama, Y. Transporters as a determinant of drug clearance and tissue distribution. *Eur. J. Pharm. Sci.* **2006**, *27*, 425–446.
34. Shitara, Y.; Maeda, K.; Ikejiri, K.; Yoshida, K.; Horie, T.; Sugiyama, Y. Clinical significance of organic anion transporting polypeptides (OATPs) in drug disposition: Their roles in hepatic clearance and intestinal absorption. *Biopharm. Drug Dispos.* **2013**, *34*, 45–78. [CrossRef]
35. Bosilkovska, M.; Samer, C.; Déglon, J.; Thomas, A.; Walder, B.; Desmeules, J.; Daali, Y. Evaluation of mutual drug-drug interaction within Geneva cocktail for cytochrome P450 phenotying using innovative dried blood sampling method. *Basic Clin. Pharmacol. Ther.* **2016**, *119*, 284–290. [CrossRef]
36. Fuhr, U.; Hsin, C.H.; Li, X.; Jabrane, W.; Sorgel, F. Assessment of pharmacokinetic drug-drug interactions in humans: In vivo probe substrates for drug metabolism and drug transporter revised. *Annu. Rev. Pharmacol. Toxicol.* **2019**, *59*, 507–536. [CrossRef]
37. Yoshida, K.; Zhao, P.; Zhang, L.; Abernethy, D.R.; Rekic, D.; Reynolds, K.S.; Galetin, A.; Huang, S.M. In vitro-ion vivo extrapolation of metabolism- and transporter-mediated drug-drug interactions-overview of basic prediction methods. *J. Pharm. Sci.* **2017**, *106*, 2209–2213. [CrossRef]
38. Gessnet, A.; Konig, J.; Fromm, M.F. Clinical aspects of transporter-mediated drug-drug interactions. *Clin. Pharmacol. Ther.* **2019**, *105*, 1386–1394. [CrossRef]
39. Müller, F.; Fromm, M.F. Transporter-mediated drug-drug interactions. *Pharmacogenomics* **2011**, *12*, 1017–1037. [CrossRef]
40. Zhang, L.; Huang, S.M.; Lesko, L.J. Transporter-mediated drug-drug interactions. *Clin. Pharmacol. Ther.* **2011**, *89*, 481–484. [CrossRef]
41. Morrissey, K.M.; Stocker, S.L.; Wittwer, M.B.; Xu, L.; Giacomini, K.M. Renal transporters in drug development. *Annu. Rev. Pharmacol. Toxicol.* **2013**, *53*, 503–529. [CrossRef]
42. Yoshida, K.; Maeda, K.; Sugiyama, Y. Hepatic and intestinal drug transporters: Prediction of pharmacokinetic effects caused by drug-drug interactions and genetic polymorphisms. *Annu. Rev. Pharmacol. Toxicol.* **2013**, *53*, 581–612. [CrossRef]
43. König, J.; Fabian Müller, F.; Fromm, M.F. Transporters and drug-drug interactions: Important determinants of drug disposition and effects. *Pharmacol. Rev.* **2013**, *65*, 944–966. [CrossRef]
44. Zientek, M.A.; Youdim, K. Reaction phenotyping: Advances in the experimental strategies used to characterize the contribution of drug-metabolizing enzymes. *Drug Metab. Dispos.* **2015**, *43*, 163–181. [CrossRef]
45. Almazroo, O.A.; Miah, M.K.; Venkataramanan, R. Drug metabolism in the liver. *Clin. Liver Dis.* **2017**, *21*, 1–20. [CrossRef]
46. Mittal, B.; Tulsyan, S.; Kumar, S.; Mittal, R.D.; Agarwal, G. Cytochrome P450 in cancer susceptibility and treatment. *Adv. Clin. Chem.* **2015**, *71*, 77–139.
47. Olsen, L.; Oostenbrink, C.; Jorgensen, F.S. Prediction of cytochrome P450 mediated metabolism. *Adv. Drug Deliv. Rev.* **2015**, *86*, 61–71. [CrossRef]
48. Achour, B.; Barber, J.; Rostami-Hodjegan, A. Expression of hepatic drug metabolizing cytochrome p450 enzymes and their intercorrelations: A meta-analysis. *Drug Metab. Dispos.* **2014**, *42*, 1349–1356. [CrossRef]

49. Wang, Q.; Jia, R.; Ye, C.; Garcia, M.; Li, J.; Hidalgo, I.J. Glucuronidation and sulfation of 7-hydroxycoumarin in liver matrices from human, dog, monkey, rat, and mouse. *In Vitro Cell Dev. Biol. Anim.* **2005**, *41*, 97–103. [CrossRef]
50. Terada, T.; Hira, D. Intestinal and hepatic drug transporters: Pharmacokinetic, pathophysiological, and pharmacogenetic roles. *J. Gastroenterol.* **2015**, *50*, 508–519. [CrossRef]
51. Ito, S.; Kusuhara, H.; Yokochi, M.; Toyoshima, J.; Inoue, K.; Yuasa, H.; Sugiyama, Y. Competitive inhibition of the luminal efflux by multidrug and toxin extrusions, but not basolateral uptake by organic cation transporter 2, is the likely mechanism underlying the pharmacokinetic drug-drug interactions caused by cimetidine in the kidney. *J. Pharmacol. Exp. Ther.* **2012**, *340*, 393–403. [CrossRef]
52. Kalliokoski, A.; Niemi, M. Impact of OATP transporters on pharmacokinetics. *Br. J. Pharmacol.* **2009**, *158*, 693–705.
53. Chang, J.H.; Ly, J.; Plise, E.; Zhang, X.; Messick, K.; Wright, M.; Cheong, J. Differential effects of rifampin and ketoconazole on the blood and liver concentration of atorvastatin in wild-type and Cyp3a and Oatp1a/b knockout mice. *Drug Metab. Dispos.* **2014**, *42*, 1067–1073.
54. Lepist, E.I.; Ray, A.S. Renal drug-drug interactions: What we have learned and where we are going. *Exp. Opin. Drug Metab. Toxicol.* **2012**, *8*, 433–448.
55. Lepist, E.-I.; Ray, A.S. Renal transporter-mediated drug-drug interactions: Are they clinically relevant? *J. Clin. Pharmacol.* **2016**, *56*, S73–S81.
56. Liang, X.; Giacomini, K.M. Transporters involved in metformin pharmacokinetics and treatment response. *J. Pharm. Sci.* **2017**, *106*, 2245–2250.
57. Stieger, B.; Mahdi, Z.M.; Jager, W. Intestinal and hepatocellular transporters: Therapeutic effects and drug interactions of herbal supplements. *Annu. Rev. Pharmacol. Toxicol.* **2017**, *57*, 399–416.
58. Benet, L.Z.; Hoener, B.A. Changes in plasma protein binding have little clinical relevance. *Clin. Pharmacol. Ther.* **2002**, *71*, 115–121.
59. Liu, X.; Wright, M.; Hop, C.E. Rational use of plasma protein and tissue binding data in drug design. *J. Med. Chem.* **2014**, *57*, 8238–8248.
60. Hochman, J.; Tang, C.; Prueksaritanont, T. Drug-drug interactions related to altered absorption and plasma protein binding: Theoretical and regulatory considerations, and an industry perspective. *J. Pharm. Sci.* **2015**, *104*, 916–929.
61. Kim, D.H. Gut microbiota-mediated drug-antibiotic interactions. *Drug Metab. Dispos.* **2015**, *43*, 1581–1589.
62. Kehrer, D.F.; Sparreboom, A.; Verweij, J.; de Bruijn, P.; Nierop, C.A.; van de Schraaf, J.; Ruijgrok, E.J.; de Jonge, M.J. Modulation of irinotecan-induced diarrhea by cotreatment with neomycin in cancer patients. *Clin. Cancer Res.* **2001**, *7*, 1136–1141.
63. Chiba, M.; Ishii, Y.; Sugiyama, Y. Prediction of hepatic clearance in human from in vitro data for successful drug development. *AAPS J.* **2009**, *11*, 262–276.
64. Watanabe, T.; Kusuhara, H.; Sugiyama, Y. Application of physiologically based pharmacokinetic modeling and clearance concept to drugs showing transporter-mediated distribution and clearance in humans. *J. Pharmacokinet. Pharmacodyn.* **2010**, *37*, 575–590.
65. Motohashi, H.; Inui, K. Multidrug and toxin extrusion family SLC47: Physiological, pharmacokinetic and toxicokinetic importance of MATE1 and MATE2-k. *Mol. Aspects Med.* **2013**, *34*, 661–668.
66. You, B.H.; Chin, Y.-W.; Kim, H.; Choi, H.S.; Choi, Y.H. *Houttuynia cordata* extract increased systemic exposure and liver concentrations of metformin through OCTs and MATEs in rats. *Phytother. Res.* **2018**, *32*, 1004–1013.
67. Han, S.Y.; Chae, H.-S.; You, B.H.; Chin, Y.-W.; Kim, H.; Choi, H.S.; Choi, Y.H. *Lonicera japonica* extract increases metformin distribution in the liver without change of systemic exposed metformin in rats. *Phytother. Res.* **2019**, *32*, 1004–1013.
68. Manohar, S.; Leung, N. Cisplatin nephrotoxicity: A review of the literature. *J. Nephrol.* **2018**, *31*, 15–25.
69. Sprowl, J.A.; van Doorn, L.; Hu, S.; van Gerven, L.; de Bruijm, P.; Li, L.; Gibson, A.A.; Mathijssen, R.H.; Sparreboom, A. Conjunctive therapy of cisplatin with the OCT2 inhibitor cimetidine: Influence on antitumor efficacy and systemic clearance. *Clin. Pharmacol. Ther.* **2013**, *94*, 585–592.
70. Frost, C.E.; Byon, W.; Song, Y.; Wang, J.; Schuster, A.E.; Boyd, R.A.; Zhang, D.; Yu, C.; Dias, C.; Shenker, A.; et al. Effect of ketoconazole and diltiazem on the pharmacokinetics of apixaban, an oral direct factor Xa inhibitor. *Br. J. Clin. Pharmacol.* **2015**, *79*, 838–846.

71. Hartter, S.; Koenen-Bergmann, M.; Sharma, A.; Nehmiz, G.; Lemke, U.; Timmer, W.; Reilly, P.A. Decrease in the oral bioavailability of dabigatran etexilate after co-medication with rifampicin. *Br. J. Clin. Pharmacol.* **2012**, *74*, 490–500.
72. Greiner, B.; Eichelbaum, M.; Fritz, P.; Kreichgauer, H.-P.; von Richter, O.; Zundler, J.; Kroemer, H.K. The role of intestinal P-glycoprotein in the interaction of digoxin and rifampin. *J. Clin. Invest.* **1999**, *104*, 147–153.
73. Sadeque, A.J.; Wandel, C.; He, H.; Shah, S.; Wood, A.J. Increased drug delivery to the brain by P-glycoprotein inhibition. *Clin. Pharmacol. Ther.* **2000**, *68*, 231–237.
74. Allred, A.J.; Bowe, C.J.; Park, J.W.; Peng, B.; Williams, D.D.; Wire, M.B.; Lee, E. Eltrombopag increases plasma rosuvastatin exposure in healthy volunteers. *Br. J. Clin. Pharmacol.* **2011**, *72*, 321–329.
75. Elsby, R.; Martin, P.; Surry, D.; Sharma, P.; Fenner, K. Solitary inhibition of the breast cancer resistance protein efflux transporter results in a clinically significant drug-drug interaction with rosuvastatin by causing up to a 2-fold increase in statin exposure. *Drug Metab. Dispos.* **2016**, *44*, 398–408.
76. Rengelshausen, J.; Goggelmann, C.; Burhenne, J.; Riedel, K.D.; Ludwig, J.; Weiss, J.; Mikus, G.; Walter-Sack, I.; Haefeli, W.E. Contribution of increased oral bioavailability and reduced nonglomerular renal clearance of digoxin to the digoxin-clarithromycin interaction. *Br. J. Clin. Pharmacol.* **2003**, *56*, 32–38.
77. Asberg, A.; Hartmann, A.; Fjeldså, E.; Bergan, S.; Holdaas, H. Bilateral pharmacokinetic interaction between cyclosporine A and atorvastatin in renal transplant recipients. *Am. J. Transplant.* **2001**, *1*, 382–386.
78. Asberg, A. Interactions between cyclosporin and lipid-lowering drugs: Implications for organ transplant recipients. *Drugs* **2003**, *63*, 367–378.
79. Maeda, K.; Ikeda, Y.; Fujita, T.; Yoshida, K.; Azuma, Y.; Haruyama, Y.; Yamane, N.; Kumagai, Y.; Sugiyama, Y. Identification of the rate-determining process in the hepatic clearance of atorvastatin in a clinical cassette microdosing study. *Clin. Pharmacol. Ther.* **2011**, *90*, 575–581.
80. Mazzu, A.L.; Lasseter, K.C.; Shamblen, E.C.; Agarwal, V.; Lettieri, J.; Sundaresen, P. Itraconazole alters the pharmacokinetics of atorvastatin to a greater extent than either cerivastatin or pravastatin. *Clin. Pharmacokinet. Ther.* **2000**, *68*, 391–400.
81. Markert, C.; Schweizer, Y.; Hellwig, R.; Wirsching, T.; Riedel, K.D.; Burhenne, J.; Weiss, J.; Mikus, G.; Haefeli, W.E. Clarithromycin substantially increases steady-state bosentan exposure in healthy volunteers. *Br. J. Clin. Pharmacol.* **2014**, *77*, 141–148.
82. Fattinger, K.; Funk, C.; Pantze, M.; Weber, C.; Reichen, J.; Stieger, B.; Meier, P.J. The endothelin antagonist bosentan inhibits the canalicular bile salt export pump: A potential mechanism for hepatic adverse reactions. *Clin. Pharmacol. Ther.* **2001**, *69*, 223–231.
83. Preston, C.L. *Stockley's Drug Interactions*, 11th ed.; Pharmaceutical Press: London, UK, 2016.
84. Prueksaritanont, T.; Chu, X.; Evers, R.; Klopfer, S.O.; Caro, L.; Kothare, P.A.; Dempsey, C.; Rasmussen, S.; Houle, R.; Chan, G.; et al. Pitavastatin is a more sensitive and selective organic anion-transporting polypeptide 1B clinical probe than rosuvastatin. *Br. J. Clin. Pharmacol.* **2014**, *78*, 587–598.
85. Jacobson, T.A. Comparative pharmacokinetic interaction profiles of pravastatin, simvastatin, and atorvastatin when coadministered with cytochrome P450 inhibitors. *Am. J. Cardiol.* **2004**, *94*, 1140–1146.
86. Simonson, S.G.; Raza, A.; Martin, P.D.; Mitchell, P.D.; Jarcho, J.A.; Brown, C.D.; Windass, A.S.; Schneck, D.W. Rosuvastatin pharmacokinetics in heart transplant recipients administered an antirejection regimen including cyclosporine. *Clin. Pharmacol. Ther.* **2004**, *76*, 167–177.
87. He, J.; Yu, Y.; Prasad, B.; Link, J.; Miyaoka, R.S.; Chen, X.; Unadkat, J.D. PET imaging of Oatp mediated hepatobiliary transport of [(11)C] rosuvastatin in the rat. *Mol. Pharm.* **2014**, *11*, 2745–2754.
88. Schneck, D.W.; Birmingham, B.K.; Zalikowski, J.A.; Mitchell, P.D.; Wang, Y.; Martin, P.D.; Lasseter, K.C.; Brown, C.D.; Windass, A.S.; Raza, A. The effect of gemfibrozil on the pharmacokinetics of rosuvastatin. *Clin. Pharmacol. Ther.* **2004**, *75*, 455–463.
89. Maeda, K.; Tian, Y.; Fujita, T.; Ikeda, Y.; Kumagai, Y.; Kondo, T.; Tanabe, K.; Nakayama, H.; Horita, S.; Kusuhara, H.; et al. Inhibitory effects of p-aminohippurate and probenecid on the renal clearance of adefovir and benzylpenicillin as probe drugs for organic anion transporter (OAT) 1 and OAT3 in humans. *Eur. J. Pharm. Sci.* **2014**, *59*, 94–103.
90. Leahey, E.B.; Bigger, J.T.; Butler, V.P.; Reiffel, J.A.; O'Connell, G.C.; Scaffidi, L.E.; Rottman, J.N. Quinidine-digoxin interaction: Time course and pharmacokinetics. *Am. J. Cardiol.* **1981**, *48*, 1141–1146.

91. Moore, K.H.; Yuen, G.J.; Raasch, R.H.; Eron, J.J.; Martin, D.; Mydlow, P.K.; Hussey, E.K. Pharmacokinetics of lamivudine administered alone and with trimethoprim-sulfamethoxazole. *Clin. Pharmacol. Ther.* **1996**, *59*, 550–558.
92. Müller, F.; Konig, J.; Hoier, E.; Mandery, K.; Fromm, M.F. Role of organic cation transporter OCT2 and multidrug and toxin extrusion proteins MATE1 and MATE2-K for transport and drug interactions of the antiviral lamivudine. *Biochem. Pharmacol.* **2013**, *86*, 808–815.
93. Grun, B.; Kiessling, M.K.; Burhenne, J.; Riedel, K.D.; Weiss, J.; Rauch, G.; Haefeli, W.E.; Czock, D Trimethoprim-metformin interaction and its genetic modulation by OCT2 and MATE1 transporters. *Br. J. Clin. Pharmacol.* **2013**, *76*, 787–796.
94. Müller, F.; Pontones, C.A.; Renner, B.; Mieth, M.; Hoier, E.; Auge, D.; Maas, R.; Zolk, O.; Fromm, M.F N1-methylnicotinamide as an endogenous probe for drug interactions by renal cation transporters: Studies on the metformin-trimethoprim interaction. *Eur. J. Clin. Pharmacol.* **2015**, *71*, 85–94.
95. Song, I.H.; Zong, J.; Borland, J.; Jerva, F.; Wynne, B.; Zamek-Gilszczynski, M.J.; Humphreys, J.E.; Bowers, G.D.; Choukour, M. The effect of dolutegravir on the pharmacokinetics of metformin in healthy subjects. *J. Acquir. Immune. Defic. Syndr.* **2016**, *72*, 400–407.
96. Li, F.; Xu, D.; Shu, N.; Zhong, Z.; Zhang, M.; Liu, C.; Ling, Z.; Liu, L.; Liu, X. Co-administration of paroxetine increased the systemic exposure of pravastatin in diabetic rats due to the decrease in liver distribution *Xenobiotica* **2015**, *45*, 794–802.
97. Grube, M.; Köck, K.; Oswald, S.; Draber, K.; Meissner, K.; Eckel, L.; Böhm, M.; Felix, S.B.; Vogelgesang, S.; Jedlitschky, G.; et al. Organic anion transporting polypeptide 2B1 is a high-affinity transporter for atorvastatin and is expressed in the human heart. *Clin. Pharmacol. Ther.* **2006**, *80*, 607–620.
98. Shin, E.; Shin, N.; Oh, J.-H.; Lee, Y.-J. High-dose metformin may increase the concentration of atorvastatin in the liver by inhibition of multidrug resistance-associated protein 2. *J. Pharm. Sci.* **2017**, *106*, 961–967.
99. Li, L.; Lei, H.; Wang, W.; Du, W.; Yuan, J.; Yuan, J.; Tu, M.; Zhou, H.; Zeng, S.; Jiang, H. Co-administration of nuciferine reduced the concentration of metformin in liver via differential inhibition of hepatic drug transporter OCT1 and MATE1. *Biopharm. Drug Dispos.* **2018**, *39*, 411–419.
100. Somogyi, A.; Stockley, C.; Keal, J.; Rolan, P.; Bochner, F. Reduction of metformin renal tubular secretion by cimetidine in man. *Br. J. Clin. Pharmacol.* **1987**, *23*, 545–551.
101. Stocker, S.L.; Morrissey, K.M.; Yee, S.W.; Castro, R.A.; Xu, L.; Dahlin, A.; Ramirez, A.H.; Roden, D.M.; Wilke, R.A.; McCarty, C.A.; et al. The effect of novel promoter variants in MATE1 and MATE2 on the pharmacokinetics and pharmacodynamics of metformin. *Clin. Pharmacol. Ther.* **2013**, *93*, 186–194.
102. Kusuhara, H.; Ito, S.; Kumagai, Y.; Jiang, M.; Shiroshita, T.; Moriyama, Y.; Inoue, K.; Yuasa, H.; Sugiuama, Y Effects of a MATE protein inhibitor, pyrimethamine, on the renal elimination of metformin at oral microdose and at therapeutic dose in healthy subjects. *Clin. Pharmacol. Ther.* **2011**, *89*, 837–844.
103. Ito, S.; Kusuhara, H.; Kuroiwa, Y.; Wu, C.; Moriyama, Y.; Inoue, K.; Kondo, T.; Yuasa, H.; Nakayama, H.; Horita, S.; et al. Potent and specific inhibition of mMate1-mediated efflux of type 1 organic cations in the liver and kidney by pyrimethamine. *J. Pharmakos. Exp. Ther.* **2010**, *333*, 341–350.
104. Choi, Y.H.; Lee, U.; Lee, B.K.; Lee, M.G. Pharmacokinetic interaction between itraconazole and metformin in rats: Competitive inhibition of metabolism of each drug by each other via hepatic and intestinal CYP3A1/2 *Br. J. Pharmacol.* **2010**, *161*, 815–829.
105. Bechmann, K.A.; Lewis, J.D. Predicting inhibitory drug–drug interactions and evaluating drug interaction reports using inhibition constants. *Ann. Pharmacother.* **2005**, *39*, 1064–1072.
106. Ma, Y.; Khojasteh, S.C.; Hop, C.E.; Erickson, H.K.; Polson, A.; Pillow, T.H.; Yu, S.F.; Wang, H.; Dragovich, P.S.; Zhang, D. Antibody drug conjugates differentiate uptake and DNA alkylation of pyrrolobenzodiazepines in tumors from organs of xenograft mice. *Drug Metab. Dispos.* **2016**, *44*, 1958–1962.
107. Zhang, D.; Yu, S.F.; Ma, Y.; Xu, K.; Dragovich, P.S.; Pillow, T.H.; Liu, L.; Del Rosario, G.; He, J.; Pei, Z.; et al. Chemical structure and concentration of intratumor catabolites determine efficacy of antibody drug conjugates. *Drug Metab. Dispos.* **2016**, *44*, 1517–1523.
108. Yamazaki, M.; Suzuki, H.; Sugiyama, Y. Recent advances in carrier-mediated hepatic uptake and biliary excretion of xenobiotics. *Pharm. Res.* **1996**, *13*, 497–513.

109. Shitara, Y.; Sugiyama, Y. Pharmacokinetic and pharmacodynamic alterations of 3-hydroxy-3-methylglutaryl coenzyme A (HMG-CoA) reductase inhibitors: Drug–drug interactions and interindividual differences in transporter and metabolic enzyme functions. *Pharmacol. Ther.* **2006**, *112*, 71–105.
110. Anitha, N.; Rao, J.; Kavimani, S.; Himabindu, V. Pharmacodynamic drug interaction of metformin with statins in rats. *J. Pharmacol. Toxicol.* **2008**, *3*, 409–413.
111. Bjornsson, E.; Jacobsen, E.I.; Kalaitzakis, E. Hepatotoxicity associated with statins: Reports of idiosyncratic liver injury post-marketing. *J. Hepatol.* **2012**, *56*, 374–380.
112. Rose, R.H.; Neuhoff, S.; Abduljalil, K.; Chetty, M.; Rostami-Hodjegan, A.; Jamei, M. Application of a physiologically based pharmacokinetic model to predict OATP1B1-related variability in pharmacodynamics of rosuvastatin. *CPT Pharmacomet. Syst. Pharmacol.* **2014**, *3*, e124.
113. Sundelin, E.; Gormsen, L.C.; Jensen, J.B.; Vendelbo, M.H.; Jakobsen, S.; Munk, O.L.; Christensen, M.; Brøsen, K.; Frøkiaer, J.; Jessen, N. Genetic polymorphisms in organic cation transporter 1 attenuates hepatic metformin exposure in humans. *Clin. Pharmacol. Ther.* **2017**, *102*, 841–848.
114. Jensen, J.B.; Sundelin, E.I.; Jakobsen, S.; Gormsen, L.C.; Munk, O.L.; Frøkier, J.; Jessen, N. [11C]-labeled metformin distribution in the liver and small intestine using dynamic positron emission tomography in mice demonstrates tissue-specific transporter dependency. *Diabetes* **2016**, *65*, 1724–1730.
115. Shu, Y.; Sheardown, S.A.; Brown, C.; Owen, R.P.; Zhang, S.; Castro, R.A.; Ianculescu, A.G.; Yue, L.; Lo, J.C.; Burchard, E.G.; et al. Effect of genetic variation in the organic cation transporter 1 (OCT1) on metformin action. *J. Clin. Invest.* **2007**, *117*, 1422–1431.
116. Vildhede, A.; Nguyen, C.; Erickson, B.K.; Kunz, R.C.; Jones, R.; Kimoto, E. Comparison of proteomic quantification approaches for hepatic drug transporters: Multiplexed global quantitation correlates with targeted proteomic quantitation. *Drug Metab. Dispos.* **2018**, *46*, 692–696.
117. Couto, N.; Al-Majdoub, Z.M.; Gibson, S.; Davies, P.J.; Achour, B.; Harwood, M.D.; Carlson, G.; Barber, J.; Rostami-Hodjegan, A.; Warhurst, G. Quantitative proteomics of clinically relevant drug-metabolizing enzymes and drug transporters and their inter-correlations in the human small intestine. *Drug Metab. Dispos.* **2020**, *48*, 407.
118. Pena, A.; Liu, P.; Derendorf, H. Microdialysis in peripheral tissues. *Adv. Drug Deliv. Rev.* **2000**, *45*, 189–216.
119. Dahyot, C.; Marchand, S.; Bodin, M.; Debeane, B.; Mimoz, O.; Couet, W. Application of basic pharmacokinetic concepts to analysis of microdialysis data: Illustration with imipenem muscle distribution. *Clin. Pharmacokinet.* **2008**, *47*, 181–189.
120. Tuntland, T.; Ethell, B.; Kosaka, T.; Blasco, F.; Zhang, R.X.; Jain, M.; Gould, T.; Hoffmaster, K. Implementation of pharmacokinetic and pharmacodynamic strategies in early research phases of drug discovery and development at Novartis Institute of Biomedical Research. *Front. Pharmacol.* **2014**, *28*, 174.
121. Guo, Y.; Chu, X.; Parrott, N.J.; Brouwer, K.L.R.; Hsu, V.; Nagar, S.; Matsson, P.; Sharma, P.; Snoeys, J.; Sugiyama, Y.; et al. Advancing predictions of tissue and intracellular drug concentrations using in vitro, imaging and physiologically based pharmacokinetic modeling approaches. *Clin. Pharmacol. Ther.* **2018**, *104*, 865–889.

Lack of Correlation between In Vitro and In Vivo Studies on the Inhibitory Effects of (-)-Sophoranone on CYP2C9 is Attributable to Low Oral Absorption and Extensive Plasma Protein Binding of (-)-Sophoranone

Yu Fen Zheng [1,†], Soo Hyeon Bae [2,3,†], Zhouchi Huang [3], Soon Uk Chae [3], Seong Jun Jo [3], Hyung Joon Shim [3], Chae Bin Lee [3], Doyun Kim [3,4], Hunseung Yoo [4] and Soo Kyung Bae [3,*]

1 School of Basic Medicine and Clinical Pharmacy, China Pharmaceutical University, 639 Longmian Road, Jiangning District, Nanjing 211198, China; 1020172557@cpu.edu.cn
2 Q-fitter, Inc., Seoul 06578, Korea; sh.bae@qfitter.com
3 College of Pharmacy and Integrated Research Institute of Pharmaceutical Sciences, The Catholic University, Korea, Bucheon 14662, Korea; hzc0826@catholic.ac.kr (Z.H.); zldtnseoz@naver.com (S.U.C.); sungjun6734@naver.com (S.J.J.); tony6533@naver.com (H.J.S.); aribri727@catholic.ac.kr (C.B.L.); doyun325@naver.com (D.K.)
4 Life Science R&D Center, SK Chemicals, 310 Pangyo-ro, Sungnam 13494, Korea; hs.yoo@sk.com
* Correspondence: baesk@catholic.ac.kr
† These authors contributed equally to this work.

Abstract: (-)-Sophoranone (SPN) is a bioactive component of *Sophora tonkinensis* with various pharmacological activities. This study aims to evaluate its in vitro and in vivo inhibitory potential against the nine major CYP enzymes. Of the nine tested CYPs, it exerted the strongest inhibitory effect on CYP2C9-mediated tolbutamide 4-hydroxylation with the lowest IC_{50} (K_i) value of 0.966 ± 0.149 μM (0.503 ± 0.0383 μM), in a competitive manner. Additionally, it strongly inhibited other CYP2C9-catalyzed diclofenac 4′-hydroxylation and losartan oxidation activities. Upon 30 min pre-incubation of human liver microsomes with SPN in the presence of NADPH, no obvious shift in IC_{50} was observed, suggesting that SPN is not a time-dependent inactivator of the nine CYPs. However, oral co-administration of SPN had no significant effect on the pharmacokinetics of diclofenac and 4′-hydroxydiclofenac in rats. Overall, SPN is a potent inhibitor of CYP2C9 in vitro but not in vivo. The very low permeability of SPN in Caco-2 cells (P_{app} value of 0.115×10^{-6} cm/s), which suggests poor absorption in vivo, and its high degree of plasma protein binding (>99.9%) may lead to the lack of in vitro–in vivo correlation. These findings will be helpful for the safe and effective clinical use of SPN.

Keywords: (-)-sophoranone; CYP2C9; potent inhibition; in vitro; in vivo; drug interaction; low permeability; high plasma protein binding

1. Introduction

(-)-Sophoranone (SPN; Figure 1), a major bioactive flavonoid isolated from the roots of *Sophora tonkinensis*, is used in traditional Chinese medicine for the treatment of acute pharyngolaryngeal infections and sore throat [1–3]. It exhibits anti-inflammatory effects by inhibiting nitric oxide production in macrophages [4] and 5-lipoxygenase activity [3]. Several studies have also demonstrated its other biological activities, such as anti-cancer [5], anti-diabetic diabetic [6], and immunomodulatory [7] activities. In our previous study, after orally administering 12.9 mg/kg SPN to rats, the maximum plasma concentration (C_{max}) was approximately 13.1 ng/mL at 60 min [8]. Thus, although conclusive results are lacking, SPN is likely to be a promising drug candidate.

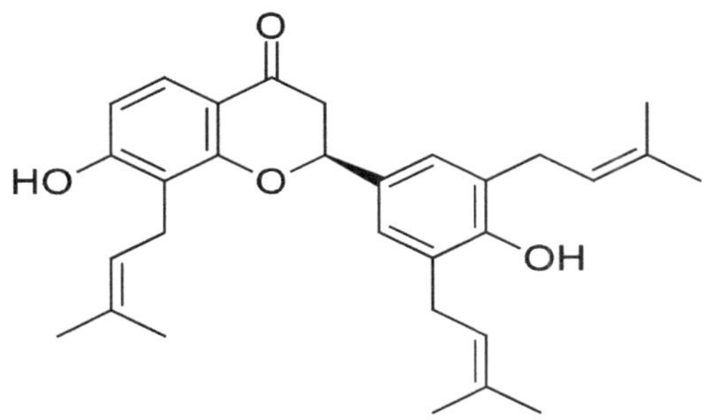

Figure 1. Chemical structure of (-)-sophoranone (SPN).

Drug–drug interactions can increase the likelihood of treatment failure or the frequency and severity of adverse events [9]. Thus, drug–drug interaction assessment is a critical component of new drug discovery and development as well as clinical practice [9,10]. The majority of known drug interactions occur because of inhibition of drug-metabolizing enzymes [11–13]. Among all drug-metabolizing enzymes, the cytochrome P450 (CYP) superfamily plays an important role in the oxidation of almost 90% of currently used drugs [14]. Among at least 57 human cytochrome P450 enzymes identified to date, 9 hepatic P450 enzymes (CYP1A2, 2A6, 2B6, 2C8, 2C9, 2C19, 2D6, 2E1, and 3A4) have shown to play predominant roles in the metabolism of drugs and other xenobiotics [12]. Therefore, the inhibitory potential of SPN on the nine major CYP enzymes should also be investigated. There are a few reports on the in vitro and in vivo inhibitory effects of SPN on CYP enzymes. In rats, oral administration of 5 g/kg *S. tonkinensis* extract over 14 days was found to increase the plasma concentrations of metoprolol, omeprazole, and bupropion. This might be attributed to the inhibition of the activities of rat CYP enzymes, CYP2D6, CYP2C19, and CYP2B6 [15]. However, these results could not directly reflect the in vivo inhibitory potential of SPN on CYP enzymes due to multiple components of the extract. Several flavonoids, including SPN, have been found to inhibit CYP3A4-mediated reactions in vitro [16].

However, currently, there is limited information about SPN's in vitro inhibitory potentials, especially on the other eight CYP enzymes, thereby warranting further in vitro and in vivo investigations to improve our understanding of drug interactions with SPN. Using human liver microsomes in this study, we evaluated SPN's potential to inhibit CYP1A2, CYP2A6, CYP2B6, CYP2C8, CYP2C9, CYP2C19, CYP2D6, CYP2E1, and CYP3A4 in a reversible and time-dependent manner. We report herein that SPN is a potent inhibitor of CYP2C9 in vitro but not in vivo. To explain this lack of correlation between in vitro and in vivo results, we performed plasma protein binding of SPN and permeability test using Caco-2 cells.

2. Materials and Methods

2.1. Chemicals and Reagents

Pooled human liver microsomes from 150 donors (75 males; 75 females) were purchased from Corning Life Sciences (Woburn, MA, USA), and (-)-sophoranone (99.7% purity; SPN) was supplied by SK Chemicals Ltd. (Sungnam, Gyeonggi-do, Korea). β-Nicotinamide adenine dinucleotide phosphate disodium salt (NADP), glucose 6-phosphate disodium salt hydrate, glucose 6-phosphate dehydrogenase, $MgCl_2$, and all chemicals including the specific substrates, its metabolites, and well-known inhibitors of nine P450s were purchased from Sigma–Aldrich Corporation (St. Louis, MO, USA), Santa Cruz Biotechnology (Dallas, TX, USA), or Cayman Chemicals (Ann Arbor, MI, USA) unless stated otherwise. The purity of all purchased compounds was higher than 97.0%. HPLC-grade acetonitrile and methanol were obtained from Burdick & Jackson Company (Morristown, NJ, USA). Caco-2 cells were supplied by the Korean Cell Line Bank (Seoul, Korea) and cultured according to the supplier's recommendations. Transwell (24-well, 6.5 mm polycarbonate inserts, 0.4-μm pore) and cell culture reagents were purchased from Corning Life Sciences. Heparinized human plasma was obtained from donors at the Severance Hospital of Yonsei University Health System (Seoul, Korea) and stored at −80 °C prior to use.

2.2. Reversible Inhibition of (-)-Sophoranone towards the Nine CYP Isoforms in Human Liver Microsomes

The inhibitory effects of SPN on CYP1A2, CYP2A6, CYP2B6, CYP2C8, CYP2C9, CYP2C19, CYP2D6, CYP2E1, and CYP3A4 were evaluated in pooled human liver microsomes through the use of specific CYP probe substrates (cocktail assay), as previously described [17,18] with a slight modification. Concentrations of each CYP probe in Table 1 were used close to their reported K_m values [17,18].

Briefly, a 90-μL incubation mixture, including pooled human liver microsomes (final concentration 0.1 mg/mL), 50 mM phosphate buffer (pH 7.4), each CYP-probe substrate cocktail set, and SPN (0–50 μM), was pre-incubated for 5 min at 37 °C. SPN was dissolved in methanol and spiked into the incubation mixture to a final concentration of 0.5% methanol. All P450-selective substrates (except coumarin due to solubility) were dissolved in methanol and serially diluted with methanol to the required concentrations, and the organic solvent was subsequently evaporated under a gentle stream of N_2 gas to minimize the effects of organic solvents on CYP activities. On the other hand, coumarin dissolved in 50 mM phosphate buffer (pH 7.4) was directly added into the mixed tube. The reaction was initiated by adding 10-μL aliquot of NADPH-generating system (1.3 mM $NADP^+$, 3.3 mM glucose 6-phosphate, 3.3 mM $MgCl_2$, and 0.4 unit/mL glucose-6-phosphate dehydrogenase) before 15 min incubation at 37 °C in a shaking water bath. After incubation, the reactions were stopped by adding 200 μL of ice-cold acetonitrile containing 2 μM chlorpropamide as an internal standard. The incubation mixtures were centrifuged (16,000× *g*, 15 min) and 5 μL of the supernatant was injected into the LC-MS/MS system. All incubations were performed in triplicate, and the data are shown as the mean ± standard deviation. Incubation samples containing well-known CYP inhibitors for each isozyme (Table 2) in parallel were included to compare inhibitory effects, all of which appear on the US FDA list of recommended or accepted in vitro inhibitors [12,19–21].

Additionally, to determine whether the inhibition of CYP2C9 by SPN was substrate specific, we also examined SPN's inhibitory effects on other CYP2C9-specific biotransformation pathways (i.e., diclofenac 4′-hydroxylation and losartan oxidation) in human liver microsomes [22,23]. Diclofenac and losartan were used at 5 μM, respectively, and other procedures were similar to those of cocktail assays.

2.3. Determination of the K_i of (-)-Sophoranone on CYP2C9 Activity in Human Liver Microsomes

Among the nine tested CYP enzymes, SPN showed the lowest IC_{50} value for CYP2C9 (Table 2). Based on the IC_{50} values, the K_i values of SPN on CYP2C9 activity were determined. Briefly, K_i values were obtained by incubating various concentrations of two CYP2C9 probe substrates (50, 100, and 150 μM tolbutamide; or 2, 5, and 10 μM diclofenac) in the presence of 0–5 μM SPN or 0–2 μM sulfaphenazole, a well-known typical CYP2C9 inhibitor. Other procedures were similar to those of the reversible inhibition studies. All incubations were performed in triplicate, and the data are shown as the mean ± standard deviation.

Table 1. Optimized mass parameters for the detection of metabolites of the nine P450-probe substrates and internal standard used in the cocktail assays.

CYPs	Probe Substrates	K_m (μM)	Metabolite	ESI [a]	Q1 Ion (*m/z*)	Q3 Ion (*m/z*)	Q1 Pre-bias (V)	CE [b] (eV)	Q3 Pre-bias (V)
1A2	Phenacetin	50	Acetaminophen	+	152	110.2	−14	−12	−19
2A6	Coumarin	5	7-Hydroxycoumarin	+	163	107	−15	−35	−15
2B6	Bupropion	50	6-Hydroxybupropion	+	256	238	−15	−35	−15
2C8	Rosiglitazone	10	*p*-Hydroxyrosiglitaonze	+	374	151	−15	−35	−15
2C9	Tolbutamide	100	4-Hydroxytolbutamide	+	287	87	−15	−35	−15
2C19	Omeprazole	20	5-Hydroxyomeprazole	+	362	214	−13	−13	−22
2D6	Dextromethorphan	5	Dextrorphan	+	258	157	−15	−35	−15
2E1	Chlorzoxazone	50	6-Hydroxychlorzoxazone	−	184	119.9	18	15	24
3A4	Midazolam	2	1′-Hydroxymidazolam	+	342	203	−15	−35	−15
Chlorpropamide (Internal standard)		2		+	277	111	−15	−20	−15
				−	275	190	15	35	15

The optimized ion spray voltage was 4 kV and a nebulizing gas flow of 3 L/min, heating gas flow of 10 L/min, an interface temperature of 300 °C, desolvation line temperature of 250 °C, heating block temperature of 400 °C, and a drying gas flow rate of 10 L/min. [a] ESI, electrospray ionization mode; [b] CE, collision energy.

Table 2. IC_{50} values of well-known CYP inhibitors and SPN in reversible inhibition studies using a cocktail assay ($n = 3$).

CYPs	IC_{50} Values (μM)		
	Well-Known Inhibitors		SPN
1A2	α-Naphthoflavone	0.0458 ± 0.00694	>50 [a]
2A6	Tryptamine	2.98 ± 0.635	>50 [a]
2B6	Ticlopidine	2.19 ± 0.513	>50 [a]
2C8	Quercetin	8.51 ± 0.958	13.6 ± 3.15
2C9	Sulfaphenazole	0.677 ± 0.109	0.966 ± 0.149
2C19	*S*-benzylnirvanol	0.215 ± 0.0228	16.8 ± 3.21
2D6	Quinidine	0.127 ± 0.0192	>50
2E1	Diethyldithiocarbamate	12.0 ± 3.67	>50 [a]
3A4	Ketoconazole	0.0404 ± 0.00821	>50

Data represent the mean ± standard deviation of triplicate. [a] The remaining activities at the highest concentration tested, 50 μM, were greater than 80%.

2.4. Time-Dependent Inactivation of (-)-Sophoranone toward the Nine CYP Isoforms in Human Liver Microsomes

Pooled human liver microsomes (1 mg/mL) were incubated with SPN (0–50 μM) for 30 min at 37 °C in the absence or presence of an NADPH-generating system (i.e., the "inactivation incubation"). After inactivation incubation, aliquots (10 μL) were transferred into fresh incubation tubes (final volume 100 μL) containing an NADPH-generating system and each P450-selective substrate cocktail set. The reaction mixtures were incubated for 15 min at 37 °C in a shaking water bath. After incubation, the reactions were stopped by adding 200 μL of ice-cold acetonitrile containing 2 μM chlorpropamide, as an internal standard. The incubation mixtures were centrifuged (16,000× *g*, 15 min) and 5 μL of the supernatant was injected into the LC-MS/MS system. All incubations were performed in triplicate, and the data are shown as the mean ± standard deviation.

2.5. Caco-2 Cell Permeability of (-)-Sophoranone

Caco-2 cell permeability was assessed to predict the oral absorption of SPN. Cell culture and transport studies were performed as previously described [24,25]. Briefly, for the bi-directional transport studies, the cells were seeded at a density of 1×10^5 cells/well, and the cell medium was replaced until they formed confluent monolayers. On the 25th day, the cell monolayers were washed with pre-warmed HBSS buffer. The bi-directional permeability assay was instigated by adding 10 μM for propranolol, or 10 μM and 50 μM for SPN in HBSS to an apical well (200 μL) for apical (A) to basolateral (B) transport or to a basolateral insert (800 μL) for the B to A transport. Before the experiment, the integrity of the cell monolayers was evaluated by measuring the transepithelial electrical resistance using a Millicell ohmmeter. After 2 h incubation at 37 °C, samples were withdrawn from both sides, respectively. All samples were stored at −80 °C until LC-MS/MS analysis, and all experiments were performed in triplicate.

The apparent permeability coefficient (P_{app}) was calculated using the following equation.

$$P_{app} = (V_r/C_0) \times (1/A) \times ([\text{Drug}]/t)$$

where, V_r is the volume of medium in the receiver chamber, C_0 is the donor compartment concentration at time zero, A is the area of the cell monolayer, t is the treatment time of the drug, and [Drug] is the drug concentration in the receiver chamber.

2.6. Effects of (-)-Sophoranone on the Pharmacokinetics of Diclofenac in Rats

In this study, we investigated whether SPN, an in vitro potent inhibitor of CYP2C9, affects the pharmacokinetics of diclofenac in rats. Male Sprague–Dawley rats (8 weeks, 270–290 g) were purchased from Orient Bio (Sungnam, Gyeonggi-do, Korea), and the protocol for pharmacokinetic interaction studies in rats was approved by the Institutional Animal Care and Use Committee (IACUC-CUK) at The Catholic University of Korea (Approval No. 2019-021, approved 31 May 2019). The procedures used for housing and handling were previously reported [18]. Before administration, rats were fasted for 12 h with free access to water. The carotid arteries of each rat were cannulated with a polyethylene tube (Clay Adams, Franklin Lakes, NJ, USA) for blood sampling. Each rat was individually housed in a rat metabolic cage and allowed to recover from anesthesia for 4–5 h prior to the start of the experiment. The rats were divided into two groups: (1) diclofenac alone (n = 6) and (2) SPN and diclofenac co-administration (n = 6). SPN was suspended in dimethylsulfoxide:PEG400:distilled water (5:60:35, *v*/*v*/*v*) and administered by oral gavage at a dose of 75 mg/kg in a volume of 5 mL/kg. Fifteen minutes after oral administration of SPN, 2 mg/kg diclofenac was dissolved in normal saline and administered by oral gavage. Approximately 0.25 mL of blood from each rat was collected into an Eppendorf tube before diclofenac dosing (0 min), and at 3, 5, 10, 15, 30, 45, 60, 90, 120, 180, 240, 360, and 480 min post-dosing. The blood samples were immediately centrifuged at 13,000× g for 5 min at 4 °C. The plasma samples were divided into two Eppendorf tubes by 50 μL and stored at −80 °C until LC-MS/MS analysis. After the experiments, the rats were euthanized with CO_2.

2.7. *Determination of the Unbound Fraction of (-)-Sophoranone in Plasma and Human Liver Microsomes*

The plasma or liver microsomal protein bindings were performed using a rapid equilibrium dialysis device and cellulose membranes with a molecular weight cutoff of 8000 (Thermo Scientific, Rockford, IL, USA) [17]. The rat and human plasma samples (200 μL) containing SPN at 10 and 50 μM, respectively, were dialyzed against a dialysis buffer, phosphate-buffered saline (PBS, 400 μL). The loaded dialysis plate was covered with sealing tape, placed on an orbital shaker at approximately 200 rpm, and incubated at 37 °C for 4 h. Thereafter, samples (100 μL) from both PBS and plasma chambers were collected and mixed with an equal volume of blank plasma and PBS, respectively. All samples were stored at −80 °C until LC-MS/MS analysis. The unbound fraction of SPN in human (or rat) plasma was calculated by dividing the SPN concentration in PBS by that in plasma.

The human liver microsomal incubation mixtures (final concentration 0.1 mg/mL) without NADPH generating system were used to determine the unbound fraction of SPN. Other procedures were similar to those of plasma protein binding assay.

2.8. *LC-MS/MS Analysis*

2.8.1. In Vitro Samples

Metabolites of nine P450-selective substrates were analyzed using a Shimadzu Nexera X2 UPLC system coupled to an LCMS-8050 triple quadruple mass spectrometer (Shimadzu Corporation, Kyoto, Japan) equipped with an electrospray ionization interface as previously described with a slight modification [17,18]. Separation was performed on a reversed-phase column (Luna C_{18}, 50 mm × 2.0 mm i.d.; 3 μm particle size; Phenomenex, Torrance, CA, USA) maintained at 40 °C. The mobile phase consisted of distilled water containing 0.1% formic acid (A) and acetonitrile containing 0.1% formic acid (B), with a flow rate of 0.5 mL/min. The gradient elution program used was as follows: (1) Mobile phase A was set to 95% at 0 min, (2) a linear gradient was run to 5% in 2.6 min, and (3) a linear gradient was run to 95% in 3.0 min and re-equilibrated for 2 min. The total run time was 5 min. The optimized compound-dependent parameters of the metabolites of the nine P450-selective substrates and the internal standard are listed in Table 1. Three-day validations were performed to confirm the effectiveness of the LC-MS/MS system for simultaneous determination of the nine P450-selective substrate metabolites at the respective ranges of 0.01–10 μM in blank microsomal incubation mixtures. We found that the precision (≤12.1%) and accuracy (95.4–110.2%) values were within acceptable ranges. Supplemental Figure S1 shows the representative LC-MS/MS chromatograms of a human liver microsomal incubation sample containing nine P450-selective metabolites and an internal standard.

The auto-optimized mass transitions were m/z 312 > 231 and m/z 437 > 207.1 for quantification of 4′-hydroxydiclofenac and losartan carboxylic acid, respectively. HPLC conditions were the same as those in the cocktail assay.

2.8.2. In Vivo Samples

The plasma concentrations of diclofenac and 4′-hydroxydiclofenac were determined by a previously reported LC-MS/MS method [26] with some modifications. Briefly, 50 μL aliquots of plasma were extracted with 300 μL aliquots of acetonitrile containing chlorpropamide (internal standard), followed by LC-MS/MS (Shimadzu Corporation). Chromatographic separation was performed on a Phenomenex Luna C_{18} column (100 × 2.00 mm; 3.0 μm). The isocratic mobile phase consisted of 0.1% formic acid in distilled water (A) and 0.1% formic acid in acetonitrile (B) (45:55, *v*/*v*), with a flow rate of 0.3 mL/min. The transitions were m/z 296.0 > 214.0 for diclofenac, m/z 312 > 231 for 4′-hydroxydiclofenac, and m/z 277 > 111 for the internal standard. The data acquisition was computed using LabSolutions LCMS Ver.5.6 (Shimadzu Corporation). The calibration curves for diclofenac and 4′-hydroxydiclofenac were linear ($r \geq 0.996$) over the concentration range of 20–5000 ng/mL.

The LC-MS/MS condition for the determination of SPN in plasma was the same with a previously reported method [27]. The calibration curve for SPN was linear ($r \geq 0.995$) over the concentration range of 1–250 ng/mL.

2.9. Analysis of Inhibition Kinetics and Pharmacokinetic Parameters

The IC_{50} values were calculated via nonlinear least-squares regression analysis from logarithmic plots of inhibitor concentration versus percentage of activity remaining after inhibition, using SigmaPlot (ver. 14.0; Systat Software Inc, Chicago, IL, USA). The K_i values were determined from the equations for a single substrate single inhibitor model and the software available in the SigmaPlot Enzyme Kinetics module. Competitive, non-competitive, uncompetitive, or mixed inhibition models were evaluated and ranked according to the best fit based on Akaike Information Criterion (AIC) values. For visual inspection, the data were presented as Dixon plots.

Pharmacokinetic parameters were calculated by a non-compartmental analysis using WinNonlin Professional software (version 5.2, Pharsight Corp., Mountain View, CA, USA) that used the total area under the plasma concentration–time curve from time zero to infinity (AUC_∞) or the last measured time (AUC_t). The logarithmic trapezoidal rule was used during the declining plasma level phase and the linear trapezoidal rule was used for the rising plasma-level phase. The peak plasma concentration (C_{max}) and time to reach C_{max} (T_{max}) were read directly from the experimental data. Statistically significant differences were recognized at $p < 0.05$.

3. Results

3.1. Reversible Inhibition of (-)-Sophoranone toward the Nine CYP Isoforms in Human Liver Microsomes

The inhibitory effects of SPN on the activities of nine CYP isozymes (CYP1A2, CYP2A6, CYP2B6, CYP2C8, CYP2C9, CYP2C19, CYP2D6, CYP2E1, and CYP3A4) in human liver microsomes are shown in Figure 2, and the IC_{50} values are listed in Table 2. The IC_{50} values for the positive controls used in the reversible inhibition studies were in an acceptable degree of accuracy with published values [12,19–21]. Of the P450 isoforms tested, SPN exerted the strongest inhibitory effect on CYP2C9-catalyzed tolbutamide hydroxylation, with an IC_{50} value of 0.966 ± 0.149 μM (Table 2). SPN showed weak inhibitory effects toward CYP2C8 and CYP2C19, with IC50 values of 13.6 ± 3.15 μM and 16.8 ± 3.21 μM, respectively. However, SPN had no apparent inhibitory effects toward the other CYPs tested (Table 2); the residual enzyme activities at the highest tested concentration (50 μM) were greater than 80%, except for CYP2D6 (53.9 ± 3.53%) and CYP3A4 (53.3 ± 4.00%) (Figure 2).

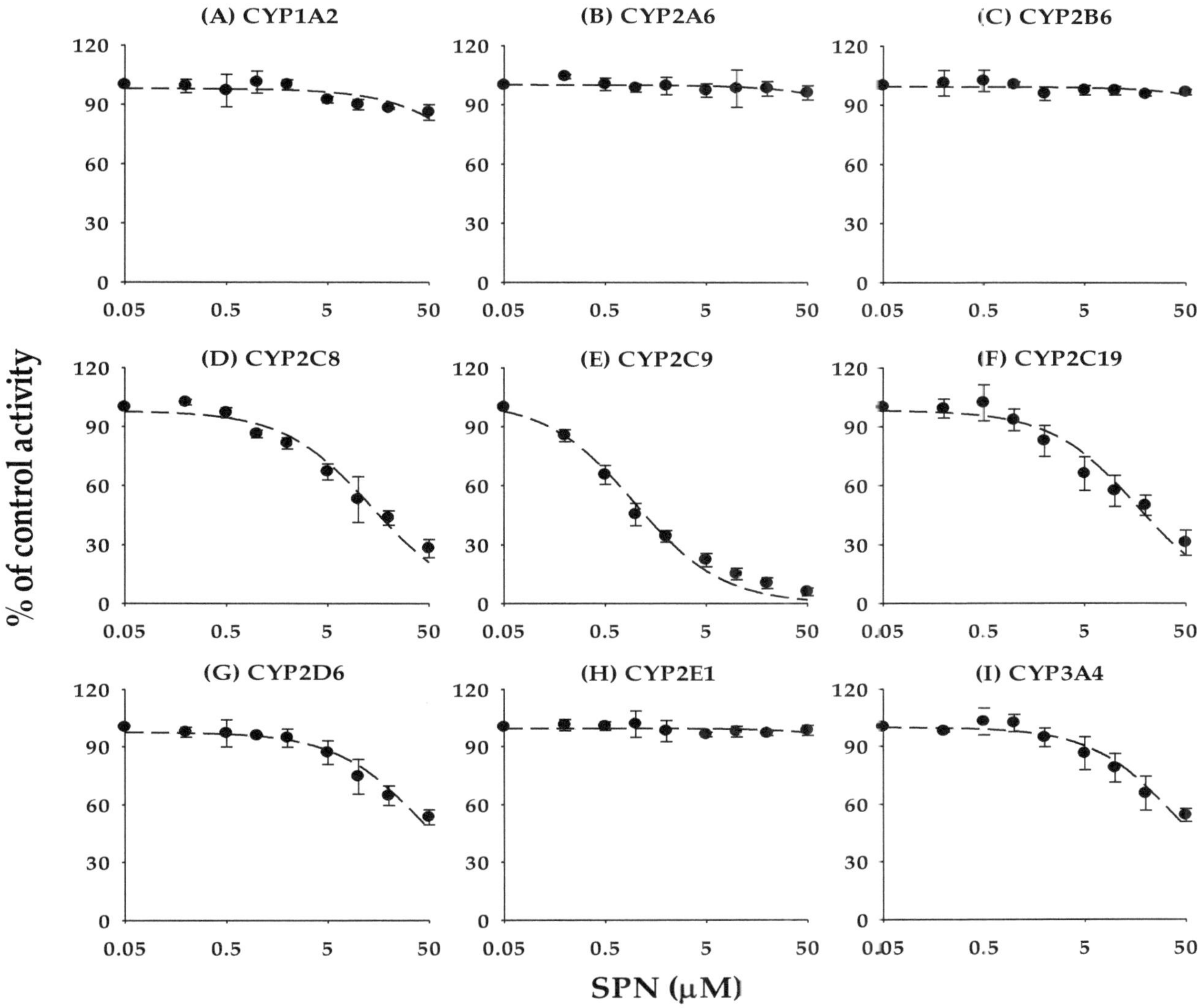

Figure 2. Inhibition curves of SPN on the nine major P450 activities in human liver microsomes using substrate cocktails including CYP1A2 for phenacetin *O*-deethylase (**A**), CYP2A6 for coumarin 7-hydroxylase (**B**), CYP2B6 for bupropion hydroxylase (**C**), CYP2C8 for rosiglitazone *p*-hydroxylase (**D**), CYP2C9 for tolbutamide 4-hydroxylase (**E**), CYP2C19 for omeprazole 5-hydroxylase (**F**), CYP2D6 for dextromethorphan *O*-demethylase (**G**), CYP2E1 for chlorzoxazone 6-hydroxylase (**H**), and CYP3A4 for midazolam 1′-hydroxylase (**I**). The activity is expressed as a percentage of remaining activity compared with the control, no containing SPN. Data are the mean ± standard deviation of triplicate incubations. The dashed lines represent the best fit to the data with non-linear regression.

To determine whether the inhibitory effects of SPN on CYP2C9 was substrate specific, we examined the inhibitory effects on other CYP2C9-specific biotransformation pathways (i.e., diclofenac 4′-hydroxylation and losartan oxidation) and found that SPN also markedly inhibited their activities, with IC_{50} values of 0.879 ± 0.0888 μM and 0.455 ± 0.0486 μM, respectively, (Figure 3).

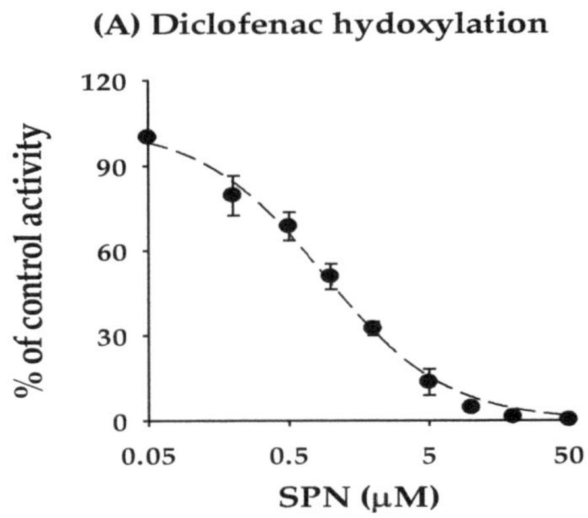

Figure 3. Inhibition curves of SPN on the CYP2C9-catalyzed diclofenac 4′-hydroxylation (**A**) and losartan oxidation (**B**) activities in human liver microsomes. Data are the mean ± standard deviation of triplicate incubations. The dashed lines represent the best fit to the data with non-linear regression.

3.2. Determination of the K_i of (-)-Sophoranone for CYP2C9 Activity

Based on the lowest IC_{50} value for CYP2C9, to characterize the type of reversible inhibition of CYP2C9 by SPN, enzyme kinetic experiments were performed in the presence of various concentrations of SPN and tolbutamide, or diclofenac. Otherwise, identical samples containing a known potent CYP2C9 inhibitor (sulfaphenazole), were included in the analysis. Representative Dixon plots of CYP2C9 inhibition by SPN and sulfaphenazole in human liver microsomes are shown in Figure 4, and the Ki values are summarized in Supplemental Table S1. Using a nonlinear regression analysis, SPN demonstrated competitive inhibition against CYP2C9-catalyzed tolbutamide hydroxylation or diclofenac hydroxylation, with calculated K_i values of 0.503 ± 0.0383 μM and 0.587 ± 0.0470 μM (Figure 4A,B). Sulphafenazole competitively inhibited CYP2C9 with a K_i value of 0.267 ± 0.0170 μM (Figure 4C), which was similar to a previously reported value [28].

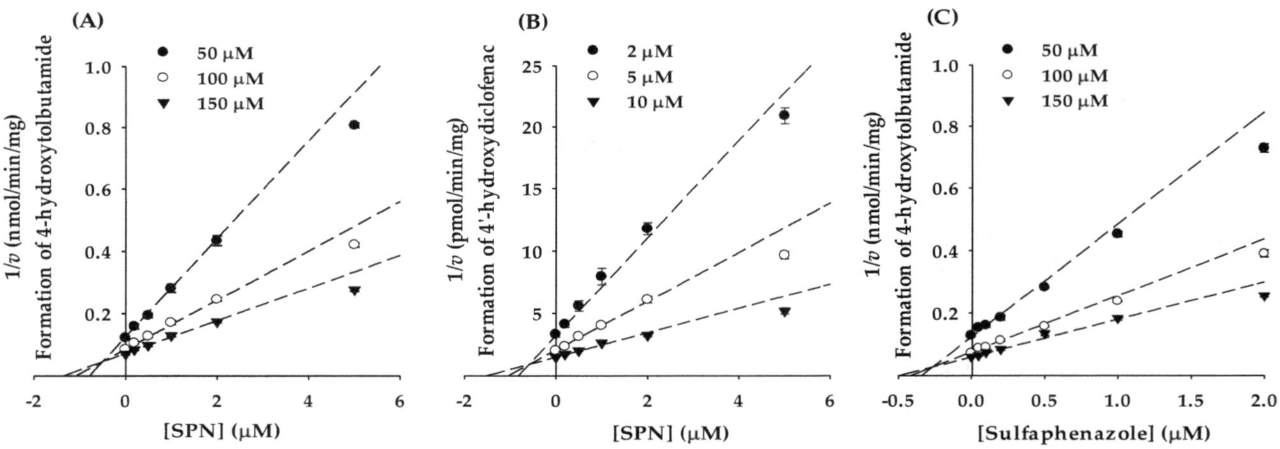

Figure 4. Dixon plots to determine K_i values of SPN on the CYP2C9 enzyme activity, using tolbutamide (**A**) or diclofenac (**B**) as substrates. The well-known inhibitor of CYP2C9, sulfaphenazole, is used as a positive control (**C**) using tolbutamide as a substrate. The concentrations of tolbutamide were determined 50 (•), 100 (○), and 150 (▼) μM, respectively; diclofenac was used at 2 (•), 5 (○), and 10 (▼) μM, respectively. v represents formation rate of 4-hydroxytolbutamide (nmol/min/mg protein) or 4′-hydroxydiclofenac (pmol/min/mg protein). Data are the mean ± standard deviation of triplicate incubations. The dashed lines of SPN (**A**,**B**) and sulfaphenazole (**C**) all fit well to competitive inhibition types.

3.3. Time-Dependent Inactivation of (-)-Sophoranone towards the Nine CYP Isoforms in Human Liver Microsomes

The IC_{50} shift method incorporating a dilution is one of the most efficient and convenient methods for evaluating time-dependent inhibitory effects. A shift in IC_{50} to a lower value ("shift") with pre-incubation indicates time-dependent inactivation [29–31]. After 30 min pre-incubation of SPN with human liver microsomes in the presence of NADPH, no obvious shift in IC_{50} was observed for inhibition of the nine CYPs (Figure 5), suggesting that SPN is not a time-dependent inactivator for the nine CYPs.

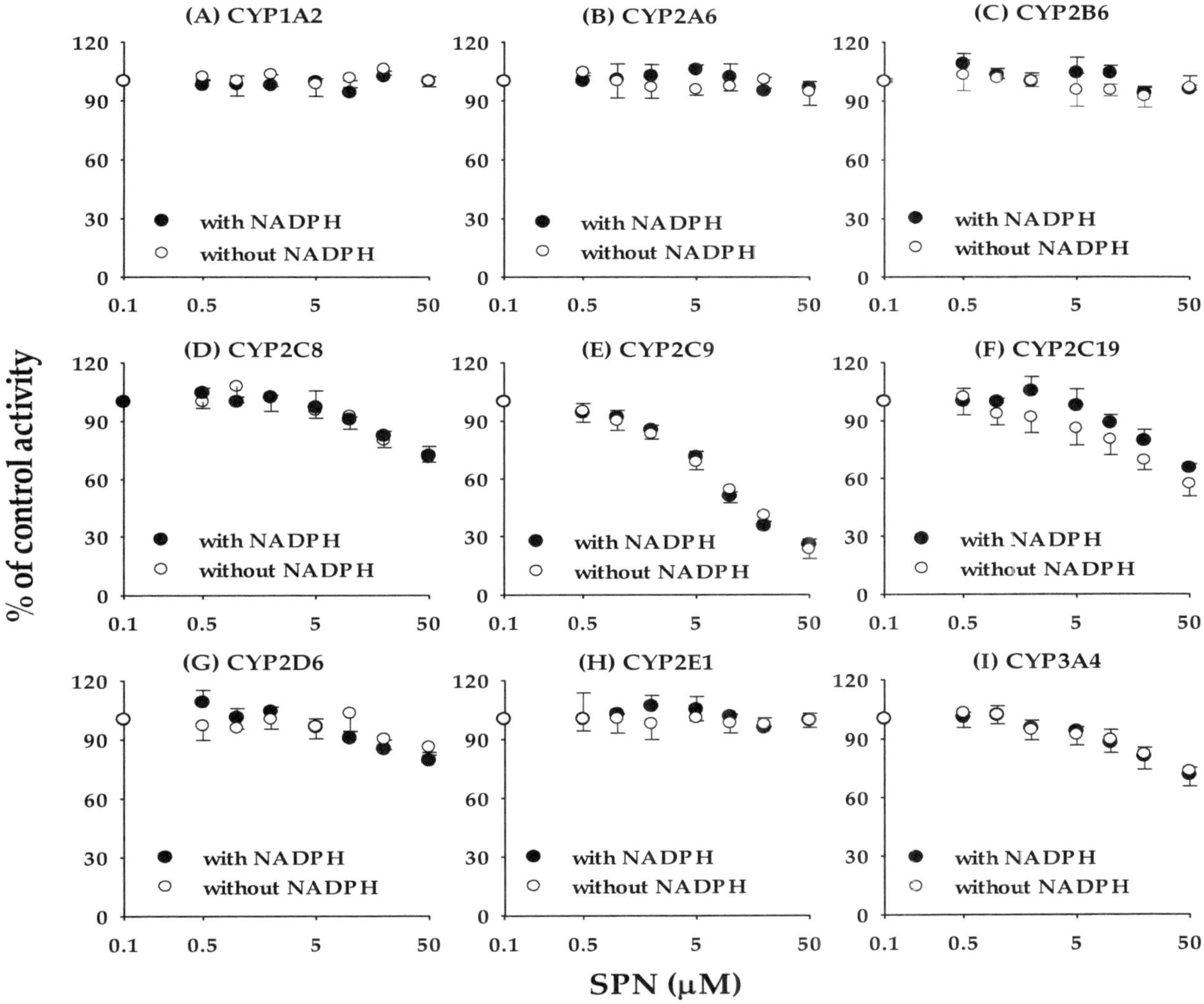

Figure 5. Time-dependent inhibition curves of SPN on the nine major P450 activities in human liver microsomes using substrate cocktails after 30 min pre-incubation with the presence (•) or absence (○) of an NADPH-generating system. Data are the mean ± standard deviation of triplicate incubations.

3.4. Caco-2 Cell Permeability of (-)-Sophoranone

A bi-directional permeability assay using Caco-2 monolayer cells was performed to predict the intestinal absorption of SPN. SPN showed very low permeability in both directions (from A-to-B and B-to-A). The calculated P_{app} values of SPN from A-to-B were $(0.115 \pm 0.0369) \times 10^{-6}$ cm/s and $(0.172 \pm 0.0488) \times 10^{-6}$ cm/s at 10 μM and 50 μM, respectively, ($n = 3$, each). These results indicated that SPN is poorly absorbed in vivo. The P_{app} values from B-to-A were $(0.101 \pm 0.00444) \times 10^{-6}$ cm/s at

10 μM (n = 3) and (0.152 ± 0.0353) × 10^{-6} cm/s at 50 μM (n = 3). SPN was not a substrate for efflux transporters, that is, P-gp and BCRP, as the efflux ratio (B-to-A/A-to-B) is less than 2. The P_{app} of propranolol, a reference high permeable compound, from A-to-B and B-to-A were (26.8 ± 3.31) × 10^{-6} cm/s and (21.5 ± 2.19) × 10^{-6} cm/s, respectively, (n = 3, each), similar to the reported values [24,25].

3.5. Effects of (-)-Sophoranone on the Pharmacokinetics of Diclofenac in Rats

We conducted pharmacokinetic studies to investigate the effects of SPN on the pharmacokinetics of diclofenac in rats. Findings in the literature on the dried *S. tonkinensis* herbs indicate that a recommended daily dose for an adult human with the body weight of 60 kg were to be 6–10 g [32], which correlated to the equivalent dose ranges in rats, 0.620–1.03 g/kg [33]. He et al. [2] reported that the average contents of SPN in various *S. tonkinensis* samples were found to be approximately 2.53 mg/g (0.0253%). Reflecting this content, the dosage in rats, 0.620–1.03 g/kg of the dried herb, might be consistent with 15.7–26.1 mg/kg in terms of SPN. Thus, in this study, the SPN dose of 75 mg/kg was used in rats, which is approximately 2.87- to 4.87-fold greater than the recommended human dose.

The mean plasma concentration-time profiles of diclofenac and 4-hydroxydiclofenac after oral administration of diclofenac (2 mg/kg) in the absence or presence of oral co-administration of SPN (75 mg/kg) in rats are illustrated in Figure 6, and the relevant pharmacokinetic parameters are shown in Table 3. The plasma levels of diclofenac and 4-hydroxydiclofenac were similar in both groups (Figure 6A,B). Likewise, no significant differences were observed in any other pharmacokinetic parameter of diclofenac and 4′-hydroxydiclofenac (Table 3). The in vivo marker for CYP2C9 activity, expressed as the molar AUC ratio of 4′-hydroxydiclofenac to diclofenac, was not significant (0.799 ± 0.167 versus 0.904 ± 0.0534; p value of 0.215) in the presence or absence of SPN (Table 3). In the treatment group with co-administration of SPN, the C_{max} of SPN was found to be 33.7 ± 14.8 ng/mL (0.0732 ± 0.0321 μM) at approximately 60–75 min post-dose (Figure 6C). Given the K_i values of SPN on CYP2C9 activity (0.503 ± 0.0383 μM for tolbutamide hydroxylation and 0.587 ± 0.0470 μM for diclofenac hydroxylation), the plasma concentrations of SPN are too low to inhibit CYP2C9-mediated metabolism of diclofenac in vivo. Overall, the co-administration of SPN did not alter the pharmacokinetics of diclofenac and 4′-hydroxydiclofenac.

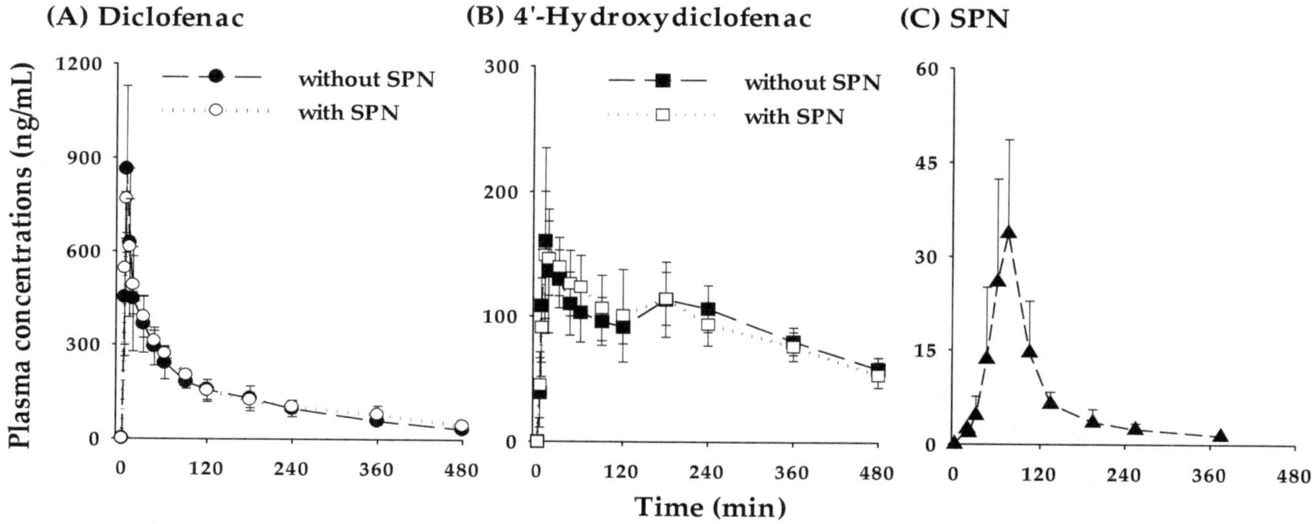

Figure 6. Mean plasma concentrations of diclofenac (**A**) and 4′-hydroxydiclofenac (**B**) after oral administration of diclofenac at a dose of 2 mg/kg without (•, n = 6) or with (○, n = 6) oral dosing of SPN (75 mg/kg) to rats. Mean plasma concentrations of SPN (**C**) after co-administration of SPN (75 mg/kg) and diclofenac (2 mg/kg) to rats (▲, n = 6). Vertical bars mean standard deviation.

Table 3. Mean (± standard deviations) pharmacokinetic parameters of diclofenac and 4′-hydroxydiclofenac after oral administration of diclofenac at a dose of 2 mg/kg without or with oral administration of SPN (75 mg/kg) to rats.

Parameters	Without SPN (n = 6)	With SPN (n = 6)
Diclofenac		
AUC_t (μg min/mL) [a]	63.8 ± 6.28	69.4 ± 2.98
AUC_∞ (μg min/mL) [b]	71.7 ± 9.16	80.8 ± 7.78
$t_{1/2}$ (min) [c]	153 ± 60.1	173 ± 41.5
C_{max} (ng/mL) [d]	882 ± 245	787 ± 104
T_{max} (min) [e]	5 (3–5)	5 (3–5)
4′-hydroxydiclofenac		
AUC_t (μg min/mL)	44.8 ± 6.38	44.5 ± 7.24
AUC_∞ (μg min/mL)	68.6 ± 12.1	67.6 ± 12.9
$t_{1/2}$ (min)	278 ± 70.0	296 ± 59.7
C_{max} (ng/mL)	180 ± 55.2	173 ± 40.8
T_{max} (min)	10 (10–30)	15 (10–30)
Metabolic conversion ratio [f]		
$AUC_{\infty,\ 4'\text{-hydroxydiclofenac}}/AUC_{\infty,\ \text{diclofenac}}$	0.904 ± 0.0534	0.799 ± 0.167

No significant differences were observed in all pharmacokinetic parameters of diclofenac and 4′-hydroxydiclofenac. [a] Total area under the plasma concentration–time curve from time zero to time last sampling time; [b] total area under the plasma concentration–time curve from time zero to infinity; [c] terminal half-life; [d] peak plasma concentration; [e] time to reach C_{max}. Median (ranges); [f] the metabolic conversion ratio, $AUC_{\infty,4'\text{-hydroxydiclofenac}}/AUC_{\infty,\text{diclofenac}}$, was calculated based on a molar basis.

3.6. Determination of the Unbound Fraction of (-)-Sophoranone in Plasma and Human Liver Microsomes

SPN was extensively bound to plasma proteins, regardless of species. The free fractions (%) of SPN at 10 and 50 μM in human plasma were 0.0457 ± 0.00612% and 0.0927 ± 0.0400%, respectively, (n = 3, each). Similarly, when 10 and 50 μM SPN were added to the rat plasma, the free fractions were 0.0380 ± 0.0102% and 0.0531 ± 0.0149%, respectively, (n = 3, each). After adding 10 and 50 μM SPN to rat and human plasma, free fractions remained relatively unchanged, suggesting that SPN has no binding saturation in plasma.

SPN also exhibited marked non-specific bindings to human liver microsomes, although to a lesser extent than those in human plasma. The unbound fractions of SPN at 10 and 50 μM were calculated to be 0.621 ± 0.0405% and 0.724 ± 0.170%, respectively (n = 3, each), at a microsomal protein concentration of 0.1 mg/mL.

4. Discussion

This study focused on the in vitro and in vivo inhibitory effects of SPN on human CYPs, especially CYP2C9. We screened the inhibitory effects of SPN on the major human CYP isoforms (CYP1A2, CYP2A6, CYP2B6, CYP2C8, CYP2C9, CYP2C19, CYP2D6, CYP2E1, and CYP3A4) in human liver microsomes. Of the nine tested CYP isoforms, SPN exerted the strongest inhibitory effect on CYP2C9 activity, with the lowest IC_{50} value of 0.966 ± 0.149 μM (Table 2; Figure 2). In addition to CYP2C9, SPN mildly inhibited several CYP enzymes, with potency ranked in the order CYP2C8 > CYP2C19; the IC_{50} values were 13.6 ± 3.15 μM and 16.8 ± 3.21 μM, respectively (Table 2; Figure 2). Although the IC_{50} values could not been calculated, SPN also appears to weakly inhibit CYP2D6 and CYP3A4; the residual enzyme activities at the highest tested concentration (50 μM) were 53.9 ± 3.53% and 53.3 ± 4.00%, respectively (Figure 2). No apparent inhibition of the other CYPs (CYP1A2, CYP2A6, CYP2B6, and CYP2E1) was observed (Figure 2). SPN also strongly inhibited other CYP2C9-catalyzed diclofenac 4′-hydroxylation and losartan oxidation activities (Figure 3). The inhibition mechanisms of SPN on CYP2C9-catalyzed tolbutamide 4-hydroxylation and diclofenac 4′-hydroxylation activities were both competitive, with K_i values of 0.503 ± 0.0383 μM and 0.587 ± 0.0470 μM, respectively. Pre-incubation of SPN for 30 min with human liver microsomes and an NADPH-generating system did not alter the inhibition potencies against the nine CYPs, suggesting that SPN is not a time-dependent inactivator.

The reversible inhibition of SPN-mediated CYP3A4 activity was less consistent with the published literature. Li et al. [16] reported that among 44 tested flavonoids, SPN inhibited CYP3A4-catalyzed bufalin 5′-hydroxylation activity with a K_i value of 2.17 ± 0.29 μM. They only focused on the in vitro inhibitory potentials of several flavonoids against CYP3A4 activity. To the best of our knowledge, to date, bufalin has not been used as the in vitro probe substrate for the CYP3A4 activity, and the reference material of 5′-hydroxybufalin is not commercially available. Because of the presence of several binding regions within the CYP3A4 active site, multiple probe substrates are often used for in vitro CYP3A4-mediated drug–drug interaction studies, including midazolam, nifedipine, and testosterone [34]. In that study, when other CYP3A4 substrates were tested, the ranges of IC_{50} values by SPN were reported to be 5.62–38.4 μM [16]. Additionally, we examined the inhibitory effect on another CYP3A4-catalyzed testosterone 6β-hydroxylation and found that SPN also inhibited the activity with an IC_{50} value of 31.5 ± 4.79 μM, which showed a higher percentage inhibition compared to midazolam (data not shown). Altogether, the in vitro CYP3A4 inhibition by SPN seemed to be substrate-specific.

Generally, alterations in the activities of hepatic CYPs through in vitro inhibition or induction represent the major mechanisms underlying pharmacokinetic drug–drug interactions [11–13]. It has been estimated that CYP2C9 is responsible for the metabolic clearance of up to 15–20% of all drugs undergoing phase I metabolism, including clinically important drugs such as *S*-warfarin, phenytoin, tolbutamide, losartan, and several anti-inflammatory drugs [23,35]. Considering that SPN is a potent CYP2C9 inhibitor in vitro, there may be potential for herb–drug interactions between SPN and CYP2C9 substrates after concomitant oral administration.

Using the in vitro reversible inhibition results, a clinical drug–drug interaction risk was initially predicted by the basic static model approach, as recommended by the EMA [36] and US FDA [37] with calculating the R_1 value ($R_1 = 1 + [I_{max,u}/K_{i,u}]$), which representing the predicted AUC ratio in the presence or absence of inhibitor. Where, $I_{max,u}$ ($C_{max,u}$) is maximal free plasma concentration of the inhibitor and $K_{i,u}$ is the unbound in vitro inhibition constant. However, little information is yet to be reported on the C_{max} values of SPN after oral administration of SPN. As stated in the Introduction, from our previous study, the C_{max} of SPN was reported to be 13.1 ng/mL in rats after oral dosing of 12.9 mg/kg SPN in rats [8]. Thus, we investigated whether SPN affects the pharmacokinetics of diclofenac and 4′-hydroxydiclofenac, produced by hepatic CYP2C9 enzyme, in rats. In the group that received co-administration of SPN (75 mg/kg), the C_{max} of SPN was found to be 33.7 ± 14.8 ng/mL (0.0732 ± 0.0321 μM) at 60–75 min (Figure 6C). These results suggest that SPN has low oral bioavailability. The calculated values of $I_{max,\,u}$ and $K_{i,u}$ for SPN used in this study were 0.0420 ± 0.0184 nM and 3.39 ± 0.258 nM (3.95 ± 0.316 nM for diclofenac 4′-hydroxylation), respectively. Considering these values, the R_1 value of SPN for the inhibition of CYP2C9 in vitro was calculated as 1.0124 (K_i, u for tolbutamide 4-hydroxylation) or 1.0106 ($K_{i,\,u}$ for diclofenac 4′-hydroxylation) which are both below the EMA and US FDA cut-off criteria of R_1, 1.02 [36,37], indicating that the potential for clinically relevant drug interaction-mediated CYP2C9 inhibition by SPN may be low and no clinical interaction studies are warranted. In our results, also no significant differences were observed in any of the other pharmacokinetic parameters of diclofenac and 4′-hydroxydiclofenac in rats in the absence or presence of oral co-administration of SPN at a dose of 75 mg/kg (Table 3). Furthermore, the molar metabolic conversion ratio, expressed as $AUC_{4'\text{-hydroxydiclofenac}}/AUC_{diclofenac}$, which indicated a causal factor for the evaluation of the capacities of CYP2C9 activity in vivo, did not show significant differences (0.799 ± 0.167 versus 0.904 ± 0.0534) in both groups (Table 3).

To explain the lack of in vitro–in vivo correlation, we assessed two factors that could limit the accuracy of in vitro models in predicting metabolic drug interactions in vivo, which were SPN's degree of plasma protein binding and its permeability in Caco-2 cells. We found that SPN was extensively bound in both human and rat plasma proteins (>99.9%) with a mean unbound fraction value of 0.0574% in the range of 10 and 50 μM. Thus, taking the plasma protein binding of SPN into account, the unbound maximum concentrations of SPN in plasma might be 0.0420 ± 0.0184 nM, which is much lower than the unbound K_i values of SPN in vitro. Some drugs that indicate in vitro–in vivo discrepancy because of high plasma protein bindings have been reported [38–40]. Tolfenamic acid strongly inhibited CYP1A2 in vitro but not in vivo because of high plasma protein binding (99.7%) [38]. Montelukast is a very potent inhibitor of CYP2C8 in vitro with K_i values ranging from 0.0092–0.15 μM [41]. However, in humans, montelukast has had no effect on the pharmacokinetics of the CYP2C8 substrates, pioglitazone [39] and rosiglitazone [40]. The high degree of protein binding of montelukast in plasma (>99.7%) is similar to that of tolfenamic acid and explicitly explains the lack of its in vivo interaction, irrespective of its strong inhibitor potency in vitro. The Caco-2 cell model is widely used to predict the absorption across the intestinal barrier, and a good correlation between its oral absorption in humans and its apparent permeability (P_{app}) across the Caco-2 cell barrier has been shown [24,25]. A recent study has provided some updated guidelines on how permeability values might correlate with human oral absorption: Low permeability (0–20% absorbed) is correlated to P_{app} values $< 1–2 \times 10^{-6}$ cm/s; moderate permeability (20–80% absorbed) to P_{app} values $< 2–10 \times 10^{-6}$ cm/s; and high permeability (80–100% absorbed) to P_{app} values $> 10 \times 10^{-6}$ cm/s [42]. Propranolol had >90% human absorption and exhibited high permeability with a P_{app} value of $(26.8 \pm 3.31) \times 10^{-6}$ cm/s in our assay. SPN exhibited a very low permeability with mean P_{app} values of 0.115×10^{-6} cm/s (0.429% of propranolol P_{app}) and 0.172×10^{-6} cm/s (0.642% of propranolol P_{app}) at 10 and 50 μM, respectively, indicating that it is poorly absorbed in vivo. SPN was not a substrate for efflux transporters, that is, P-gp and BCRP, as the efflux ratio (B-to-A/A-to-B) is less than 2.

Overall, SPN is a potent inhibitor of CYP2C9 in vitro but not in vivo. This apparent discrepancy is due to the extensive plasma protein binding and very low permeability of SPN, which resulted in poor oral absorption. These approaches could help in making more reliable in vitro–in vivo extrapolations about the risk of in vivo inhibition potential. In conclusion, these findings have provided useful information on the safe and effective use of SPN in clinical practice.

Author Contributions: Conceptualization, Y.F.Z., S.H.B., and S.K.B.; methodology, Z.H., S.U.C., C.B.L., and D.K.; software, Z.H. and S.U.C.; validation, Y.F.Z., Z.H., S.U.C., C.B.L., S.J.J., and H.J.S.; formal analysis, Y.F.Z., S.U.C., and S.J.J.; investigation, Z.H., C.B.L., D.K., and H.Y.; resources, D.K. and H.Y.; data curation, Y.F.Z., S.H.B., and S.K.B.; writing—original draft preparation, Y.F.Z. and S.H.B.; writing—review and editing, S.H.B. and S.K.B.; visualization, S.J.J. and H.J.S.; supervision, S.K.B.; project administration, S.K.B.; funding acquisition, S.K.B. All authors have read and agreed to the published version of the manuscript.

Previous Presentation of Information: A portion of the information in this manuscript has been presented as a poster in a conference previously: Soo Hyun Jang, Yu Fen Zheng, Chae Bin Lee, Soo Kyung Bae. 2019. Cytochrome P450 2C9 inhibition by sophoranone in human liver microsomes. 15th Euro-Global Summit on Toxicology and Applied Pharmacology, Berlin, Germany.

References

1. Ding, P.L.; He, C.M.; Cheng, Z.H.; Chen, D.F. Flavonoids rather than alkaloids as the diagnostic constituents to distinguish *Sophorae Flavescentis Radix* from *Sophorae Tonkinensis Radix* et Rhizoma: An HPLC fingerprint study. *Chin. J. Nat. Med.* **2018**, *16*, 951–960. [CrossRef]
2. He, C.M.; Cheng, Z.H.; Chen, D.F. Qualitative and quantitative analysis of flavonoids in *Sophora tonkinensis* by LC/MS and HPLC. *Chin. J. Nat. Med.* **2013**, *11*, 690–698. [CrossRef]
3. Yoo, H.; Kang, M.; Pyo, S.; Chae, H.S.; Ryu, K.H.; Kim, J.; Chin, Y.W. SKI3301, a purified herbal extract from *Sophora tonkinensis*, inhibited airway inflammation and bronchospasm in allergic asthma animal models in vivo. *J. Ethnopharmacol.* **2017**, *206*, 298–305. [CrossRef]
4. Lee, J.W.; Lee, J.H.; Lee, C.; Jin, Q.; Lee, D.; Kim, Y.; Hong, J.T.; Lee, M.K.; Hwang, B.Y. Inhibitory constituents of *Sophora tonkinensis* on nitric oxide production in RAW 264.7 macrophages. *Bioorg. Med. Chem. Lett.* **2015**, *25*, 960–962. [CrossRef]

5. Kajimoto, S.; Takanashi, N.; Kajimoto, T.; Xu, M.; Cao, J.; Masuda, Y.; Aiuchi, T.; Nakajo, S.; Ida, Y.; Nakaya, K Sophoranone, extracted from a traditional Chinese medicine Shan Dou Gen, induces apoptosis in human leukemia U937 cells via formation of reactive oxygen species and opening of mitochondrial permeability transition pores. *Int. J. Cancer* **2002**, *99*, 879–890. [CrossRef]
6. Yang, X.; Deng, S.; Huang, M.; Wang, J.; Chen, L.; Xiong, M.; Yang, J.; Zheng, S.; Ma, X.; Zhao, P.; et al Chemical constituents from *Sophora tonkinensis* and their glucose transporter 4 translocation activities. *Bioorg. Med. Chem. Lett.* **2017**, *27*, 1463–1466. [CrossRef] [PubMed]
7. Atta-Ur-Rahman; Haroone, M.S.; Tareen, R.B.; Mohammed Ahmed Hassan, O.M.; Jan, S.; Abbaskhan, A.; Asif, M.; Gulzar, T.; Al-Majid, A.M.; Yousuf, S.; et al. Secondary metabolites of Sophora mollis subsp. griffithii (Stocks) Ali. *Phytochem. Lett.* **2012**, *5*, 613–616. [CrossRef]
8. Jang, S.M.; Bae, S.H.; Choi, W.K.; Park, J.B.; Kim, D.; Min, J.S.; Yoo, H.; Kang, M.; Ryu, K.H.; Bae, S.K. Pharmacokinetic properties of trifolirhizin, (-)-maackiain, (-)-sophoranone and 2-(2,4-dihydroxyphenyl)-5,6-methylenedioxybenzofuran after intravenous and oral administration of *Sophora tonkinensis* extract in rats. *Xenobiotica* **2015**, *45*, 1092–1104. [CrossRef] [PubMed]
9. Rekić, D.; Reynolds, K.S.; Zhao, P.; Zhang, L.; Yoshida, K.; Sachar, M.; Piquette Miller, M.; Huang, S.M.; Zineh, I. Clinical drug-drug interaction evaluations to inform drug use and enable drug access. *J. Pharm. Sci.* **2017**, *106*, 2214–2218. [CrossRef]
10. Bjornsson, T.D.; Callaghan, J.T.; Einolf, H.J.; Fischer, V.; Gas, L.; Grimm, S.; Kao, J.; King, S.P.; Miwa, G.; Ni, L.; et al. The conduct of in vitro and in vivo drug-drug interaction studies: A pharmaceutical research and manufactures of America (PhRMA) perspective. *Drug Metab. Dispos.* **2003**, *31*, 815–832. [CrossRef]
11. Lin, J.H.; Lu, A.Y. Inhibition and induction of cytochrome P450 and the clinical implications. *Clin. Pharmacokinet.* **1998**, *35*, 361–390. [CrossRef] [PubMed]
12. Peng, Y.; Wu, H.; Zhang, X.; Zhang, F.; Qi, H.; Zhong, Y.; Wang, Y.; Sang, H.; Wang, G.; Sun, J. A comprehensive assay for nine major cytochrome P450 enzymes activities with 16 probe reactions on human liver microsomes by a single LC/MS/MS run to support reliable in vitro inhibitory drug-drug interaction evaluation. *Xenobiotica* **2015**, *45*, 961–977. [CrossRef]
13. Wienkers, L.C.; Heath, T.G. Predicting in vivo drug interactions from in vitro drug discovery data. *Nat. Rev. Drug Discov.* **2005**, *4*, 825–833. [CrossRef] [PubMed]
14. Chen, Q.; Zhang, T.; Wang, J.F.; Wei, D.Q. Advances in human cytochrome P450 and personalized medicine. *Curr. Drug Metab.* **2011**, *12*, 436–444. [CrossRef] [PubMed]
15. Cai, J.; Ma, J.; Xu, K.; Gao, G.; Xiang, Y.; Lin, C. Effect of Radix Sophorae Tonkinensis on the activity of cytochrome P450 isoforms in rats. *Int. J. Clin. Exp. Med.* **2015**, *8*, 9737–9743.
16. Li, Y.; Ning, J.; Wang, Y.; Wang, C.; Sun, C.; Huo, X.; Yu, Z.; Feng, L.; Zhang, B.; Tian, X.; et al. Drug interaction study of flavonoids toward CYP3A4 and their quantitative structure activity relationship (QSAR) analysis for predicting potential effects. *Toxicol. Lett.* **2018**, *294*, 27–36. [CrossRef]
17. Cho, D.Y.; Bae, S.H.; Lee, J.K.; Kim, Y.W.; Kim, B.T.; Bae, S.K. Selective inhibition of cytochrome P450 2D6 by Sarpogrelate and its active metabolite, M-1, in human liver microsomes. *Drug Metab. Dispos.* **2014**, *42*, 33–39. [CrossRef]
18. Zheng, Y.F.; Bae, S.H.; Choi, E.J.; Park, J.B.; Kim, S.O.; Jang, M.J.; Park, G.H.; Shin, W.G.; Oh, E.; Bae, S.K. Evaluation of the in vitro/in vivo drug interaction potential of BST204, a purified dry extract of ginseng, and its four bioactive ginsenosides through cytochrome P450 inhibition/induction and UDP-glucuronosyltransferase inhibition. *Food Chem. Toxicol.* **2014**, *68*, 117–127. [CrossRef]
19. Li, G.; Huang, K.; Nikolic, D.; van Breemen, R.B. High-throughput cytochrome P450 cocktail inhibition assay for assessing drug-drug and drug-botanical interactions. *Drug Metab. Dispos.* **2015**, *43*, 1670–1678. [CrossRef]
20. Kim, H.J.; Lee, H.; Ji, H.K.; Lee, T.; Liu, K.H. Screening of ten cytochrome P450 enzyme activities with 12 probe substrates in human liver microsomes using cocktail incubation and liquid chromatography-tandem mass spectrometry. *Biopharm. Drug Dispos.* **2019**, *40*, 101–111. [CrossRef]
21. Valicherla, G.R.; Mishra, A.; Lenkalapelly, S.; Jillela, B.; Francis, F.M.; Rajagopalan, L.; Srivastava, P. Investigation of the inhibition of eight major human cytochrome P450 isozymes by a probe substrate cocktail in vitro with emphasis on CYP2E1. *Xenobiotica* **2019**, *49*, 1396–1402. [CrossRef] [PubMed]
22. Kumar, V.; Wahlstrom, J.L.; Rock, D.A.; Warren, C.J.; Gorman, L.A.; Tracy, T.S. CYP2C9 inhibition: Impact of probe selection and pharmacogenetics on in vitro inhibition profiles. *Drug Metab. Dispos.* **2006**, *34*, 1966–1975. [CrossRef] [PubMed]

23. Yasar, U.; Tybring, G.; Hidestrand, M.; Oscarson, M.; Ingelman-Sundberg, M.; Dahl, M.L.; Eliasson, E. Role of CYP2C9 polymorphism in losartan oxidation. *Drug Metab. Dispos.* **2001**, *29*, 1051–1056. [PubMed]
24. Elsby, R.; Surry, D.D.; Smith, V.N.; Gray, A.J. Validation and application of Caco-2 assays for the in vitro evaluation of development candidate drugs as substrates or inhibitors of P-glycoprotein to support regulatory submissions. *Xenobiotica* **2008**, *38*, 1140–1164. [CrossRef] [PubMed]
25. Markowska, M.; Oberle, R.; Juzwin, S.; Hsu, C.P.; Gryszkiewicz, M.; Streeter, A.J. Optimizing Caco-2 cell monolayers to increase throughput in drug intestinal absorption analysis. *J. Pharmacol. Toxicol. Methods* **2001**, *46*, 51–55. [CrossRef]
26. Cho, M.A.; Yoon, J.G.; Kim, V.; Kim, H.; Lee, R.; Lee, M.G.; Kim, D. Functional characterization of pharmcogenetic variants of human cytochrome P450 2C9 in Korean populations. *Biomol. Ther. (Seoul)* **2019**, *27*, 577–583. [CrossRef] [PubMed]
27. Yoo, H.; Ryu, K.H.; Bae, S.K.; Kim, J. Simultaneous determination of trifolirhizin, (-)-maackiain, (-)-sophoranone, and 2-(2,4-dihydroxyphenyl)-5,6-methylenedioxybenzofuran from Sophora tonkinensis in rat plasma by liquid chromatography with tandem mass spectrometry and its application to a pharmacokinetic study. *J. Sep. Sci.* **2014**, *37*, 3235–3244. [CrossRef]
28. Bourrié, M.; Meunier, V.; Berger, Y.; Fabre, G. Cytochrome P450 isoform inhibitors as a tool for the investigation of metabolic reactions catalyzed by human liver microsomes. *J. Pharmacol. Exp. Ther.* **1996**, *277*, 321–332.
29. Obach, R.S.; Walsky, R.L.; Venkatakrishnan, K. Mechanism-based inactivation of human cytochrome P450 enzymes and the prediction of drug-drug interactions. *Drug Metab. Dispos.* **2006**, *35*, 246–255. [CrossRef]
30. Parkinson, A.; Kazmi, F.; Buckley, D.B.; Yerino, P.; Paris, B.L.; Holsapple, J.; Toren, P.; Otradovec, S.M.; Ogilvie, B.W. An evaluation of the dilution method for identifying metabolism-dependent inhibitors of cytochrome P450 enzymes. *Drug Metab. Dispos.* **2011**, *39*, 1370–1387. [CrossRef]
31. Stresser, D.M.; Mao, J.; Kenny, J.R.; Jones, B.C.; Grime, K. Exploring concepts of in vitro time-dependent CYP inhibition assays. *Expert Opin. Drug Metab. Toxicol.* **2014**, *10*, 157–174. [CrossRef] [PubMed]
32. Xu, L.; Wang, W. Herbs for clearing heat. In *Chinese Materia Medica: Combinations and Applications*, 1st ed.; Donica Publishing Ltd.: St. Albans, UK, 2002; p. 115.
33. US Food and Drug Administration. Guidance for Industry: Estimating the Maximum Safe Starting Dose in Initial Clinical Trials for Therapeutics in Adult Healthy Volunteer. 2005. Available online: https://www.fda.gov/media/72309/download (accessed on 31 March 2020).
34. Foti, R.S.; Rock, D.A.; Wienkers, L.C.; Wahlstrom, J.L. Selection of alternative CYP3A4 probe substrates for clinical drug interaction studies using in vitro data and in vivo simulation. *Drug Metab. Dispos.* **2010**, *38*, 981–987. [CrossRef] [PubMed]
35. Van Booven, D.; Marsh, S.; McLeod, H.; Carrillo, M.W.; Sangkuhl, K.; Klein, T.E.; Altman, R.B. Cytochrome P450 2C9-CYP2C9. *Pharmacogenet. Genom.* **2010**, *20*, 277–281. [CrossRef] [PubMed]
36. European Medicine Agency. Guideline on the Investigation of Drug Interactions. 2012. Available online: https://www.ema.europa.eu/en/documents/scientific-guideline/guideline-investigation-drug-interactions-revision-1_en.pdf (accessed on 31 March 2020).
37. US Food and Drug Administration. Guidance for industry: In Vitro Drug Interaction Studies-Cytochrome P450 Enzyme-and Transporter-Mediated Drug Interactions. 2020. Available online: https://www.fda.gov/media/134582/download (accessed on 31 March 2020).
38. Karjalainen, M.J.; Neuvonen, P.J.; Backman, J.T. Tolfenamic acid is a potent CYP1A2 inhibitor in vitro but does not interact in vivo: Correction for protein binding is needed for data interpretation. *Eur. J. Clin. Pharmacol.* **2007**, *63*, 829–836. [CrossRef] [PubMed]
39. Jaakkola, T.; Backman, J.T.; Neuvonen, M.; Niemi, M.; Neuvonen, P.J. Montelukast and zafirlukast do not affect the pharmacokinetics of the CYP2C8 substrate pioglitazone. *Eur. J. Clin. Pharmacol.* **2006**, *62*, 503–509. [CrossRef] [PubMed]
40. Kim, K.A.; Park, P.W.; Kim, K.R.; Park, J.Y. Effect of multiple doses of montelukast on the pharmacokinetics of rosiglitazone, a CYP2C8 substrate, in humans. *Br. J. Clin. Pharmacol.* **2006**, *63*, 339–345. [CrossRef]
41. Walsky, R.L.; Obach, R.S.; Gaman, E.A.; Gleeson, J.P.; Proctor, W.R. Selective inhibition of human cytochrome P4502C8 by montelukast. *Drug Metab. Dispos.* **2005**, *33*, 413–418. [CrossRef]
42. Press, B.; di Grandi, D. Permeability for intestinal absorption: Caco-2 assay and related issues. *Curr. Drug Metab.* **2008**, *9*, 893–900. [CrossRef]

Effect of Ticagrelor, a Cytochrome P450 3A4 Inhibitor on the Pharmacokinetics of Tadalafil in Rats

Young-Guk Na †, Jin-Ju Byeon †, Hyun Wook Huh, Min-Ki Kim, Young G. Shin, Hong-Ki Lee * and Cheong-Weon Cho *

College of Pharmacy and Institute of Drug Research and Development, Chungnam National University, 99, Daehak-ro, Yuseong-gu, Daejeon 34134, Korea

* Correspondence: dvmlhk@gmail.com (H.-K.L.); chocw@cnu.ac.kr (C.-W.C.) +82-42-821-5934 (C.-W.C.)

† These authors contributed equally to this work.

Abstract: Tadalafil is a cytochrome P450 (CYP) 3A4 substrate. Because there are few data on drug-drug interactions, it is advisable to take sufficient consideration when co-administering tadalafil with CYP3A4 inducers or inhibitors. This study was conducted to assess the effect of ticagrelor, a CYP3A4 inhibitor, on the pharmacokinetic properties of tadalafil after oral administration to rats. A total of 20 Sprague–Dawley male rats were randomly divided into the non-pretreated group and ticagrelor-pretreated group, and tadalafil was orally administered to each group after pretreatment with or without ticagrelor. Blood samples were collected at predetermined time points after oral administration of tadalafil. As a result, systemic exposure of tadalafil in the ticagrelor-pretreated group was significantly increased compared to the non-pretreated group (1.61-fold), and the clearance of tadalafil in the ticagrelor-pretreated group was significantly reduced than the non-pretreated group (37%). The prediction of the drug profile through the one-compartment model could explain the differences of pharmacokinetic properties of tadalafil in the non-pretreated and ticagrelor-pretreated groups. This study suggests that ticagrelor reduces a CYP3A-mediated tadalafil metabolism and that tadalafil and a combination regimen with tadalafil and ticagrelor requires dose control and specific pharmacotherapy.

Keywords: tadalafil; ticagrelor; drug-drug interaction; pharmacokinetics; plasma concentration; CYP3A4

---

1. Introduction

Erectile dysfunction (ED), the most prevalent complaint in males, is the persistent inability to maintain an erection [1]. Various factors, such as age and presence of cardiovascular diseases, influence the incidence of ED [2,3]. Particularly, vascular diseases, such as coronary artery disease (CAD), are related to a high prevalence of ED [4–6]. It has been reported that 42% of patients between the ages of 40 and 60 years are affected by this condition [7–9]. In addition, a high rate of ED prevalence (~75%) has been investigated in CAD patients [10,11]. The most commonly prescribed oral drugs for ED are the 5-phosphodiesterase (PDE5) inhibitors, and the drugs for CAD are the platelet aggregation inhibitor [12,13]. Therefore, PDE5 may be co-administered to CAD patients already receiving platelet aggregation inhibitors.

Tadalafil (Cialis®), the approved PDE5 inhibitor, is used in the treatment of ED and is one of the most frequently prescribed PDE5 inhibitors [14]. In addition, tadalafil exhibits a longer clinical efficacy (up to 36 h) than sildenafil or vardenafil [15,16]. Because of the long duration of action, a once-a-day dose regimen improves the life quality of patients. Tadalafil is classified as a cytochrome P450 (CYP) 3A4 substrate and is mainly metabolized by CYP3A4 to catechol, which is extensively bound to form methyl catechol glucuronide, a major circulating metabolite of tadalafil through methylation [17].

Ticagrelor (Brilinta®), the platelet aggregation inhibitor, belongs to $P2Y_{12}$ receptor antagonists and is used for the treatment of CAD [18,19]. It provides the superior and more sustained inhibition of platelet aggregation than clopidogrel, another $P2Y_{12}$ receptor antagonist [20]. Recent studies have reported that ticagrelor acts as an inhibitor of CYP3A4 [21,22]. When ticagrelor was co-administered with atorvastatin, ticagrelor acted as a CYP inhibitor, increasing the maximal plasma concentration of atorvastatin and the area under the plasma concentration-time curve from 0 to infinity by 23% and 36%, respectively [23]. Therefore, drug-drug interaction by co-administration of tadalafil and ticagrelor can inhibit the metabolism of CYP3A4 substrates, such as tadalafil. Despite the possibility of co-administration, the pharmacokinetic interactions between ticagrelor and tadalafil are still uncertain.

Because ticagrelor is an inhibitor of CYP3A4 that accounts for about 15–30% of the total CYP enzyme in humans, the co-administration potentially affects efficacy and safety by altering tadalafil exposure [24]. In healthy male volunteers, the plasma concentrations of tadalafil have been shown to increase with CYP3A4 inhibitors, such as ritonavir [25]. Although tadalafil is well tolerated, patients have experienced side effects, such as headaches, stomachaches, back pain, muscle aches, nasal congestion, redness, limb pain, dizziness, or blurred vision due to the high exposure of tadalafil [26,27]. In other studies, the side effects were increased when doses of tadalafil were higher, indicating that side effects were somewhat related to blood concentration of tadalafil [28,29]. Thus, the combination of tadalafil with ticagrelor also warranted investigation and a drug-drug interaction study should be conducted. However, pharmacokinetic interactions between tadalafil and ticagrelor have not been reported in vivo models.

The objective of our study was to evaluate the effect of ticagrelor on the plasma concentration-time profiles of tadalafil in rats. This study was performed with a parallel design consisting of a non-pretreated group and a ticagrelor-pretreated group. The ticagrelor-pretreated group received oral administration of ticagrelor for seven days of the pretreatment period to inhibit CYP3A. Tadalafil was then orally administered on the seventh day. The non-compartment analysis was performed to analyze the pharmacokinetic profile and the one-compartment model was successfully applied to compare the pharmacokinetics between the two groups. This study assumed that potential drug-drug interactions between ticagrelor and tadalafil could have a clinical impact on the patients.

2. Materials and Methods

2.1. Chemicals and Reagents

Tadalafil, ticagrelor, and paclitaxel (internal standard (IS)) were kindly obtained from Korea United Pharma Inc. (Seoul, Korea). Dimethyl sulfoxide, formic acid, and polyethylene glycol 400 (PEG 400) were purchased from Sigma–Aldrich (St. Louis, MO, USA). Acetonitrile and methanol were purchased from J.T. Baker (Phillipsburg, NJ, USA). Analytical grade reagents were used throughout this study. Overall, distilled water was used.

2.2. LC-MS/MS Analysis of Tadalafil

The concentrations of tadalafil were analyzed by a liquid chromatography tandem-mass spectrometry (LC-MS/MS) system equipped with Agilent 1290 series and Agilent 6495 Triple Quad LC/MS (Agilent Technologies, Santa Clara, CA, USA). A YMC-Triart C18 column (50 × 2.0 mm, 1.9 μm; YMC Inc., Wilmington, NC, USA) was used. The mobile phase was a mixture of 0.2% formic acid in acetonitrile and 0.2% formic acid in distilled water (50:50, *v/v*), and the flow rate was 0.4 mL/min. The temperature of the column and autosampler were set as 30 °C and 4 °C, respectively. The positive ion mode using Agilent jet stream electrospray ionization (AJS-ESI) was applied to record the scan mass spectra. The ion transitions of tadalafil and IS were set as 390.4→268.1 m/z and 876.4→308.1 m/z, respectively, and detected with a multiple reaction monitoring (MRM) mode. The collision energies for tadalafil and IS were 10 V and 30 V, respectively. The cell accelerator voltage was 5 V and the dwell time was set as 200 ms. The source parameters were set as follows: Gas temperature 200 °C, gas flow

14 L/min, nebulizer 20 psi, sheath gas heater 250 °C, sheath gas flow 11 L/min, capillary 3000 V, and nozzle voltage 1500 V.

In this analysis, the most abundant ion transition of tadalafil (390.4→268.1 m/z) was selected to determine the lowest limit of quantification (LLOQ), and the LLOQ of tadalafil was 3 ng/mL. The range of calibration curve of tadalafil was set to 3–6670 ng/mL. The curve was written with a weighted linear regression (1/x) and showed excellent linearity with $R^2 > 0.997$. The method has shown accurate and reproducible results within acceptable tolerances (less than 20% coefficient of variation (CV) at LLOQ and less than 15% CV at all other concentrations) [30]. The acquired LC-MS/MS data were processed with Agilent analysis software (Agilent MassHunter Quantitative Software Version B.07.00, Agilent Technologies, Santa Clara, CA, USA).

2.3. *Animals*

All animal experiments were carried out in accordance with the protocol (No. CNU-01167) and the "Guidelines in Use of Animal" approved by Chungnam National University Institutional Animal Care and Use Committee (Daejeon, Korea, 2019). Male Sprague–Dawley rats (aged 7–8 weeks, bodyweight 250–300 g) were purchased from Nara-Biotec (Seoul, Korea). All animals were housed in a dark-light cycle of 12 h at 22 °C and were allowed free access to water and food.

2.4. *Pharmacokinetic Study*

The experiment was performed in a parallel design. A total of 20 rats were randomly divided into two groups. The control group, Group N (n = 10, non-pretreated rats), was orally administered for 7 days only with the vehicle (normal saline/polyethylene glycol 400/dimethyl sulfoxide = 40:20:20). Group T (n = 10, ticagrelor-pretreated rats), an experimental group, received 10 mg/kg of ticagrelor in the vehicle once a day for 7 days orally. Thereafter, on the seventh day, tadalafil (2 mg/kg) was orally administered 30 min after the final administration of the vehicle or ticagrelor. Doses of all samples were calculated according to the weight of the rats and administered using gavage. The dose of ticagrelor and tadalafil given to rats were determined by converting the human doses (90 mg for ticagrelor and 20 mg for tadalafil) to animal doses with body surface area, according to the United States Food and Drug Administration guidelines [31]. Blood (0.3 mL) was collected from the retro-orbital plexus or the jugular vein at predetermined time-points (0, 0.33, 0.67, 1, 1.5, 2, 4, 6, 8, 12, and 24 h) after the oral administration. Samples were centrifuged at 15,000× *g* for 5 min at 4 °C. The plasma was collected and stored at −20 °C until the concentration of tadalafil was analyzed by LC-MS/MS.

2.5. *Sample Preparation for LC-MS/MS Analysis*

Protein precipitation was applied to extract tadalafil from plasma. Briefly, 200 μL of acetonitrile (0.2 *v/v*% formic acid) containing 500 ng/mL of IS was added to 20 μL of the plasma sample. After shaking for 5 min, the mixture was centrifuged at 15,000× *g* for 5 min. The supernatant (150 μL) was transferred and 5 μL of the sample was injected into the LC-MS/MS.

2.6. *Pharmacokinetic Data Analysis*

Pharmacokinetic data were analyzed based on the non-compartment analysis of WinNonlin software 8.1 (Pharsight Corp., Sunnyvale, CA, USA). The maximum plasma concentration of tadalafil (maximum concentration (C_{max})) and the time to reach the maximal plasma concentration (T_{max}) of tadalafil were determined from the plasma concentration-time profiles. The area under the plasma concentration vs time curve from 0 to 24 h ($AUC_{0–24}$) was calculated by the linear trapezoidal rule and the area under the plasma concentration vs time curve from 0 h to infinite time ($AUC_{0–\infty}$) was estimated by extrapolating time to infinity. The elimination half-life ($T_{1/2}$) and apparent total clearance (CL/F) were determined from the ln 2/elimination rate constant and dose/$AUC_{0–\infty}$, respectively [32].

2.7. Pharmacokinetic Modeling

Pharmacokinetic modeling of the plasma concentration-time profile of tadalafil was performed using a one-compartment model to investigate the absorption and elimination rates. The parameters of the one-compartment model of tadalafil were estimated based on data from Group N and Group T.

In this model, the shift of the tadalafil amount in the gut compartment and the central compartment is described by the following equations [33]:

$$\frac{dG}{dt} = -K_a \cdot G$$

$$\frac{dC}{dt} = K_a \cdot G - K_e \cdot C$$

where G and C represent the amount of tadalafil in the gut compartment and the central compartment, respectively. K_a indicates the absorption rate constant from the gut compartment to the central compartment. K_e indicates the elimination rate constant from the central compartment to the gut compartment. Each equation was applied to both Group N and Group T data through the classic model of WinNolin software 8.1 (Pharsight Corp., Sunnyvale, CA, USA).

Predicted plasma concentrations of tadalafil (Con_{pred}) using the one-compartment model were estimated by the following equation [34]:

$$Con_{pred} = C/(V/F)$$

where *V/F* indicates the central volume of distribution of tadalafil.

The fold error versus concentration or time was calculated using the following equation [35]:

$$Fold\ error = \frac{Con_{pred} - Con_{obs}}{Con_{obs}}$$

where Con_{pred} indicates the predicted concentration of tadalafil from the one-compartment pharmacokinetic modeling and Con_{obs} indicates the observed concentration of tadalafil from the pharmacokinetic experiment. The fold error within ±2-fold is an acceptable range [35].

2.8. Statistical Analysis

Values are represented as mean ± standard deviation (SD). A student's t-test was applied for statistical significance of differences ($p < 0.05$) and the statistical analysis was performed using GraphPad Prism 8 software (GraphPad Software Inc., La Jolla, CA, USA).

3. Results and Discussion

3.1. Pharmacokinetic Data

The purpose of our study was to assess the effect of ticagrelor on plasma concentration-time profiles of tadalafil in rats. Drug-drug interactions may occur when CYP inducers or inhibitors are co-administered with the drug metabolized by the CYP enzyme. Several studies have demonstrated that ticagrelor is a CYP3A4 inhibitor and tadalafil is a CYP3A4 substrate [23,25]. Therefore, potential drug-drug interactions between ticagrelor and tadalafil can occur, affecting the pharmacokinetic profile, the efficacy for treatment of erectile dysfunction, and the frequency of side effects.

To identify the potential drug-drug interactions between ticagrelor and tadalafil in rats, ticagrelor was administered once a day for seven days to inhibit CYP3A in rats only for Group T. On the last day of the study, Group N and Group T received 2 mg/kg tadalafil via oral administration to assess the pharmacokinetics effect of ticagrelor on tadalafil. The plasma concentrations of ticagrelor were sufficient to competitively inhibit CYP3A, and the effects of CYP3A inhibition on systemic exposure of tadalafil could be determined [36].

The pharmacokinetic profiles of tadalafil for Group N and Group T are shown in Figure 1. The parameters of the non-compartment analysis are listed in Table 1. The non-compartmental analysis is the model-independent method, which is based on the time course of drug concentrations. Pharmacokinetic parameters from the non-compartmental analysis are mainly used to evaluate drug exposure in oral administration of a drug. The systemic exposure of tadalafil was increased in Group T compared with Group N. Group T showed higher C_{max}, AUC_{0-24}, and $AUC_{0-\infty}$ than the C_{max}, AUC_{0-24}, and $AUC_{0-\infty}$ of Group N. These results showed significant increases in the values of AUC_{0-24} (1.61-fold, $p < 0.05$) and $AUC_{0-\infty}$ (1.66-fold, $p < 0.05$). The C_{max} of Group T slightly increased 1.15-fold compared to that of Group N, but there was no significant difference ($p = 0.3332$). The ratio of ACU_{0-24} and $AUC_{0-\infty}$ between Group N and Group T exceeded the range of 0.8–1.25, where no pre-specified pharmacological effect was observed [37].

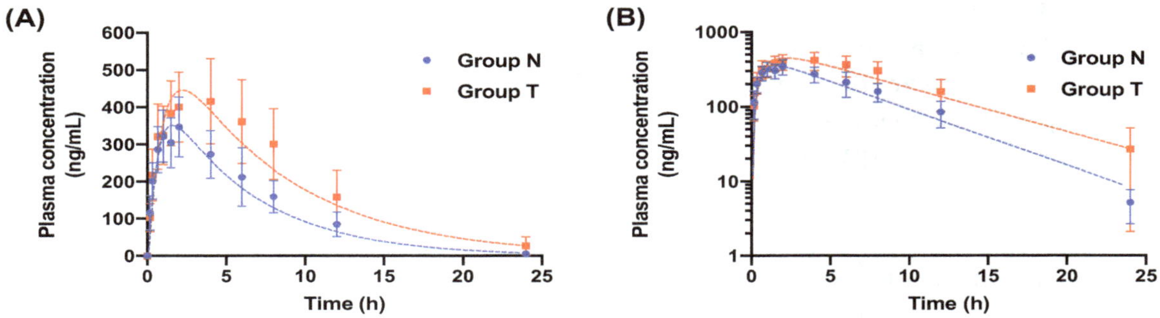

Figure 1. Plasma concentration-time profiles of tadalafil after oral administration to non-pretreated rats (Group N) and ticagrelor-pretreated rats (Group T). Values are represented as mean ± SD (n = 10). Dotted marks and dashed lines indicate the observed plasma concentration and the fitted pharmacokinetic profile from the one-compartment model, respectively. (**A**) Linear scale; (**B**) log scale.

Table 1. Non-compartment analysis parameters of tadalafil after oral administration to non-pretreated rats (Group N) and ticagrelor-pretreated rats (Group T). Values are represented as mean ± SD (n = 10).

Parameters	Group N	Group T	Ratio [a]	p-Value
C_{max} (ng/mL)	375.94 ± 72.81	432.71 ± 119.79	1.15	0.3332
AUC_{0-24} (ng·h/mL)	3046.88 ± 732.50	4895.74 ± 1592.87	1.61	0.0124
$AUC_{0-\infty}$ (ng·h/mL)	3070.95 ± 743.01	5095.04 ± 1800.30	1.66	0.0134
T_{max} (h)	1.45 ± 0.50	3.22 ± 1.30	2.22	0.0030
$T_{1/2}$ (h)	3.15 ± 0.23	4.47 ± 0.89	1.42	0.0018
CL/F (L/h/kg)	0.68 ± 0.15	0.43 ± 0.13	0.63	0.0035

[a] Ratio = $\frac{Value\ of\ Group\ T}{Value\ of\ Group\ N}$; maximum concentration (C_{max}); area under the plasma concentration vs. time curve from 0 to 24 h (AUC_{0-24}); area under the plasma concentration vs. time curve from 0 to infinity ($AUC_{0-\infty}$);time to reach maximal concentration (T_{max}); half-life ($T_{1/2}$); apparent total clearance (CL/F).

As a result of CYP inhibition by ticagrelor, the plasma concentration of tadalafil decreased more slowly after co-administration of ticagrelor and tadalafil than after tadalafil alone. T_{max}, $T_{1/2}$, and CL/F showed statistically significant differences between Groups T and Group N. In the case of T_{max}, the absorption of tadalafil in Group T was delayed (T_{max} of 3.22 ± 1.30 h) compared to that in Group N (T_{max} of 1.45 ± 0.50 h) ($p < 0.005$). Thus, the tadalafil plasma concentration remained high until 8 h. This result indicated that the reduced metabolism of tadalafil by CYP3A inhibition caused the absorption of the drug for a longer period of time [38]. In particular, Group T showed an increased $T_{1/2}$ compared to Group N ($p < 0.005$) and the CL/F value of Group T was significantly lower than that of Group N ($p < 0.005$). These results showed that the inhibition of hepatic CYP3A metabolism and the reduction of the first pass effect increased the exposure of tadalafil [39].

In general, the non-compartment analysis parameters of tadalafil showed statistically significant differences between Group N and Group T (Figure 2). In the present study, co-administration with ticagrelor increased tadalafil exposure and affected the AUC_{0-24}, $AUC_{0-\infty}$, T_{max}, and half-life of tadalafil. In particular, the half-life of tadalafil increased from 3.15 h in Group N to 4.47 h in Group T, resulting in the increased AUC_{0-24} (1.61-fold), $AUC_{0-\infty}$ (1.66-fold), and T_{max} (2.22-fold). In addition, the result of 37% reduction of tadalafil clearance in Group T compared with Group N supported our findings. These data suggest that ticagrelor inhibits tadalafil metabolism due to drug-drug interaction with tadalafil.

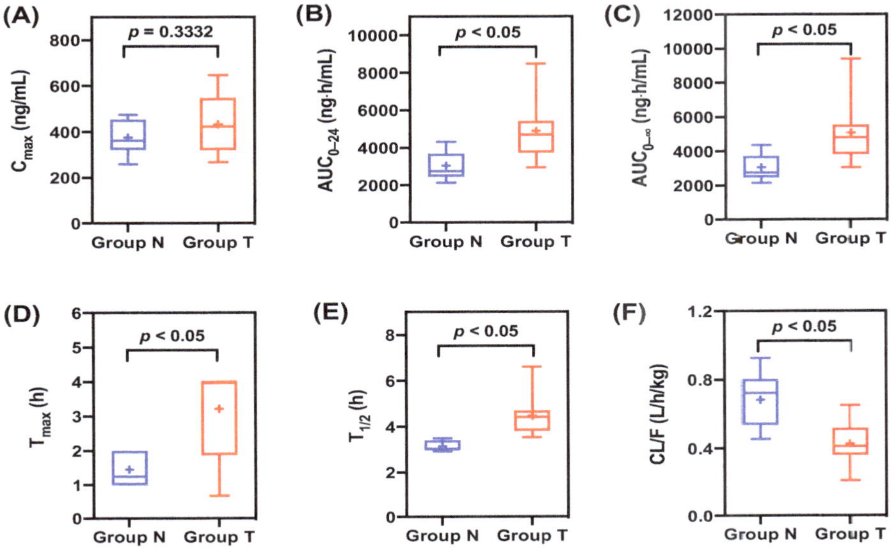

Figure 2. Comparisons of the non-compartment analysis parameters of tadalafil from non-pretreated rats (Group N) and ticagrelor-pretreated rats (Group T). Boxes mean 25th and 75th percentiles of data and whiskers mean 5th and 95th percentiles of data. The median and mean values are displayed as a solid line (–) and a plus mark (+) in boxes, respectively. (**A**) C_{max}; (**B**) AUC_{0-24}; (**C**) $AUC_{0-\infty}$; (**D**) T_{max}; (**E**) $T_{1/2}$; (**F**) CL/F. Maximum concentration (C_{max}); area under the plasma concentration vs. time curve from 0 to 24 h (AUC_{0-24}); area under the plasma concentration vs. time curve from 0 to infinity ($AUC_{0-\infty}$);time to reach maximal concentration (T_{max}); half-life ($T_{1/2}$); apparent total clearance (CL/F).

3.2. Pharmacokinetic Modeling

The one-compartment model was successfully applied to describe each group in terms of the plasma concentration-time profile after a single oral administration of 2 mg/kg tadalafil. Among the various compartment models, the one-compartment model, which is the simplest and best suited to the observed pharmacokinetic profile of tadalafil, was used to compare the observed pharmacokinetic profile with the fitted pharmacokinetic profile. The one-compartment modeling supports the results of the non-compartment analysis that changed by the co-administration of ticagrelor. The modeling-based comparison allows for greater confidence in the metabolic inhibition effect by comparing the observed pharmacokinetic profile with the fitted pharmacokinetic profile, as well as by matching with the parameters of the non-compartment analysis. Additionally, the model-based approach was used to evaluate a more specific and quantified absorption, elimination, and distribution of tadalafil in vivo.

As shown in Figure 1, the dashed lines and dotted marks mean the predicted plasma concentration and observed plasma concentration, respectively. The dashed lines showed similar patterns to the dotted marks. Figure 3 indicates the residual plot of the fold error versus time or observed plasma concentration. It shows the acceptable residual values (fold error <2) at most of the analyzed points, which indicates that the one-compartment model is suitable for the explanation of the plasma concentration profile of tadalafil [35,40].

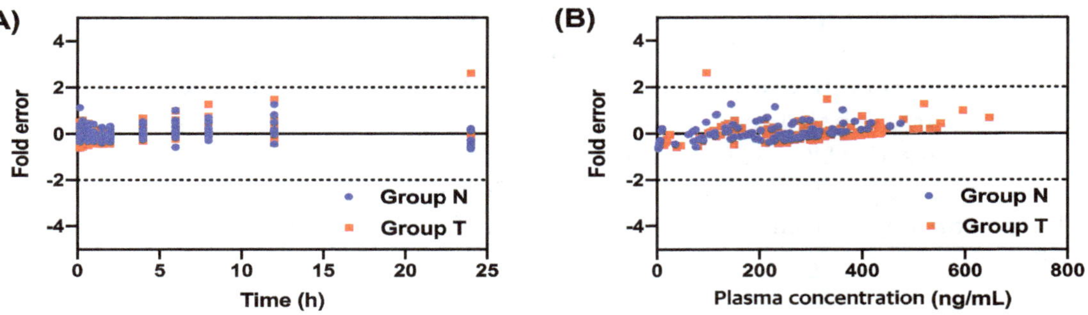

Figure 3. Residual plots written with the pharmacokinetic modeling values of non-pretreated rats (Group N) and ticagrelor-pretreated rats (Group T). (**A**) Fold error vs. time; (**B**) fold error vs. plasma concentration.

Table 2 lists the parameters of the one-compartment model. In the one-compartment model, K_e and V/F were decreased significantly in Group T compared to Group N. The K_e of Group T (0.13 ± 0.03 h^{-1}) were decreased compared with that of Group N (0.17 ± 0.05 h^{-1}) ($p < 0.05$). Moreover, the V/F of Group T (3.36 ± 0.95 L/kg) was significantly decreased compared with that of Group N (4.39 ± 0.78 L/kg) ($p < 0.05$). These reductions led to a decrease in the clearance of tadalafil. In addition, the K_a of Group T was also decreased, but there was no statistical significance ($p = 0.1933$) (Figure 4). However, this slight reduction was due to the delay in absorption, and it is clear that the absorption increased because of the high C_{max}. These results were consistent with those from the non-compartment analysis, indicating that the more absorption and the low clearance caused the increased exposure of tadalafil.

Table 2. The one-compartment model parameters of tadalafil in non-pretreated rats (Group N) and ticagrelor-pretreated rats (Group T). Values are represented as mean ± SD (n = 10).

Parameters	Group N	Group T	Ratio [a]	*p*-Value
K_a (1/h)	1.71 ± 0.91	1.14 ± 0.73	0.67	0.1933
K_e (1/h)	0.17 ± 0.03	0.13 ± 0.03	0.77	0.0166
V/F (L/kg)	4.39 ± 0.76	3.36 ± 0.95	0.77	0.0438

[a] Ratio = $\frac{Value\ of\ Group\ T}{Value\ of\ Group\ N}$; Absorption rate constant from the gut compartment to the central compartment (K_a); elimination rate constant from the central compartment to the gut compartment (K_e); the central volume of distribution (V/F).

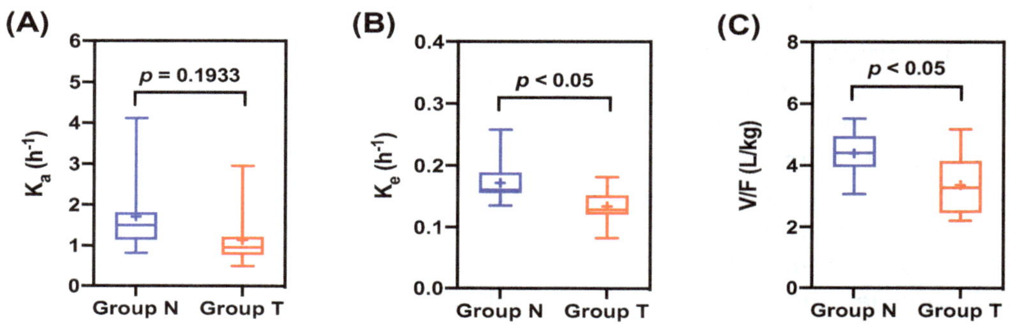

Figure 4. Comparisons of the one-compartment model parameters of tadalafil in non-pretreated rats (Group N) and ticagrelor-pretreated rats (Group T). Boxes mean 25th and 75th percentiles of data and whiskers mean 5th and 95th percentiles of data. The median and mean values are displayed as a solid line (–) and a plus mark (+) in boxes, respectively. (**A**) K_a; (**B**) K_e; (**C**) V/F. Absorption rate constant from the gut compartment to the central compartment (K_a); elimination rate constant from the central compartment to the gut compartment (K_e); the central volume of distribution (V/F).

In addition, the results from the modeling indicate that ticagrelor is a weak CYP3A inhibitor. The weak inhibitor is defined as a substance that increases the AUC value of the CYP substrate by

1.25-fold to 2-fold, or that it reduces the clearance of the CYP substrate by 20–50%, and ticagrelor is also classified as this inhibitor [22,41]. Changes in the AUC (1.61-fold) and clearance (37%) of tadalafil by co-administration with ticagrelor were within the range, supporting the above classification. Therefore, we inferred that ticagrelor acts as a weak CYP3A inhibitor, affecting the pharmacokinetic profiles of tadalafil, a CYP3A substrate. Furthermore, co-administration of tadalafil with ticagrelor or other CYP3A inhibitors, such as ketoconazole and diltiazem, would also be expected to increase tadalafil exposure [42].

In a clinical aspect, tadalafil shows robust safety and tolerability [12]. However, the co-administration of tadalafil with ticagrelor to elderly men may cause unexpected side effects. The half-life of tadalafil in normal healthy men is reported to be approximately 17.5 h after administration, whereas that of elderly men is about 21.6 h [43]. This half-life in elderly men is likely to increase further due to co-administration with ticagrelor, which may increase the incidence of side effects, such as headaches and dyspepsia. In addition, patients receiving nitrate medication for treatment of angina are recommended to postpone the nitrate treatment for at least 48 h after administration of tadalafil, but this may need to be longer to prevent serious hypotension [44]. Therefore, most patients receiving these drugs are older, so co-administration of tadalafil should be carefully considered.

4. Conclusions

In our study, the plasma concentration-time profile of tadalafil was significantly changed by co-administration with ticagrelor. A ticagrelor-inhibited CYP3A-mediated tadalafil metabolism and the systemic exposure of tadalafil increased by pretreatment with ticagrelor. Co-administration of tadalafil with ticagrelor increased the AUC of tadalafil by approximately 61% and decreased the clearance of tadalafil by 37%. These results suggest that the co-administration of tadalafil and ticagrelor may need dose control and specific drug therapy to avoid side effects from drug-drug interactions. Therefore, CAD patients receiving ticagrelor should be closely monitored when administering tadalafil concomitantly. For further studies, an additional experiment is expected to identify the variation of clinical efficacy of tadalafil by co-administration with ticagrelor, a CYP3A4 inhibitor.

Author Contributions: Conceptualization, Y.-G.N.; methodology, Y.-G.N. and J.-J.B.; software, Y.-G.N. and J.-J.B.; validation, H.-W.H. and J.-J.B.; formal analysis, J.-J.B. and H.-W.H.; investigation, Y.-G.N. and J.-J.B.; resources, M.-K.K.; data curation, Y.-G.N.; writing—original draft preparation, Y.-G.N. and J.-J.B.; writing—review and editing, Y.-G.S., H.-K.L., and C.-W.C.; supervision, C.-W.C.

Acknowledgments: The materials were kindly supported by Korea United Pharma Inc.

References

1. Hatzimouratidis, K.; Amar, E.; Eardley, I.; Giuliano, F.; Hatzichristou, D.; Montorsi, F.; Vardi, Y.; Wespes, E. Guidelines on male sexual dysfunction: Erectile dysfunction and premature ejaculation. *Eur. Urol.* **2010**, *57*, 804–814. [CrossRef] [PubMed]
2. Laumann, E.O.; Nicolosi, A.; Glasser, D.B.; Paik, A.; Gingell, C.; Moreira, E.; Wang, T. Sexual problems among women and men aged 40–80 y: Prevalence and correlates identified in the global study of sexual attitudes and behaviors. *Int. J. Import. Res.* **2005**, *17*, 39–57. [CrossRef] [PubMed]
3. Dégano, I.R.; Marrugat, J.; Grau, M.; Salvador-González, B.; Ramos, R.; Zamora, A.; Martí, R.; Elosua, R. The association between education and cardiovascular disease incidence is mediated by hypertension, diabetes, and body mass index. *Sci. Rep.* **2017**, *7*, 12370. [CrossRef] [PubMed]
4. Gandaglia, G.; Briganti, A.; Jackson, G.; Kloner, R.A.; Montorsi, F.; Montorsi, P.; Vlachopoulos, C. A systematic review of the association between erectile dysfunction and cardiovascular disease. *Eur. Urol.* **2014**, *65*, 968–978. [CrossRef] [PubMed]
5. Montorsi, P.; Ravagnani, P.M.; Galli, S.; Rotatori, F.; Briganti, A.; Salonia, A.; Dehò, F.; Montorsi, F. Common grounds for erectile dysfunction and coronary artery disease. *Curr. Opin. Urol.* **2004**, *14*, 361–365. [CrossRef] [PubMed]
6. Jackson, G.; Boon, N.; Eardley, I.; Kirby, M.; Dean, J.; Hackett, G.; Montorsi, P; Montorsi, F.; Vlachopoulos, C.; Kloner, R.; et al. Erectile dysfunction and coronary artery disease prediction: Evidence-based guidance and consensus. *Int. J. Clin. Pract.* **2010**, *64*, 848–857. [CrossRef]

7. Schwarz, E.R.; Rastogi, S.; Kapur, V.; Sulemanjee, N.; Rodriguez, J.J. Erectile dysfunction in heart failure patients. *J. Am. Coll. Cardiol.* **2006**, *48*, 1111–1119. [CrossRef]
8. Speel, T.G.; Van Langen, H.; Meuleman, E.J. The risk of coronary heart disease in men with erectile dysfunction. *Eur. Urol.* **2003**, *44*, 366–371. [CrossRef]
9. Montorsi, P.; Ravagnani, P.M.; Galli, S.; Rotatori, F.; Veglia, F.; Briganti, A.; Salonia, A.; Deho, F.; Rigatti, P.; Montorsi, F.; et al. Association between erectile dysfunction and coronary artery disease. Role of coronary clinical presentation and extent of coronary vessels involvement: The COBRA trial. *Eur. Heart J.* **2006**, *27*, 2632–2639. [CrossRef]
10. Kloner, R.A.; Mullin, S.H.; Shook, T.; Matthews, R.; Mayeda, G.; Burstein, S.; Peled, H.; Pollick, C.; Choudhary, R.; Rosen, R.; et al. Erectile dysfunction in the cardiac patient: How common and should we treat? *J. Urol.* **2003**, *170*, S46–S50. [CrossRef]
11. Nascimento, E.R.; Maia, A.C.; Pereira, V.; Soares-Filho, G.; Nardi, A.E.; Silva, A.C. Sexual dysfunction and cardiovascular diseases: A systematic review of prevalence. *Clinics* **2013**, *68*, 1462–1468. [CrossRef]
12. Coward, R.M.; Carson, C.C. Tadalafil in the treatment of erectile dysfunction. *Ther. Clin. Risk Manag.* **2008**, *4*, 1315–1330. [CrossRef]
13. Clappers, N.; Brouwer, M.A.; Verheugt, F.W. Antiplatelet treatment for coronary heart disease. *Heart* **2007**, *93*, 258–265. [CrossRef]
14. Huang, S.A.; Lie, J.D. Phosphodiesterase-5 (PDE5) inhibitors in the management of erectile dysfunction. *Pharm. Ther.* **2013**, *38*, 407–419.
15. Gong, B.; Ma, M.; Xie, W.; Yang, X.; Huang, Y.; Sun, T.; Luo, Y.; Huang, J. Direct comparison of tadalafil with sildenafil for the treatment of erectile dysfunction: A systematic review and meta-analysis. *Int. Urol. Nephrol.* **2017**, *49*, 1731–1740. [CrossRef]
16. Blount, M.A.; Beasley, A.; Zoraghi, R.; Sekhar, K.R.; Bessay, E.P.; Francis, S.H.; Corbin, J.D. Binding of tritiated sildenafil, tadalafil, or vardenafil to the phosphodiesterase-5 catalytic site displays potency, specificity, heterogeneity, and cGMP stimulation. *Mol. Pharmacol.* **2004**, *66*, 144–152. [CrossRef]
17. Rezvanfar, M.A.; Rahimi, H.R.; Abdollahi, M. ADMET considerations for phosphodiesterase-5 inhibitors. *Expert Opin. Drug Metab. Toxicol.* **2012**, *8*, 1231–1245. [CrossRef]
18. Na, Y.G.; Byeon, J.J.; Wang, M.; Huh, H.W.; Son, G.H.; Jeon, S.H.; Bang, K.H.; Kim, S.J.; Lee, H.J.; Lee, H.K.; et al. Strategic approach to developing a self-microemulsifying drug delivery system to enhance antiplatelet activity and bioavailability of ticagrelor. *Int. J. Nanomed.* **2019**, *14*, 1193–1212. [CrossRef]
19. Son, G.H.; Na, Y.G.; Huh, H.W.; Wang, M.; Kim, M.K.; Han, M.G.; Byeon, J.J.; Lee, H.K.; Cho, C.W. Systemic design and evaluation of ticagrelor-loaded nanostructured lipid carriers for enhancing bioavailability and antiplatelet activity. *Pharmaceutics* **2019**, *11*, E222. [CrossRef]
20. Bliden, K.P.; Tantry, U.S.; Storey, R.F.; Jeong, Y.H.; Gesheff, M.; Wei, C.; Gurbel, P.A. The effect of ticagrelor versus clopidogrel on high on-treatment platelet reactivity: Combined analysis of the ONSET/OFFSET and RESPOND studies. *Am. Heart J.* **2011**, *162*, 160–165. [CrossRef]
21. Teng, R.; Butler, K. The effect of ticagrelor on the metabolism of midazolam in healthy volunteers. *Clin. Ther.* **2013**, *35*, 1025–1037. [CrossRef]
22. Zhou, D.; Andersson, T.B.; Grimm, S.W. In vitro evaluation of potential drug-drug interactions with ticagrelor: Cytochrome P450 reaction phenotyping, inhibition, induction, and differential kinetics. *Drug Metab. Dispos.* **2011**, *39*, 703–710. [CrossRef]
23. Teng, R.; Mitchell, P.D.; Butler, K.A. Pharmacokinetic interaction studies of co-administration of ticagrelor and atorvastatin or simvastatin in healthy volunteers. *Eur. J. Clin. Pharmacol.* **2013**, *69*, 477–487. [CrossRef]
24. Klein, K.; Zanger, U.M. Pharmacogenomics of cytochrome P450 3A4: Recent progress toward the "missing heritability" problem. *Front. Genet.* **2013**, *4*, 1–12. [CrossRef]
25. Garraffo, R.; Lavrut, T.; Ferrando, S.; Durant, J.; Rouyrre, N.; MacGregor, T.R.; Sabo, J.P.; Dellamonica, P. Effect of tipranavir/ritonavir combination on the pharmacokinetics of tadalafil in healthy volunteers. *J. Clin. Pharmacol.* **2011**, *51*, 1071–1078. [CrossRef]
26. Fraunfelder, F.W. Visual side effects associated with erectile dysfunction agents. *Am. J. Oppthalmol.* **2005**, *140*, 723–724. [CrossRef]

27. Montorsi, F.; Verheyden, B.; Meuleman, E.; Jünemann, K.P.; Moncada, I.; Valiquette, L.; Casabe, A.; Pacheco, C.; Denne, J.; Knight, J.; et al. Long-term safety and tolerability of tadalafil in the treatment of erectile dysfunction. *Eur. Urol.* **2004**, *45*, 339–345. [CrossRef]
28. Porst, H.; Giuliano, F.; Glina, S.; Ralph, D.; Casabé, A.R.; Elion-Mboussa, A.; Shen, W.; Whitaker, J.S. Evaluation of the efficacy and safety of once-a-day dosing of tadalafil 5 mg and 10 mg in the treatment of erectile dysfunction: Results of a multicenter, randomized, double-blind, placebo-controlled trial. *Eur. Urol.* **2006**, *50*, 351–359. [CrossRef]
29. Hatzichristou, D.; Gambla, M.; Rubio-Aurioles, E.; Buvat, J.; Brock, G.B.; Spera, G.; Rose, L.; Lording, D.; Liang, S. Efficacy of tadalafil once daily in men with diabetes mellitus and erectile dysfunction. *Diabet. Med.* **2008**, *25*, 138–146. [CrossRef]
30. Tiwari, G.; Tiwari, R. Bioanalytical method validation: An updated review. *Pharm. Methods* **2010**, *1*, 25–38. [CrossRef]
31. US Food and Drug Administration. Guidance for Industry and Reviewers: Estimating the Maximum Safe Starting Dose in Initial Clinical Trials for Therapeutics in Adult Healthy Volunteers. 2005. Available online: https://www.fda.gov/regulatory-information/search-fda-guidance-documents/estimating-maximum-safe-starting-dose-initial-clinical-trials-therapeutics-adult-healthy-volunteers (accessed on 24 August 2018).
32. Bang, K.H.; Na, Y.G.; Huh, H.W.; Hwang, S.J.; Kim, M.S.; Kim, M.; Lee, H.K.; Cho, C.W. The delivery strategy of paclitaxel nanostructured lipid carrier coated with platelet membrane. *Cancers* **2019**, *11*, 807. [CrossRef]
33. Kim, M.S.; Baek, I.H. Effect of dronedarone on the pharmacokinetics of carvedilol following oral administration to rats. *Eur. J. Pharm. Sci.* **2018**, *111*, 13–19. [CrossRef]
34. Kim, J.S.; Kim, M.S.; Baek, I.H. Enhanced bioavailability of tadalafil after intranasal administration in beagle dogs. *Pharmaceutics* **2018**, *10*, 187. [CrossRef]
35. Sjögren, E.; Thorn, H.; Tannergren, C. In silico modeling of gastrointestinal drug absorption: Predictive performance of three physiologically based absorption models. *Mol. Pharm.* **2016**, *13*, 1763–1778. [CrossRef]
36. Teng, R. Ticagrelor: Pharmacokinetic, pharmacodynamic and pharmacogenetic profile: An update. *Clin. Pharmacokinet.* **2015**, *54*, 1125–1138. [CrossRef]
37. Kothare, P.A.; Seger, M.E.; Northrup, J.; Mace, K.; Mitchell, M.I.; Linnebjerg, H. Effect of exenatide on the pharmacokinetics of a combination oral contraceptive in healthy women: An open-label, randomised, crossover trial. *BMC Clin. Pharmacol.* **2012**, *12*, 8. [CrossRef]
38. Doligalski, C.T.; Tong Logan, A.; Silverman, A. Drug interactions: A primer for the gastroenterologist. *Gastroenterol. Hepatol.* **2012**, *8*, 376–383.
39. Jetter, A.; Kinzig-Schippers, M.; Walchner-Bonjean, M.; Hering, U.; Bulitta, J.; Schreiner, P.; Sörgel, F.; Fuhr, U. Effects of grapefruit juice on the pharmacokinetics of sildenafil. *Clin. Pharmacol. Ther.* **2002**, *71*, 21–29. [CrossRef]
40. Lee, D.S.; Kim, S.J.; Choi, G.W.; Lee, Y.B.; Cho, H.Y. Pharmacokinetic–pharmacodynamic model for the testosterone-suppressive effect of leuprolide in normal and prostate cancer rats. *Molecules* **2018**, *23*, 909. [CrossRef]
41. Wagner, C.; Pan, Y.; Hsu, V.; Grillo, J.A.; Zhang, L.; Reynolds, K.S.; Sinha, V.; Zhao, P. Predicting the effect of cytochrome P450 inhibitors on substrate drugs: Analysis of physiologically based pharmacokinetic modeling submissions to the US Food and Drug Administration. *Clin. Pharmacokinet.* **2015**, *54*, 117–127. [CrossRef]
42. Teng, R.; Butler, K. Effect of the CYP3A inhibitors, diltiazem and ketoconazole, on ticagrelor pharmacokinetics in healthy volunteers. *J. Drug Assess.* **2013**, *2*, 30–39. [CrossRef]
43. Fransis, S.H.; Corbin, J.D. Molecular mechanisms and pharmacokinetics of phosphodiesterase-5 antagonists. *Curr. Urol. Rep.* **2003**, *4*, 457–465. [CrossRef]
44. Kloner, R.A.; Hutter, A.M.; Emmick, J.T.; Mitchell, M.I.; Denne, J.; Jackson, G. Time course of the interaction between tadalafil and nitrates. *J. Am. Coll. Cardiol.* **2003**, *42*, 1855–1860. [CrossRef]

12

BCS Class IV Oral Drugs and Absorption Windows: Regional-Dependent Intestinal Permeability of Furosemide

Milica Markovic [1], Moran Zur [1], Inna Ragatsky [1], Sandra Cvijić [2] and Arik Dahan [1,*]

[1] Department of Clinical Pharmacology, School of Pharmacy, Faculty of Health Sciences, Ben-Gurion University of the Negev, Beer-Sheva 8410501, Israel; milica@post.bgu.ac.il (M.M.); moranfa@post.bgu.ac.il (M.Z.); inna.ragatsky@gmail.com (I.R.)

[2] Department of Pharmaceutical Technology and Cosmetology, Faculty of Pharmacy, University of Belgrade, Vojvode Stepe 450, 11221 Belgrade, Serbia; sandra.cvijic@pharmacy.bg.ac.rs

* Correspondence: arikd@bgu.ac.il

Abstract: Biopharmaceutical classification system (BCS) class IV drugs (low-solubility low-permeability) are generally poor drug candidates, yet, ~5% of oral drugs on the market belong to this class. While solubility is often predictable, intestinal permeability is rather complicated and highly dependent on many biochemical/physiological parameters. In this work, we investigated the solubility/permeability of BCS class IV drug, furosemide, considering the complexity of the entire small intestine (SI). Furosemide solubility, physicochemical properties, and intestinal permeability were thoroughly investigated in-vitro and in-vivo throughout the SI. In addition, advanced in-silico simulations (GastroPlus®) were used to elucidate furosemide regional-dependent absorption pattern. Metoprolol was used as the low/high permeability class boundary. Furosemide was found to be a low-solubility compound. Log D of furosemide at the three pH values 6.5, 7.0, and 7.5 (representing the conditions throughout the SI) showed a downward trend. Similarly, segmental-dependent in-vivo intestinal permeability was revealed; as the intestinal region becomes progressively distal, and the pH gradually increases, the permeability of furosemide significantly decreased. The opposite trend was evident for metoprolol. Theoretical physicochemical analysis based on ionization, pK_a, and partitioning predicted the same trend and confirmed the experimental results. Computational simulations clearly showed the effect of furosemide's regional-dependent permeability on its absorption, as well as the critical role of the drug's absorption window on the overall bioavailability. The data reveals the absorption window of furosemide in the proximal SI, allowing adequate absorption and consequent effect, despite its class IV characteristics. Nevertheless, this absorption window so early on in the SI rules out the suitability of controlled-release furosemide formulations, as confirmed by the in-silico results. The potential link between segmental-dependent intestinal permeability and adequate oral absorption of BCS Class IV drugs may aid to develop challenging drugs as successful oral products.

Keywords: BCS class IV drugs; segmental-dependent intestinal permeability; intestinal absorption; oral drug delivery; biopharmaceutics; physiologically-based pharmacokinetic (PBPK) modeling; furosemide

1. Introduction

The biopharmaceutical classification system (BCS) developed by Amidon et al. revealed that the solubility/dissolution of the drug and its intestinal permeability are the two key factors that dictate drug absorption following oral administration [1,2]. Drug solubility in the gastrointestinal milieu may change in different intestinal segments, e.g., due to pH changes, in a fairly predictable manner; depending on the pKa, the solubility of acidic drugs may increase as the luminal pH rises in more distal regions of the small intestine, and vice versa for basic drugs [3–5]. On the other hand, time- and segmental-dependent intestinal permeability is more complicated and harder to predict [1]. Mechanisms contributing to segmental-dependent permeability throughout the gastrointestinal tract (GIT) include different morphology along the GIT, variable intestinal mucosal cell differentiation, changes in the drug concentration (in case of carrier-mediated transport), modulation of tight junction permeability, and luminal contents and properties, e.g., pH, transporter expression, variability in the structure/composition of the intestinal membrane itself, and more [6–11].

The four BCS classes highlight the limiting factors of the absorption process: (1) Class I, high-solubility high-permeability drugs, indicate the easier and straightforward development process, and complete absorption is expected; (2) Class II, low-solubility high-permeability drugs, indicate that a solubility/dissolution limitation is expected; (3) Class III, high-solubility low-permeability drugs, indicate that the intestinal absorption of this class of drugs will be limited by the permeability rate; and (4) Class IV, low-solubility low-permeability drugs [12]. Since Class IV drugs suffer from inadequate solubility and permeability, they have very poor oral bioavailability and are inclined to exhibit very large inter- and intrasubject variability. Therefore, unless the drug dose is very low, they are generally poor oral drug candidates. Yet, according to some estimates, ~5% of the world's top oral drugs belong to this class [13–15]. In some cases, this is due to the absorption window, which is often critical for the success or failure of a certain drug. In order to gather information about the drug absorption window, extensive work and thorough analysis of luminal conditions and drug absorption is needed, within different locations throughout the GIT. Here, we present such analysis for BCS class IV drug, furosemide [16].

Furosemide is a powerful loop diuretic and is indicated for treating edematous conditions associated with heart, renal, and hepatic failure, as well as for the treatment of hypertension [17,18]. Drug therapy with furosemide is often complex, due to apparent erratic oral systemic availability and unpredictable responses to an administered dose [19]. Even though furosemide is a class IV drug, it is a very common and widely prescribed drug on the market.

In this work, we aimed to investigate the reason for apparent success of furosemide as a marketed product, despite its poor biopharmaceutical properties, and classification as BCS class IV drug, in order to allow development of future class IV compounds. We posit that segmental-dependent permeability of furosemide may contribute to its absorption complexity and provide a certain absorption window in which the drug has suitable permeability and, hence, gets absorbed. For this reason, we investigated the in-vivo intestinal permeability of furosemide throughout different segments of the small intestine. Solubility studies, as well as theoretical physicochemical analysis of furosemide and advanced modern in-silico GastroPlus® simulations, were performed, in order to elucidate the mechanistic reasons behind the experimental results. Furosemide data were compared to the β-blocker metoprolol, the Food and Drug Administration (FDA) reference drug for the low/high permeability class boundary. Overall, this experimental setup allowed us to reveal important insights on the performance of furosemide, despite its unfavorable drug-like properties, and discuss extrapolation of these insights to other BCS class IV drug candidates.

2. Methods

2.1. Materials

Furosemide, metoprolol, phenol red, potassium chloride, potassium phosphate monobasic, potassium phosphate dibasic, sodium chloride, acetic acid, maleic acid, *n*-octanol, and trifluoroacetic acid (TFA) were all purchased from Sigma Chemical Co. (St. Louis, MO, USA). Acetonitrile and water, ultra-performance liquid chromatography (UPLC) grade were purchased from Merck KGaA, Darmstadt, Germany. Remaining chemicals were of analytical reagent grade.

2.2. Solubility Studies

The pH-dependent solubility studies were performed using the shake flask method, as previously reported [20–23]. The equilibrium solubility of furosemide was determined at both 37 °C and at room temperature (25 °C), in phosphate buffer pH 7.5, acetate buffer pH 4.0, and maleate buffer pH 1.0. Surplus quantity of furosemide was introduced to glass vials holding buffer solutions with different pH; the pH of those solutions was measured following drug addition to the buffers and, consequently, placed in the shaking incubator (100 rpm) at 37 °C. The vials were centrifuged (10,000 rpm, 10 min), and the supernatant was instantly analyzed by UPLC. The dose number for furosemide was calculated using the established equation: $D_0 = M/V_0/C_s$; M being the highest single-unit dose strength of furosemide (taken as 80 mg [24]), V_0 is the initial volume of water (250 mL), and C_s is the solubility at each pH; the drug is considered highly soluble if the $D_0 < 1$.

2.3. Evaluation of Octanol-Buffer Partition Coefficients (Log D)

Furosemide and metoprolol experimental octanol-buffer partition coefficients (Log D) were studied at pH 6.5, 7.0, and 7.5 using the shake-flask method [8,11]. Drug solutions in octanol-saturated phosphate buffer (pH 6.5, 7.0, 7.5) were equilibrated at 37 °C for 48 h. The octanol and water phase were divided via centrifugation, and the drug content in the water phase was quantified using UPLC; the furosemide/metoprolol concentration in the octanol phase was determined by mass balance.

2.4. Physicochemical Analysis

The theoretical fraction extracted into octanol (f_e) was calculated using the following equation [25,26].

$$f_e = \frac{f_u P}{1 + f_u P},$$

in which P represents the octanol-water partition coefficient of the unionized drug form, and f_u is the fraction unionized of the drug at a certain pH. Experimental Log P values were taken from the literature for both furosemide (2.29) [27] and metoprolol (2.19) [28]. The f_u versus pH was plotted according to the Henderson-Hasselbalch equation, using the pK_a literature values: 9.68 for metoprolol [29] and 3.8 for furosemide [24].

2.5. Rat Single-Pass Intestinal Perfusion

Effective permeability coefficient (P_{eff}) of furosemide versus metoprolol in various intestinal segments was assessed using the single-pass rat intestinal perfusion (SPIP) in-vivo model. The murine studies were completed according to the approved protocol by Ben-Gurion University of the Negev Animal Use and Care Committee (Protocol IL-08-01-2015). The animals (male Wistar rats weighing 230–260 g, Harlan, Israel) were housed and handled according to Ben-Gurion University of the Negev Unit for Laboratory Animal Medicine Guidelines. All animals were fasted overnight (12–18 h) with free access to water; rats were randomly allocated to different experimental groups. The intestinal perfusion study was performed according to the previous reports [7,9,30–32]. Animals were anesthetized via intramuscular injection of 1 mL/kg ketamine-xylazine solution (9%:1%) and placed on a heated (37 °C) surface (Harvard Apparatus Inc., Holliston, MA, USA); the rat abdomen was uncovered via a midline incision (~3 cm). Permeability (P_{eff}) was measured in proximal jejunum (starting 2 cm lower from the ligament of Treitz), mid-small intestine (SI) segment (isolated between the end of the upper and the beginning of the lower segments), and distal segment of the ileum (ending 2 cm above the cecum) accounting for the complexity of the entire SI [7]. Intestinal segments were cannulated on both ends and perfused with drug-free buffer. Working solutions containing furosemide (320 μg/mL), metoprolol (400 μg/mL), and phenol red (a non-absorbable marker for water flux measurements) were prepared with potassium phosphate monobasic and sodium phosphate dibasic, to achieve pH of 6.5, 7.0 and 7.5; osmolarity (290 mOsm/L) and ionic strength in all buffers was maintained throughout the study.

Drug solutions were incubated in a 37 °C water bath. Steady-state environment was ensured by perfusing the drug-containing buffer for 1 h, followed by additional 1 h of perfusion, during which sampling was done every 10 min. The pH of the collected samples was measured in the outlet sample to verify that there was no pH change throughout the perfusion. All samples were assayed by UPLC. The length of each perfused intestinal segment was measured in the end of the experiment. The effective permeability (P_{eff}; cm/s) through the rat SI wall was calculated according to the following equation:

$$P_{eff} = \frac{-Q\ln\left(C'_{out}/C'_{in}\right)}{2\pi RL},$$

in which Q is the perfusion buffer flow rate (0.2 mL/min); C'_{out}/C'_{in} is the ratio of the outlet/inlet drug concentration adjusted for water transport; R is the radius of the intestinal segment (conventionally used as 0.2 cm); and L is the exact length of the perfused SI segment as was measured at the experiment endpoint [7,33,34].

2.6. Analytical Methods

Concentration of furosemide and metoprolol was evaluated using an UPLC instrument Waters Acquity UPLC H-Class (Milford, MA, USA), with a photodiode array detector and Empower software. Furosemide and metoprolol were separated on Acquity UPLC XTerra C18 3.5 μm 4.6 mm × 250 mm column (Waters Co., Milford, MA, USA). Gradient mobile phase, going from 70:30% to 90:10% *v/v* 0.1% trifluoroacetic acid in water/acetonitrile, respectively, on a flow rate of 1 mL/min (25 °C). The inter- and intraday coefficients of variation were < 1.0% and 0.5%, respectively.

2.7. Statistics

Solubility studies were performed in four replicates; Log D studies were performed in six replicates, whereas animal perfusion studies were $n = 4$. Values are expressed as means ± standard deviation (SD). To determine statistically significant differences among the experimental groups, a 2-tailed nonparametric Mann–Whitney U test for 2-group comparison was used; $p < 0.05$ was termed significant.

2.8. In-Silico Simulations

Computer simulations of furosemide absorption and concomitant plasma concentrations following oral administration in humans were conducted using GastroPlus™ software package (v. 9.7.0009, 2019, Simulations Plus Inc., Lancaster, CA, USA). The required input data regarding drug physicochemical and pharmacokinetic properties were experimentally determined, taken from literature or in-silico predicted. Human permeability values throughout the SI were calculated from the experimental rat single-pass intestinal perfusion data, using the software integrated "permeability converter". Drug disposition was best described by three-compartmental pharmacokinetic model, whereas the relevant parameters (clearance (*CL*), volume of distribution (*Vd*) and distribution constants between central and peripheral compartments) were estimated using PKPlus software module, based on the in-vivo plasma concentration data for an intravenous (i.v.) bolus dose [35]. The application of three-compartmental model to describe furosemide pharmacokinetics has already been reported in literature [36,37]. Graphical data from literature were digitized using DigIt™ program (version 1.0.4, 2001–2008, Simulations Plus, Inc., Lancaster, CA, USA). Physiological parameters were the software default values representing fasted state physiology of a healthy human representative.

The software simulates drug absorption from the GIT using the integrated Advanced Compartment Absorption and Transit (ACAT) GIT model that consists of nine compartments (stomach, duodenum, two segments of jejunum, three segments of ileum, caecum, and ascendant colon). These compartments are linked in series, and the amount of drug dissolved and absorbed from each compartment is calculated by the system of differential equations. More details on the ACAT model can be found in the literature [38,39]. Regarding the fact that furosemide is a poorly-soluble drug, the model accounted for the effect of bile salt on drug solubility and diffusion coefficient. Drug dissolution rate under physiological conditions was predicted using the software default Johnson dissolution equation (based on modified Nernst-Bruner equation) [40].

The validity of the model (i.e., the selection of input values) was validated by comparison of the prediction results (bioavailability (F), maximum plasma concentration (C_{max}), time to reach C_{max} (t_{max}), and area under the plasma concentration-time curve ($AUC_{0-\infty}$)) with published data from the in-vivo studies for peroral (p.o.) drug administration. Percent prediction error (%PE) between the predicted and mean in-vivo observed data from a clinical study was calculated using the following equation:

$$\%PE = \frac{(\text{Observed value} - \text{Predicted value}) \times 100}{\text{Observed value}}.$$

In the next step, the generated model was used to mechanistically interpret furosemide regional absorption pattern, and to estimate the outcomes for various hypothetical drug dissolution scenarios (illustrating drug dissolution from immediate-release (IR) and controlled-release (CR) oral formulations) In the last case, hypothetical dissolution profiles were used as additional inputs to describe drug release rate in-vivo, and the selected dosage form was "CR dispersed" to allow input of the tabulated dissolution data.

3. Results

The solubility values obtained for furosemide at 37 °C and at room temperature (25 °C) are summarized in Table 1, as well as the corresponding dose number (D_0). Furosemide showed pH-dependent solubility, in accordance with its acidic nature. It can be seen that, while, at pH 7.5, furosemide has suitable solubility (as evident by D_0 lower than 1), at the lower pH values, 1.0 and 4.0, it is poorly soluble. When taking 80 mg as the highest dose strength, although $D_0 < 1$ was obtained at pH 7.5, at pH 1.0 and 4.0, the D_0 is higher than 1; hence, furosemide was found to be a low-solubility compound according to the BCS.

Table 1. Furosemide solubility values (μg/mL) at the tree pH values 1.0, 4.0, and 7.5, at 37 °C (upper panel), and at room temperature (25 °C; lower panel), as well as the corresponding dose number (D_0) calculated for an 80-mg dose. Data presented as mean ± SD; $n = 6$.

	At 37 °C	
pH	**Solubility (μg/mL)**	**Corresponding D_0**
1	19.4 ± 3.7	16.5
4	65.5 ± 9.0	4.8
7.5	8340.1 ± 81.6	0.04
	At 25 °C	
pH	**Solubility (μg/mL)**	**Corresponding D_0**
1	40.3 ± 16.2	7.9
4	56.7 ± 12.2	5.6
7.5	8550.6 ± 149.4	0.04

Octanol-buffer partition coefficient values of furosemide and metoprolol at the three pH values 6.5, 7.0, and 7.5 (representing the conditions throughout the small intestine) are presented in Figure 1. Both drugs presented a clear pH-dependent Log D values across the studied pH range, with opposite trends; while furosemide's partitioning decreases as the pH rises, metoprolol shows higher partitioning into octanol at higher pH (metoprolol is the acceptable reference drug for the low/high permeability class boundary). In addition, furosemide's Log D at pH 6.5 was higher than that of metoprolol at the same pH; this is a surprising finding since Log D may sometimes be used as a surrogate for passive permeability. Indeed, at higher pH values (7.0 and 7.5), metoprolol Log D increases, while furosemide decreases, and metoprolol Log D becomes higher than furosemide.

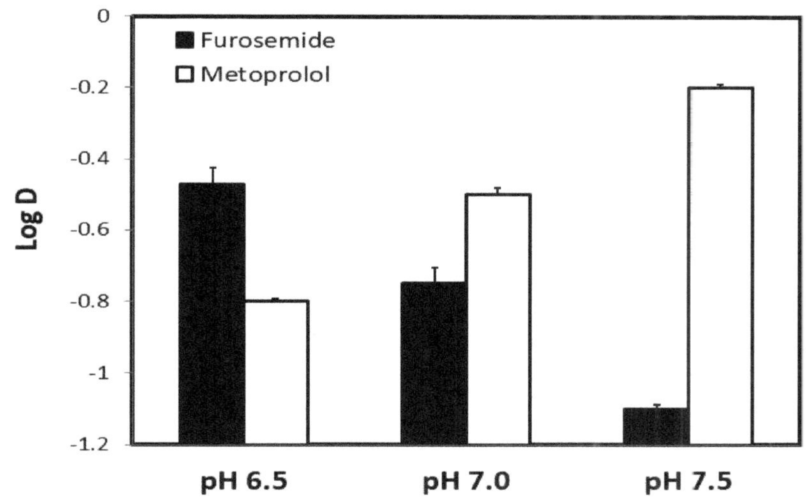

Figure 1. The octanol-buffer partition coefficients, Log D, for furosemide and metoprolol at the three pH values 6.5, 7.0, and 7.5. Data are presented as the mean ± S.D.; $n = 6$ in each experimental group.

Furosemide and metoprolol physicochemical properties are presented in Table 2. Figure 2 presents furosemide versus metoprolol theoretical fraction unionized (f_u) and fraction extracted into octanol (f_e) as a function of pH. The plots have a standard sigmoidal shape, with opposite trends for furosemide vs. metoprolol. The f_e vs. pH plot follows the same pattern to the f_u plot, only with a shift to the right (higher pH values) for acidic drug (furosemide), and to the left (lower pH values) for basic (metoprolol) drugs. The shift magnitude in both cases equals $\text{Log}(P - 1)$ at the midpoint of the f_e and f_u curves [25,26]. The experimental drug octanol-buffer partitioning at the three pH values (6.5, 7.0, and 7.5) are illustrated in Figure 2, as well, and it can be seen that they were in excellent agreement with the theoretical plots.

Table 2. Physicochemical parameters and chemical structure of furosemide and metoprolol.

Drug	Chemical Structure	pK_a	Log P	PSA
Furosemide	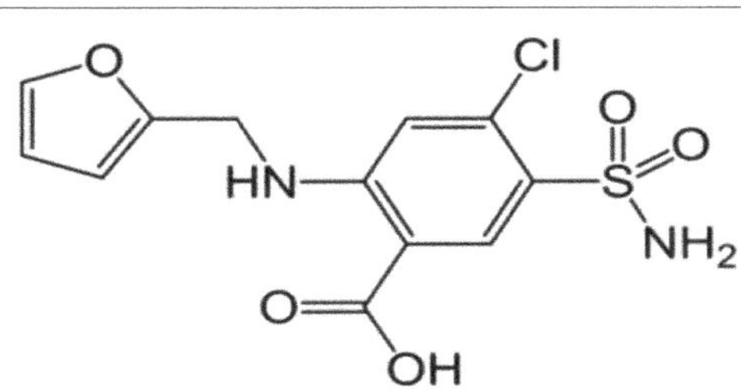	3.8	2.3	127.7
Metoprolol	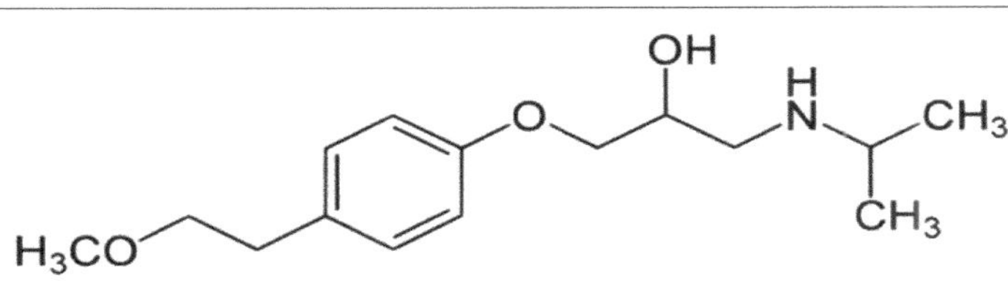	9.7	2.2	53.2

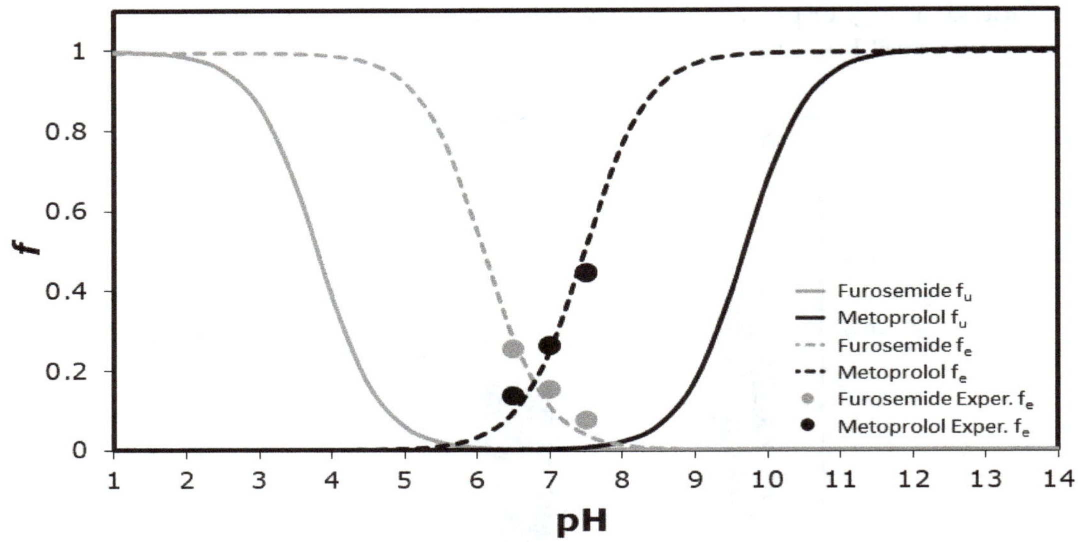

Figure 2. The theoretical fraction unionized (f_u) and fraction extracted into octanol (f_e) plots as a function of pH for furosemide and metoprolol, as well as experimental buffer-octanol partitioning of the drugs in the three pH values 6.5, 7.0, and 7.5 ($n = 5$).

The effective permeability coefficient (P_{eff}, cm/sec) values of furosemide and metoprolol determined using the single-pass intestinal perfusion (SPIP) rat model, in three intestinal segments, namely proximal jejunum (pH 6.5), mid small intestine (pH 7.0), and distal ileum (pH 7.5), are presented in Figure 3. It can be seen that significant regional-dependent permeability of furosemide throughout the small intestine was evident: the permeability of furosemide gradually decreases, while the permeability of metoprolol gradually increases, as the SI segments become more distal.

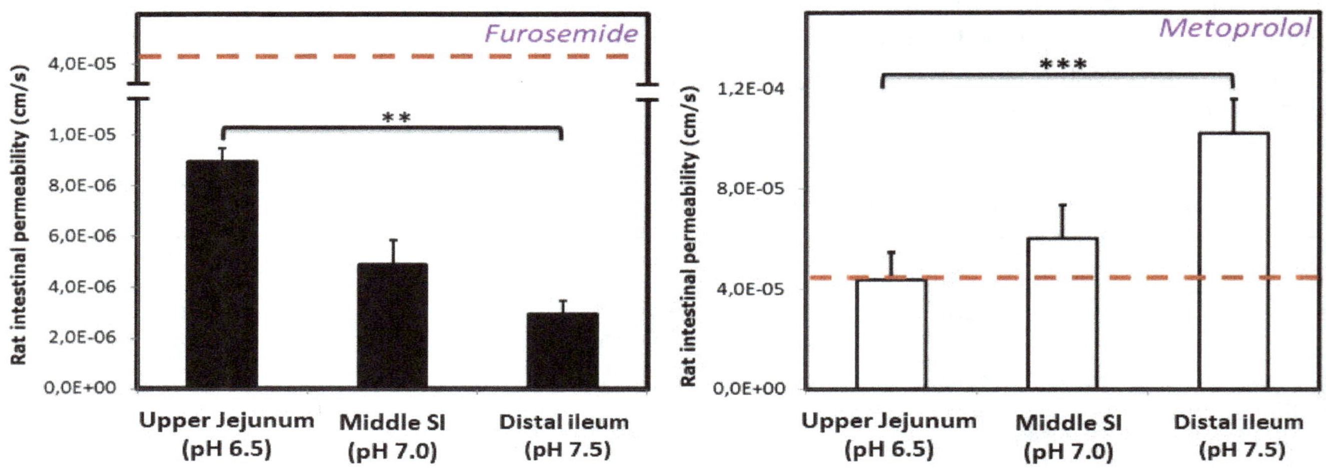

Figure 3. Effective permeability values (P_{eff}; cm/s) obtained for furosemide and metoprolol after in-situ single pass perfusion to the rat proximal jejunum at pH 6.5, mid-small intestine at pH 7.0, and to the distal ileum at pH 7.5. Mean ± S.D.; $n = 4$ in each experimental group; ** $p < 0.01$, *** $p < 0.001$.

The input data regarding drug physicochemical and pharmacokinetic properties, used for in-silico simulations, are presented in Table 3. The simulated furosemide plasma concentration profile following p.o. administration is depicted in Figure 4, along with the mean profiles observed in the in-vivo studies. In addition, the observed and model predicted pharmacokinetic parameters are compared in

Table 4. The presented data demonstrate that the generated model adequately describes furosemide absorption and disposition. The course of the predicted plasma profile fairly resembles the observed data. However, certain variations are observed between the mean in-vivo data from different studies referring to the same drug dose (Figure 4, Table 4). Indeed, it has been reported that furosemide oral absorption is highly variable between individuals, e.g., C_{max} varied three-fold, and t_{max} varied five-fold [36,37,41]; moreover, individual AUC values for 40 mg furosemide oral dose varied between 1.57 and 3.76 μg·h/mL (more than two-fold) [36,37,41], and even larger AUC values were observed in another study with the same drug dose (2.23–6.10 μg·h/mL) [42], indicating that, regardless of the high PE(%) values in Table 4, the model predicted value of 3.66 μg·h/mL is not an overestimate of the extent of drug absorption. In addition, extensive intrasubject variability was observed for orally dosed furosemide, and these variations were attributed to the absorption process (i.e., day to day variations in physiological factors) since the repeated i.v. doses showed only marginal intrasubject variability [36,37,41]. Considering pronounced inter- and intraindividual variability in furosemide oral absorption, the simulated profile can be seen as a reasonable estimate (Figure 4). Moreover, the predicted fraction of oral drug absorption (cc. 52%) is in accordance with the values reported in the literature [36,37].

Table 3. The selected input parameters for furosemide absorption GastroPlus® simulation.

Parameter	Value	Source
Molecular weight (g/mol)	330.75	/
Log D (pH 7.5)	−1.0818	experimental values
Solubility at 37 °C (μg/mL)	19.4 (pH 1.0) 65.5 (pH 4.0) 8340.1 (pH 7.5)	
pK_a (acid)	3.8	[24]
Human effective permeability, P_{eff} (cm/s)	0.4043×10^{-4} (duodenum, jejunum) 0.2246×10^{-4} (ileum 1 and 2) 0.1392×10^{-4} (ileum 3, caecum, colon)	values converted using GastroPlus™ integrated "permeability converter" based on experimental rat perfusion data
Diffusion coefficient (cm^2/s)	0.7289×10^{-5}	GastroPlus™ calculated value (based on molecular weight)
Mean precipitation time (s)	900	GastroPlus™ default values
Particle density (g/mL)	1.2	
Particle radius (μm)	25	
Blood/plasma concentration ratio	1	
Plasma fraction unbound (%)	1	[24]
Clearance, CL (L/h/kg)	0.121	calculated using GastroPlus™ PKPlus module, based on the i.v. data [35]
Volume of distribution, Vd (L/kg)	0.043	
Distribution constant k_{12} (1/h)	0.964	
Distribution constant k_{21} (1/h)	1.614	
Distribution constant k_{13} (1/h)	0.925	
Distribution constant k_{32} (1/h)	0.708	
Regional pH in the GIT	1.3; 6.0; 6.2; 6.4; 6.6; 6.9; 7.4; 6.4; 6.8	GastroPlus™ default values for stomach, duodenum, jejunum 1, jejunum 2, ileum 1, ileum 2, ileum 3, caecum, and ascendant colon
Regional volume of fluid in the GIT (mL)	46.56; 40.54; 150.00; 119.30; 91.71; 68.88; 48.57; 46.44; 49.21	
Regional transit time in the GIT (h)	0.25; 0.26; 0.93; 0.74; 0.58; 0.42; 0.29; 4.13; 12.38	

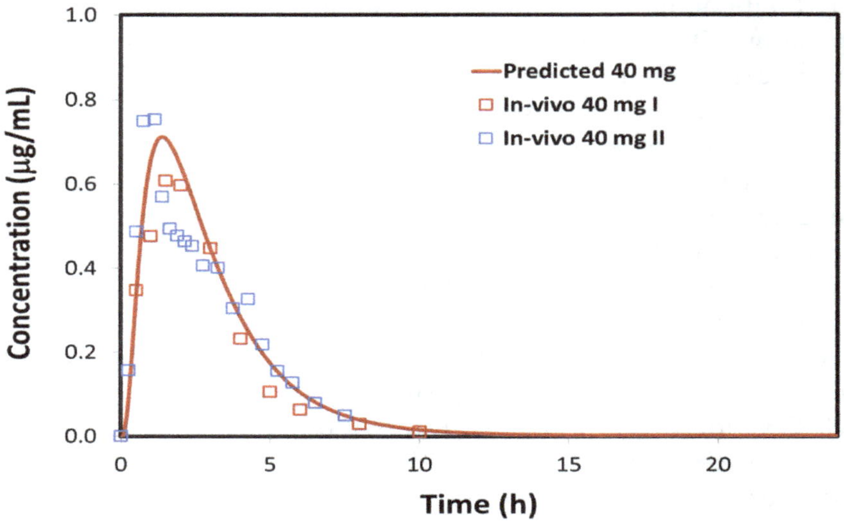

Figure 4. GastroPlus® simulated (line) versus mean observed (markers) plasma concentration profiles following p.o. administration of furosemide. Mean observed values represent 40 mg immediate-release (IR) tablet profile I [43] and 40 mg IR tablet profile II [37].

Table 4. Comparison between GastroPlus® simulated and in-vivo observed furosemide pharmacokinetic parameters following p.o. drug administration.

40 mg p.o. Dose					
Parameter	**In-Vivo I [a]**	**In-Vivo II [b]**	**Predicted**	**PE(%) I**	**PE(%) II**
C_{max} (µg/mL)	0.61	0.75	0.71	−17.14	5.54
t_{max} (h)	1.5	1.12	1.36	9.33	−22.22
$AUC_{0\rightarrow\infty}$ (µg·h/mL)	2.13	2.44	3.66	−71.25	−50.06
$AUC_{0\rightarrow 24\,h}$ (µg·h/mL)	2.11	2.33	2.52	−19.25	−8.15
F (%)	NA	NA	52.2	NA	NA

[a] Refers to the mean plasma profile from [43] (40 mg IR tablet); [b] refers to the mean plasma profile from [37] (40 mg IR tablet); NA, not available/not applicable.

The predicted furosemide dissolution and absorption profiles following an IR oral formulation (IR tablet) are illustrated in Figure 5. The generated profiles clearly indicate that drug permeability is the limiting factor for absorption under fasted state GIT conditions. Namely, although furosemide is a low-solubility drug, due to ionization at the elevated pH conditions in the proximal SI, drug dissolution from an IR formulation is expected to be fast (>85% in 30 min). Therefore, furosemide absorption from an IR formulation is mainly governed by poor permeability. The predicted regional-dependent absorption distribution (Figure 6) further highlights the role of furosemide segmental absorption on the overall drug bioavailability. As implied by the regional-dependent permeability data, but also considering the surface area available for absorption, furosemide absorption predominantly happens in the proximal parts of the SI (76.6% of the total amount absorbed into the enterocytes), and only a minor fraction of drug (23.2% of the total amount absorbed into the enterocytes) passes into systemic circulation through mid and distal GIT regions.

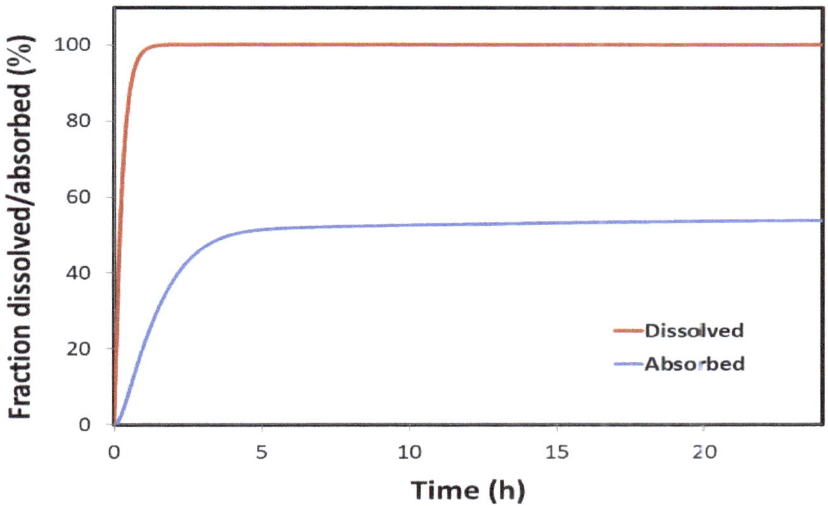

Figure 5. GastroPlus® simulated dissolution and absorption profiles following p.o. administration of 40 mg furosemide dose (dissolution profile was simulated using the software default Johnson equation).

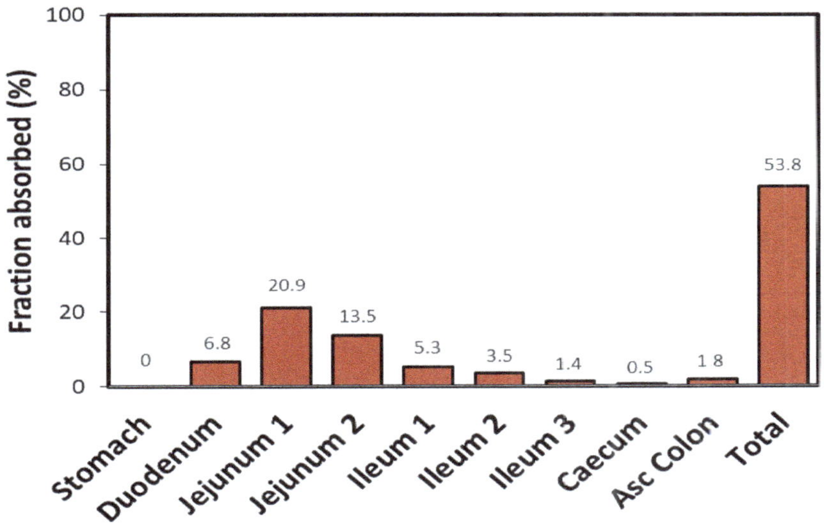

Figure 6. GastroPlus® simulated regional absorption of furosemide following p.o. administration of 40 mg drug dose (the simulated values refer to the fraction of drug dose that entered into the enterocytes).

The prediction results corresponding to various dissolution scenarios are presented in Figure 7b–d and Table 5. According to the simulated data, furosemide release rate from an oral formulation highly impacts the concomitant absorption process, whereas prolonged drug release rate leads to marked delay in the rate and extent of drug absorption. The estimated pharmacokinetic parameters (Table 5) indicate that furosemide bioavailability would show more than a 10-fold decrease in case the complete drug dissolution is achieved within 24 h in comparison to 15 min. A similar trend is observed for C_{max} and AUC values (17.75- and 17.38-fold decrease, respectively), while t_{max} would be prolonged (about two-fold). It is interesting to note that t_{max} increases with decrease in drug dissolution up to some point, but further decrease in drug dissolution (e.g., 85% in more than 6 h) would not cause additional delay in peak plasma concentration. This is because, after cc. 2 h, the drug leaves proximal parts of the intestine, where majority of furosemide absorption takes place, and, later on, in mid and especially distal intestine, only a small fraction of drug can be absorbed, as illustrated in Figure 7d.

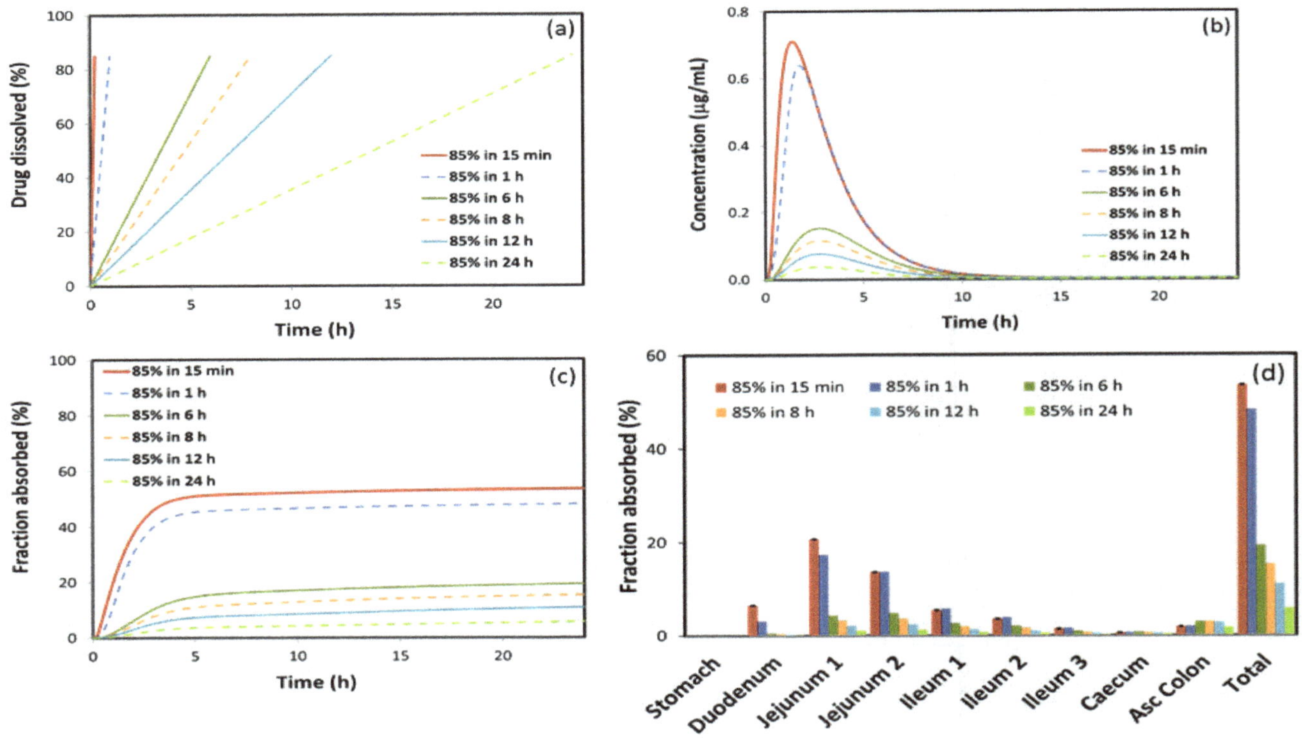

Figure 7. GastroPlus® simulated furosemide dissolution profiles (**a**); and (**b**) the corresponding simulated plasma profiles; (**c**) absorption profiles; and (**d**) regional absorption distribution.

Table 5. GastroPlus® predicted pharmacokinetic parameters for different furosemide virtual dissolution profiles from 40 mg p.o. dosage forms.

Dissolution	C_{max} (μg/mL)	t_{max} (h)	$AUC_{0\rightarrow\infty}$ (μg·h/mL)	F (%)
85% in 15 min	0.71	1.36	3.65	51.91
85% in 1 h	0.64	1.76	3.71	46.35
85% in 6 h	0.15	2.80	0.80	16.64
85% in 8 h	0.11	2.80	0.61	12.73
85% in 12 h	0.08	2.80	0.41	8.65
85% in 24 h	0.04	2.80	0.21	4.36

4. Discussion

BCS class IV drugs (e.g., sulfamethoxazole, ritonavir, paclitaxel, and furosemide) exhibit numerous unfavorable characteristics (low solubility and permeability, high presystemic metabolism, efflux transport), which make their oral drug delivery challenging. In addition to this, class IV drugs often demonstrate inter/intra-subject variability. Indeed, following oral administration, the absorption and bioavailability of furosemide are highly variable (37–51%) [35,41]. It has been suggested that this variability is highly depend on the absorption process [41], which in turn is dependent on drug aqueous solubility and intestinal permeability following oral administration [1,44]. It has also been hypothesized that variable gastric/intestinal first-pass metabolism can be a factor in causing incomplete and irregular furosemide absorption in humans [45]. Despite the unfavorable class IV drug characteristics, furosemide was shown to be exceptionally useful and successful marketed drug product for the treatment of edema [17]. For this reason, we decided to investigate furosemide's solubility and in-vivo regional-dependent permeability throughout the GIT, as main parameters that guide absorption of oral drugs.

It was shown that a correlation between human P_{eff} in the jejunum and physicochemical parameters advocates that there is a high pH-dependent influence on the passive intestinal permeability in-vivo [46]. Indeed, furosemide in-vivo permeability data demonstrate a downward trend towards the distal intestinal segments as the pH gradually increases, a trend that can be expected for acidic drugs, since the pH in the intestinal lumen gradually increases towards distal SI regions (Figure 3). Many BCS class IV drugs are substrates for efflux transporters [47]. There is some evidence that furosemide might be a substrate for efflux transporters [48,49]; thus, such permeability trend could also be influenced by the P-glycoprotein (P-gp) transporter in which expression levels are increased from proximal to distal SI segments [6,50–52]. Since metoprolol's intestinal permeability is passive and does not involve carrier-mediated absorption, it exhibited pH-dependent intestinal permeability, with reverse tendency compared to furosemide; as a basic drug, metoprolol showed upward increase in permeability towards distal SI segments with rising pH values (Figure 3). At any point throughout the SI, furosemide exhibited significantly lower permeability than the benchmark (metoprolol's jejunum permeability), which confirms its BCS low-permeability classification and incomplete absorption. Despite the fact that furosemide is a low-permeability drug, the higher permeability in the proximal intestinal regions provides a window for furosemide absorption, and we posit that this is one of the main reasons for furosemide's sufficient bioavailability and success as a marketed drug. Theoretical f_u and f_e as a function of pH were found to be in excellent correlation to these in-vivo data. In addition, in-silico modeling indicated that furosemide dissolution from an IR formulation would be fairly complete before the drug leaves proximal SI (Figure 5), although the drug is generally classified as low-soluble, enabling timely delivery of the dissolved drug to the distinct absorption site. Complete furosemide dissolution under physiological conditions is also confirmed by the experimental solubility results (Table 1).

Furosemide Log D studies showed higher partition coefficient in comparison to metoprolol at pH 6.5, whereas, in the in-vivo intestinal perfusion experiment, furosemide showed significantly lower jejunum permeability than metoprolol (Figure 1). A possible reason for this difference in the partitioning and in-vivo permeability can be the polar surface area (PSA) of both drugs [53]. A sigmoidal relationship between the fraction absorbed following oral administration and the dynamic polar surface area was reported in the past [54–56]. It was shown that orally administered drugs with large PSA (>120) are hardly absorbed by the passive transcellular route, while drugs with a small PSA (<60) are almost completely absorbed [55,56]. This is in agreement with our results, as furosemide has much higher PSA (127.7) than metoprolol (53.2) [54,55]. Another reason for the difference in the partitioning and in-vivo permeability may be the presence of active efflux transport involved in the intestinal permeability. The influence of efflux transport at pH 6.5 (proximal intestinal segments) could decrease furosemide's permeability in-vivo, which was not accounted for in the octanol partitioning studies.

The Log P value of furosemide (2.3) is in the close proximity to that of metoprolol (2.2), pointing to high permeability (Table 2). However, the Log P calculation is based on the unionized drug fraction, and, since furosemide has acidic nature it is likely that, once it passes the acidic stomach environment, it will mostly be in ionized form (the pH throughout the GIT varies from 5.9–6.3 in the proximal SI to 7.4–7.8 in distal SI segments; pH in the colon is fluctuating between pH 5–8 [57]); therefore the high furosemide Log P is not in correspondence with permeability in-vivo. Thus, we posit that no single parameter can be used for measuring the drug absorption process, but rather, a combination of physicochemical parameters and in-vitro and in-vivo findings, as well as careful consideration of inclusion criteria prior to making decisions. Despite the high Log P value for furosemide, it was indeed confirmed that furosemide is a BCS class IV drug, based on both the solubility data (Table 1) and the intestinal permeability (Figure 3).

Suitable formulation is the main approach to create an efficacious drug product for the administration of BCS class IV drugs [47]. Absorption windows in the proximal intestinal segments can restrict the oral drug bioavailability and can be a significant limitation for the development of CR drug formulation. The underlying reasons are mechanistically explained by our in-silico results (Figure 7). As mentioned, furosemide permeability results revealed acceptable permeability in the proximal segments of the SI, which is presumably the reason why furosemide has appropriate drug bioavailability, despite being a BCS class IV drug. However, since CR products release the drug over 12–24 h, mostly in the colon, (transit time throughout the small intestine is 3–4 h [58]), the fact that furosemide is mainly absorbed from proximal SI segments, (with decreased permeability at distant GIT segments) prevents the formulation of furosemide as a CR product, as shown previously [21,59,60]. However, we believe that formulations based on gastro-retentive dosage forms (GRDF) can be shown as prosperous for furosemide [61]. There are several similar examples in the literature where absorption window occurs in the upper GI, and this has been used to create GDRF formulations to improve the drug absorption, such as riboflavin [62] and levodopa [59,63].

Several types of bariatric surgeries (specifically Roux-en-Y gastric bypass and mini bypass) result in bypassing the upper SI. In cases where the absorption window is indeed in this upper SI region, the absorption following the bariatric surgery can be hampered vastly, since the actual segment responsible for the majority of absorption is bypassed [64–66].

5. Conclusions

Regional-dependent permeability throughout the small intestine was evident for furosemide. The permeability of furosemide gradually decreases throughout the small intestine as a function of the pH change in the intestinal lumen. However, at any point throughout the small intestine, furosemide exhibited significantly lower permeability than the benchmark of metoprolol's permeability in the jejunum, which may explain the incomplete absorption of the drug. We propose that, for a drug to be classified as BCS low-permeability, its intestinal permeability should not match/exceed the low/high class benchmark anywhere throughout the intestinal tract, as well as is not restricted necessarily to the jejunum. Nevertheless, low-permeable drugs should not be treated as 'unfavorable' by default; instead, therapeutic potential and suitable formulation strategies should be considered on a case-by-case basis, taking into account the overall results of in-vitro, in-vivo, and in-silico testing, throughout the entire gastrointestinal tract.

Author Contributions: M.M., M.Z., I.R., S.C. and A.D. worked on conceptualization, methodology, investigation, analyzed the data, and outlined the manuscript. S.C. worked on software investigation. Writing: S.C., A.D. and M.M. prepared the original draft of the article, and M.Z. and I.R. contributed to the writing-review and editing of the full version. All authors have read and agreed to the published version of the manuscript.

References

1. Amidon, G.L.; Lennernäs, H.; Shah, V.P.; Crison, J.R. A theoretical basis for a biopharmaceutic drug classification: The correlation of in vitro drug product dissolution and in vivo bioavailability. *Pharm. Res.* **1995**, *12*, 413–420. [CrossRef]
2. Dahan, A.; Miller, J.M.; Amidon, G.L. Prediction of solubility and permeability class membership: Provisional BCS classification of the world's top oral drugs. *AAPS J.* **2009**, *11*, 740–746. [CrossRef]
3. Dahan, A.; Beig, A.; Lindley, D.; Miller, J.M. The solubility-permeability interplay and oral drug formulation design: Two heads are better than one. *Adv. Drug Deliv. Rev.* **2016**, *101*, 99–107. [CrossRef]
4. Dahan, A.; Miller, J.M. The solubility-permeability interplay and its implications in formulation design and development for poorly soluble drugs. *AAPS J.* **2012**, *14*, 244–251. [CrossRef]
5. Miller, J.M.; Beig, A.; Carr, R.A.; Webster, G.K.; Dahan, A. The solubility-permeability interplay when using cosolvents for solubilization: Revising the way we use solubility-enabling formulations. *Mol. Pharm.* **2012**, *9*, 581–590. [CrossRef]
6. Dahan, A.; Amidon, G.L. Segmental dependent transport of low permeability compounds along the small intestine due to P-Glycoprotein: The role of efflux transport in the oral absorption of BCS class III drugs *Mol. Pharm.* **2009**, *6*, 19–28. [CrossRef]
7. Dahan, A.; West, B.T.; Amidon, G.L. Segmental-dependent membrane permeability along the intestine following oral drug administration: Evaluation of a triple single-pass intestinal perfusion (TSPIP) approach in the rat. *Eur. J. Pharm. Sci.* **2009**, *36*, 320–329. [CrossRef]

8. Fairstein, M.; Swissa, R.; Dahan, A. Regional-dependent intestinal permeability and BCS classification: Elucidation of pH-related complexity in rats using pseudoephedrine. *AAPS J.* **2013**, *15*, 589–597. [CrossRef]
9. Lozoya-Agullo, I.; Zur, M.; Beig, A.; Fine, N.; Cohen, Y.; Gonzalez-Alvarez, M.; Merino-Sanjuan, M.; Gonzalez-Alvarez, I.; Bermejo, M.; Dahan, A. Segmental-dependent permeability throughout the small intestine following oral drug administration: Single-pass vs. Doluisio approach to in-situ rat perfusion. *Int. J. Pharm.* **2016**, *515*, 201–208. [CrossRef]
10. Markovic, M.; Zur, M.; Dahan, A.; Cvijić, S. Biopharmaceutical characterization of rebamipide: The role of mucus binding in regional-dependent intestinal permeability. *Eur. J. Pharm. Sci.* **2020**, *152*, 105440. [CrossRef]
11. Zur, M.; Hanson, A.S.; Dahan, A. The complexity of intestinal permeability: Assigning the correct BCS classification through careful data interpretation. *Eur. J. Pharm. Sci.* **2014**, *51*, 11–17. [CrossRef]
12. U.S. Department of Health and Human Services, Food and Drug Administration; Center for Drug Evaluation and Research (CDER). *Waiver of In-Vivo Bioavailability and Bioequivalence Studies for Immediate-Release Solid Oral Dosage Forms Based on a Biopharmaceutics Classification System; Guidance for Industry*; Center for Drug Evaluation and Research (CDER): Silver Spring, MD, USA, 2017.
13. Dahan, A.; Wolk, O.; Kim, Y.H.; Ramachandran, C.; Crippen, G.M.; Takagi, T.; Bermejo, M.; Amidon, G.L. Purely in silico BCS classification: Science based quality standards for the world's drugs. *Mol. Pharm.* **2013**, *10*, 4378–4390. [CrossRef]
14. Takagi, T.; Ramachandran, C.; Bermejo, M.; Yamashita, S.; Yu, L.X.; Amidon, G.L. A provisional biopharmaceutical classification of the top 200 oral drug products in the United States, Great Britain, Spain, and Japan. *Mol. Pharm.* **2006**, *3*, 631–643. [CrossRef]
15. Wolk, O.; Agbaria, R.; Dahan, A. Provisional in-silico biopharmaceutics classification (BCS) to guide oral drug product development. *Drug Des. Dev. Ther.* **2014**, *8*, 1563–1575. [CrossRef]
16. Lindenberg, M.; Kopp, S.; Dressman, J.B. Classification of orally administered drugs on the World Health Organization model list of essential medicines according to the biopharmaceutics classification system. *Eur. J. Pharm. Biopharm.* **2004**, *58*, 265–278. [CrossRef]
17. Furosemide Tablets, United States Pharmacopeia Label. Available online: https://www.accessdata.fda.gov/drugsatfda_docs/label/2016/018487s043lbl.pdf (accessed on 11 July 2020).
18. Ellison, D.H.; Felker, G.M. Diuretic Treatment in Heart Failure. *N. Engl. J. Med.* **2017**, *377*, 1964–1975. [CrossRef]
19. Hammarlund-Udenaes, M.; Benet, L.Z. Furosemide pharmacokinetics and pharmacodynamics in health and disease—An update. *J. Pharmacokinet. Biopharm.* **1989**, *17*, 1–46. [CrossRef]
20. Dahan, A.; Wolk, O.; Zur, M.; Amidon, G.L.; Abrahamsson, B.; Cristofoletti, R.; Groot, D.W.; Kopp, S.; Langguth, P.; Polli, J.E.; et al. Biowaiver monographs for immediate-release solid oral dosage forms: Codeine phosphate. *J. Pharm. Sci.* **2014**, *103*, 1592–1600. [CrossRef]
21. Markovic, M.; Zur, M.; Fine-Shamir, N.; Haimov, E.; González-Álvarez, I.; Dahan, A. Segmental-dependent solubility and permeability as key factors guiding controlled release drug product development. *Pharmaceutics* **2020**, *12*, 295. [CrossRef]
22. Zur, M.; Cohen, N.; Agbaria, R.; Dahan, A. The biopharmaceutics of successful controlled release drug product: Segmental-dependent permeability of glipizide vs. metoprolol throughout the intestinal tract. *Int. J. Pharm.* **2015**, *489*, 304–310. [CrossRef]
23. Zur, M.; Gasparini, M.; Wolk, O.; Amidon, G.L.; Dahan, A. The low/high BCS permeability class boundary: Physicochemical comparison of metoprolol and labetalol. *Mol. Pharm.* **2014**, *11*, 1707–1714. [CrossRef]
24. Granero, G.E.; Longhi, M.R.; Mora, M.J.; Junginger, H.E.; Midha, K.K.; Shah, V.P.; Stavchansky, S.; Dressman, J.B.; Barends, D.M. Biowaiver monographs for immediate release solid oral dosage forms: Furosemide. *J. Pharm. Sci.* **2010**, *99*, 2544–2556. [CrossRef] [PubMed]
25. Wagner, J.G.; Sedman, A.J. Quantitaton of rate of gastrointestinal and buccal absorption of acidic and basic drugs based on extraction theory. *J. Pharmacokinet. Biopharm.* **1973**, *1*, 23–50. [CrossRef]
26. Winne, D. Shift of pH-absorption curves. *J. Pharmacokinet. Biopharm.* **1977**, *5*, 53–94. [CrossRef]
27. Berthod, A.; Carda-Broch, S.; Garcia-Alvarez-Coque, M.C. Hydrophobicity of ionizable compounds. A theoretical study and measurements of diuretic octanol–water partition coefficients by countercurrent chromatography. *Anal. Chem.* **1999**, *71*, 879–888. [CrossRef]

28. Henchoz, Y.; Guillarme, D.; Martel, S.; Rudaz, S.; Veuthey, J.L.; Carrupt, P.A. Fast log P determination by ultra-high-pressure liquid chromatography coupled with UV and mass spectrometry detections. *Anal. Bioanal. Chem.* **2009**, *394*, 1919–1930. [CrossRef]
29. Teksin, Z.S.; Hom, K.; Balakrishnan, A.; Polli, J.E. Ion pair-mediated transport of metoprolol across a three lipid-component PAMPA system. *J. Control. Release Off. J. Control. Release Soc.* **2006**, *116*, 50–57. [CrossRef]
30. Lozoya-Agullo, I.; Gonzalez-Alvarez, I.; Zur, M.; Fine-Shamir, N.; Cohen, Y.; Markovic, M.; Garrigues, T.M.; Dahan, A.; Gonzalez-Alvarez, M.; Merino-Sanjuán, M.; et al. Closed-loop doluisio (colon, small intestine) and single-pass intestinal perfusion (colon, jejunum) in rat—Biophysical model and predictions based on Caco-2. *Pharm. Res.* **2017**, *35*, 2. [CrossRef]
31. Lozoya-Agullo, I.; Zur, M.; Fine-Shamir, N.; Markovic, M.; Cohen, Y.; Porat, D.; Gonzalez-Alvarez, I.; Gonzalez-Alvarez, M.; Merino-Sanjuan, M.; Bermejo, M.; et al. Investigating drug absorption from the colon: Single-pass vs. Doluisio approaches to in-situ rat large-intestinal perfusion. *Int. J. Pharm.* **2017**, *527*, 135–141. [CrossRef]
32. Lozoya-Agullo, I.; Zur, M.; Wolk, O.; Beig, A.; Gonzalez-Alvarez, I.; Gonzalez-Alvarez, M.; Merino-Sanjuan, M.; Bermejo, M.; Dahan, A. In-situ intestinal rat perfusions for human Fabs prediction and BCS permeability class determination: Investigation of the single-pass vs. the Doluisio experimental approaches. *Int. J. Pharm.* **2015**, *480*, 1–7. [CrossRef]
33. Dahan, A.; Miller, J.M.; Hilfinger, J.M.; Yamashita, S.; Yu, L.X.; Lennernas, H.; Amidon, G.L. High-permeability criterion for BCS classification: Segmental/pH dependent permeability considerations. *Mol. Pharm.* **2010**, *7*, 1827–1834. [CrossRef]
34. Wolk, O.; Markovic, M.; Porat, D.; Fine-Shamir, N.; Zur, M.; Beig, A.; Dahan, A. Segmental-dependent intestinal drug permeability: Development and model validation of in silico predictions guided by in vivo permeability values. *J. Pharm. Sci.* **2019**, *108*, 316–325. [CrossRef]
35. Kelly, M.R.; Cutler, R.E.; Forrey, A.W.; Kimpel, B.M. Pharmacokinetics of orally administered furosemide. *Clin. Pharmacol. Ther.* **1974**, *15*, 178–186. [CrossRef]
36. Benet, L.Z. Pharmacokinetics/pharmacodynamics of furosemide in man: A review. *J. Pharmacokinet. Biopharm.* **1979**, *7*, 1–27. [CrossRef]
37. Hammarlund, M.M.; Paalzow, L.K.; Odlind, B. Pharmacokinetics of furosemide in man after intravenous and oral administration. Application of moment analysis. *Eur. J. Clin. Pharmacol.* **1984**, *26*, 197–207. [CrossRef]
38. Agoram, B.; Woltosz, W.S.; Bolger, M.B. Predicting the impact of physiological and biochemical processes on oral drug bioavailability. *Adv. Drug Deliv. Rev.* **2001**, *50*, S41–S67. [CrossRef]
39. Lin, L.; Wong, H. Predicting oral drug absorption: Mini review on physiologically-based pharmacokinetic models. *Pharmaceutics* **2017**, *9*, 41. [CrossRef]
40. Lu, A.T.K.; Frisella, M.E.; Johnson, K.C. Dissolution modeling: Factors affecting the dissolution rates of polydisperse powders. *Pharm. Res.* **1993**, *10*, 1308–1314. [CrossRef]
41. Grahnén, A.; Hammarlund, M.; Lundqvist, T. Implications of intraindividual variability in bioavailability studies of furosemide. *Eur. J. Clin. Pharmacol.* **1984**, *27*, 595–602. [CrossRef]
42. Waller, E.S.; Hamilton, S.F.; Massarella, J.W.; Sharanevych, M.A.; Smith, R.V.; Yakatan, G.J.; Doluisio, J.T. Disposition and absolute bioavailability of furosemide in healthy males. *J. Pharm. Sci.* **1982**, *71*, 1105–1108. [CrossRef]
43. Beermann, B.; Midskov, C. Reduced bioavailability and effect of furosemide given with food. *Eur. J. Clin. Pharmacol.* **1986**, *29*, 725–727. [CrossRef]
44. Dahan, A.; Lennernäs, H.; Amidon, G.L. The fraction dose absorbed, in humans, and high jejunal human permeability relationship. *Mol. Pharm.* **2012**, *9*, 1847–1851. [CrossRef]
45. Lee, M.G.; Chiou, W.L. Evaluation of potential causes for the incomplete bioavailability of furosemide: Gastric first-pass metabolism. *J. Pharm. Biopharm.* **1983**, *11*, 623–640. [CrossRef]
46. Dahlgren, D.; Lennernas, H. Intestinal permeability and drug absorption: Predictive experimental, computational and in vivo approaches. *Pharmaceutics* **2019**, *11*, 411. [CrossRef]
47. Ghadi, R.; Dand, N. BCS class IV drugs: Highly notorious candidates for formulation development. *J. Control. Release Off. J. Control. Release Soc.* **2017**, *248*, 71–95. [CrossRef]

48. Flanagan, S.D.; Cummins, C.L.; Susanto, M.; Liu, X.; Takahashi, L.H.; Benet, L.Z. Comparison of furosemide and vinblastine secretion from cell lines overexpressing multidrug resistance protein (P-glycoprotein) and multidrug resistance-associated proteins (MRP1 and MRP2). *Pharmacology* **2002**, *64*, 126–134. [CrossRef]
49. Takahashi, M.; Washio, T.; Suzuki, N.; Igeta, K.; Fujii, Y.; Hayashi, M.; Shirasaka, Y.; Yamashita, S. Characterization of gastrointestinal drug absorption in cynomolgus monkeys. *Mol. Pharm.* **2008**, *5*, 340–348. [CrossRef]
50. Cao, X.; Yu, L.X.; Barbaciru, C.; Landowski, C.P.; Shin, H.C.; Gibbs, S.; Miller, H.A.; Amidon, G.L.; Sun, D. Permeability dominates in vivo intestinal absorption of P-gp substrate with high solubility and high permeability. *Mol. Pharm.* **2005**, *2*, 329–340. [CrossRef]
51. Englund, G.; Rorsman, F.; Rönnblom, A.; Karlbom, U.; Lazorova, L.; Gråsjö, J.; Kindmark, A.; Artursson, P. Regional levels of drug transporters along the human intestinal tract: Co-expression of ABC and SLC transporters and comparison with Caco-2 cells. *Eur. J. Pharm. Sci.* **2006**, *29*, 269–277. [CrossRef]
52. Zimmermann, C.; Gutmann, H.; Hruz, P.; Gutzwiller, J.-P.; Beglinger, C.; Drewe, J. Mapping of multidrug resistance gene 1 and multidrug resistance-associated protein isoform 1 to 5 mRNA expression along the human intestinal tract. *Drug Metab. Dispos.* **2005**, *33*, 219. [CrossRef]
53. Winiwarter, S.; Bonham, N.M.; Ax, F.; Hallberg, A.; Lennernäs, H.; Karlén, A. Correlation of human jejunal permeability (in vivo) of drugs with experimentally and theoretically derived parameters. A multivariate data analysis approach. *J. Med. Chem.* **1998**, *41*, 4939–4949. [CrossRef]
54. Clark, D.E. Rapid calculation of polar molecular surface area and its application to the prediction of transport phenomena. 1. Prediction of intestinal absorption. *J. Pharm. Sci.* **1999**, *88*, 807–814. [CrossRef]
55. Palm, K.; Luthman, K.; Ungell, A.-L.; Strandlund, G.; Beigi, F.; Lundahl, P.; Artursson, P. Evaluation of dynamic polar molecular surface area as predictor of drug absorption: Comparison with other computational and experimental predictors. *J. Med. Chem.* **1998**, *41*, 5382–5392. [CrossRef]
56. Ertl, P.; Rohde, B.; Selzer, P. Fast calculation of molecular polar surface area as a sum of fragment-based contributions and its application to the prediction of drug transport properties. *J. Med. Chem.* **2000**, *43*, 3714–3717. [CrossRef]
57. Koziolek, M.; Grimm, M.; Becker, D.; Iordanov, V.; Zou, H.; Shimizu, J.; Wanke, C.; Garbacz, G.; Weitschies, W. Investigation of pH and temperature profiles in the GI tract of fasted human subjects using the intellicap(®) system. *J. Pharm. Sci.* **2015**, *104*, 2855–2863. [CrossRef]
58. Davis, S.S.; Hardy, J.G.; Fara, J.W. Transit of pharmaceutical dosage forms through the small intestine. *Gut* **1986**, *27*, 886–892. [CrossRef]
59. Streubel, A.; Siepmann, J.; Bodmeier, R. Drug delivery to the upper small intestine window using gastroretentive technologies. *Curr. Opin. Pharmacol.* **2006**, *6*, 501–508. [CrossRef]
60. Clear, N.J.; Milton, A.; Humphrey, M.; Henry, B.T.; Wulff, M.; Nichols, D.J.; Anziano, R.J.; Wilding, I. Evaluation of the Intelisite capsule to deliver theophylline and frusemide tablets to the small intestine and colon. *Eur. J. Pharm. Sci. Off. J. Eur. Fed. Pharm. Sci.* **2001**, *13*, 375–384. [CrossRef]
61. Darandale, S.S.; Vavia, P.R. Design of a gastroretentive mucoadhesive dosage form of furosemide for controlled release. *Acta Pharm. Sin. B* **2012**, *2*, 509–517. [CrossRef]
62. Kagan, L.; Lapidot, N.; Afargan, M.; Kirmayer, D.; Moor, E.; Mardor, Y.; Friedman, M.; Hoffman, A. Gastroretentive accordion pill: Enhancement of riboflavin bioavailability in humans. *J. Control. Release Off. J. Control. Release Soc.* **2006**, *113*, 208–215. [CrossRef]
63. Klausner, E.A.; Eyal, S.; Lavy, E.; Friedman, M.; Hoffman, A. Novel levodopa gastroretentive dosage form: In-vivo evaluation in dogs. *J. Control. Release* **2003**, *88*, 117–126. [CrossRef]
64. Israel, S.; Elinav, H.; Elazary, R.; Porat, D.; Gibori, R.; Dahan, A.; Azran, C.; Horwitz, E. Case report of increased exposure to antiretrovirals following sleeve gastrectomy. *Antimicrob. Agents Chemother.* **2020**, *64*. [CrossRef]
65. Porat, D.; Dahan, A. Medication management after bariatric surgery: Providing optimal patient care. *J. Clin. Med.* **2020**, *9*, 1511. [CrossRef]
66. Porat, D.; Markovic, M.; Zur, M.; Fine-Shamir, N.; Azran, C.; Shaked, G.; Czeiger, D.; Vaynshtein, J.; Replyanski, I.; Sebbag, G.; et al. Increased paracetamol bioavailability after sleeve gastrectomy: A crossover pre- vs. post-operative clinical trial. *J. Clin. Med.* **2019**, *8*, 1949. [CrossRef]

13

Drug–Drug Interactions Involving Intestinal and Hepatic CYP1A Enzymes

Florian Klomp [1], Christoph Wenzel [2], Marek Drozdzik [3] and Stefan Oswald [1,*]

1 Institute of Pharmacology and Toxicology, Rostock University Medical Center, 18057 Rostock, Germany; florian.klomp@uni-rostock.de
2 Department of Pharmacology, Center of Drug Absorption and Transport, University Medicine Greifswald, 17487 Greifswald, Germany; Christoph.Wenzel@med.uni-greifswald.de
3 Department of Experimental and Clinical Pharmacology, Pomeranian Medical University, 70-111 Szczecin, Poland; marek.drozdzik@pum.edu.pl
* Correspondence: stefan.oswald@med.uni-rostock.de

Abstract: Cytochrome P450 (CYP) 1A enzymes are considerably expressed in the human intestine and liver and involved in the biotransformation of about 10% of marketed drugs. Despite this doubtless clinical relevance, CYP1A1 and CYP1A2 are still somewhat underestimated in terms of unwanted side effects and drug–drug interactions of their respective substrates. In contrast to this, many frequently prescribed drugs that are subjected to extensive CYP1A-mediated metabolism show a narrow therapeutic index and serious adverse drug reactions. Consequently, those drugs are vulnerable to any kind of inhibition or induction in the expression and function of CYP1A. However, available in vitro data are not necessarily predictive for the occurrence of clinically relevant drug–drug interactions. Thus, this review aims to provide an up-to-date summary on the expression, regulation, function, and drug–drug interactions of CYP1A enzymes in humans.

Keywords: cytochrome P450; CYP1A1; CYP1A2; drug–drug interaction; expression; metabolism; regulation

---

1. Introduction

The oral bioavailability of many drugs is determined by first-pass metabolism taking place in human gut and liver. In this regard, a considerable fraction of the administered dose is presystemically eliminated by intestinal and hepatic phase I and/or phase II drug metabolism Consequently, only a minor fraction of the administered dose reaches the central compartment and in turn the site of action. Thus, alterations of the aforementioned presystemic metabolism in terms of inhibition or induction of the involved metabolizing enzymes may result in two unwanted clinical scenarios: (1) increased drug exposure as caused by enzyme inhibition with an increased risk of side effects up to drug-related toxicity, and (2) subtherapeutic drug levels due to induction of the respective metabolizing enzymes, which may threaten the therapeutic drug effects [1,2].

During the last decades, it was clearly demonstrated that major cytochrome P450 (CYP) enzymes such as CYP3A4, CYP2C9/19, and CYP2D6 play a major role in first-pass metabolism of drugs [3–5]. Here, extensive pharmacokinetic and pharmacogenetic studies have been conducted and identified these enzymes as crucial determinants in the pharmacokinetics and, in turn, for efficacy and safety of their substrates [6–9]. However, beside these major enzymes, the information about other CYPs that are considerably expressed in the human intestine or liver and significantly involved in the metabolism of frequently used drugs is much more limited. Examples for these somewhat "under-investigated" enzymes are CYP1A1 and CYP1A2, which are involved in the metabolism of about 10% of the drugs on the market [10,11]. Despite their clinical relevance, considerably fewer studies related to human pharmacokinetics and drug–drug interactions compared to the above-mentioned major enzymes have so far been published. For example, Medline search (via PubMed®) on "human pharmacokinetics" and certain enzymes listed 6379 entries for CYP3A4, 2902 for CYP2C9/19, and 2794 for CYP2D6, but "only" 734 and 1749 have been found for CYP1A1 and CYP1A2, respectively (assessed 22 October, 2020). Thus, the aim of this mini review article is to provide an up-to-date overview about the current knowledge on the expression, regulation, and clinically relevant drug–drug interactions of CYP1A1 and CYP1A2 in humans.

2. Expression

CYP1A1 and CYP1A2 belong to the CYP1 gene family; they are highly conserved and located on chromosome 15 [10,12]. CYP1A2 is constitutively expressed at high levels in human liver, whereas CYP1A1 was shown to be expressed at markedly lower levels in the organ but is also found in extrahepatic tissues including lung, intestine, prostate, kidney and placenta [11,13–19]. However, data on the protein abundance of hepatic CYP1A1 are conflicting; some studies demonstrated its absence in human liver, while others could clearly quantify the enzymatic protein [14,16,18,20–23]. In particular, recent mass spectrometry-based studies have demonstrated a substantial abundance of CYP1A1 in the human liver ranging from 0.5 to 9 pmol/mg microsomal protein [18,23].

In general, the available data on CYP1A1/2 expression are somewhat limited. There are sporadic studies on intestinal or hepatic CYP1A1 and/or CYP1A2 gene expression or protein abundance that are partly inconsistent and conflicting (Table 1). To overcome this limitation counteracting reliable conclusions, especially on the role of intestinal and hepatic CYP1A1, comprehensive information about gene and protein expression of CYP1A1 and CYP1A2 in intestinal and hepatic tissues from the same individuals are needed. So far, only one study from our group is available that included intestinal and hepatic tissue samples in parallel from organ donors, in order to overcome the known issue of high inter-subject variability in the expression of metabolizing enzymes [24]. However, this study only considered CYP1A2, but not CYP1A1.

Table 1. Overview of available data on mRNA expression and protein abundance of cytochrome P450 (CYP) 1A1 and CYP1A2 in the human intestine and liver (+, gene/protein expression was shown; -, not investigated n.d., not detectable; PTC, proteomics; WB, Western blot). Data are ranked in chronological order (publication date).

Liver				**Small Intestine**				
CYP1A1		**CYP1A2**		**CYP1A1**		**CYP1A2**		
Gene	**Protein (Method)**	**Gene**	**Protein (Method)**	**Gene**	**Protein (Method)**	**Gene**	**Protein (Method)**	**Reference**
-	n.d. (WB)	-	+ (WB)	-	-	-	-	[20]
+	-	+	+ (WB)	-	-	-	-	[13]
-	+ (WB)	-	-	-	-	-	-	[25]
-	-	-	-	+	+ (WB)	n.d.	-	[26]
-	-	-	-	-	+ (WB)	-	-	[27]
+	-	+	-	+	-	n.d.	-	[15]
+	n.d. (WB)	+	+ (WB)	-	-	-	-	[21]
-	+ (WB)	-	+ (WB)	-	-	-	-	[14]
-	+ (WB)	-	-	-	+ (WB)	-	-	[16]
+	-	+	-	+	-	n.d.	-	[17]
-	-	+	+ (PTC)	-	-	-	-	[28]
-	+ (PTCs)	-	+ (PTC)	-	-	-	-	[23]
-	-	-	+ (PTC)	-	-	-	n.d. (PTC)	[29]
-	-	-	-	-	+ (PTC)	-	–, traces (PTC)	[30]
-	-	+	+ (PTC)	-	-	n.d.	n.d. (PTC)	[24]
-	-	-	+ (PTC)	-	-	-	-	[31]
-	-	-	-	+	-	n.d.	-	[32]
-	n.d. (PTC)	-	+ (PTC)	-	n.d. (PTC)	-	n.d. (PTC)	[22]
-	+ (PTC)	-	+ (PTC)	-	-	-	-	[18]

Compared to CYP3A4 and CYP2C9, which are the most abundant intestinal CYP enzymes [16,24], CYP1A1 expression is rather little in the intestine and highly variable as well [16,30] (Figure 1). Paine et al. were able to detect CYP1A1 enzyme in only three of 31 investigated human jejunal samples at a range of 3.6 to 7.7 pmol/mg (Western blotting), while Miyauchi et al. using the targeted proteomics approach found CYP1A1 in 15 out of 28 analyzed human small intestinal samples (range: 0.07–2.3 pmol/mg) [16,30]. In parallel, also Shrivas et al. found CYP1A1 only in three out of 32 human liver microsomal samples using global proteomics [23]. Those findings indicate a substantial inter-subject variability in CYP1A1 protein that is most likely attributed to the individual lifestyle, including exposure to different diets or smoking, which were already shown to be important determinants of variability in the expression as well as the metabolic function of CYP1A enzymes [13,21,27,33]. In addition, experimental conditions may have partly contributed to the observed variability.

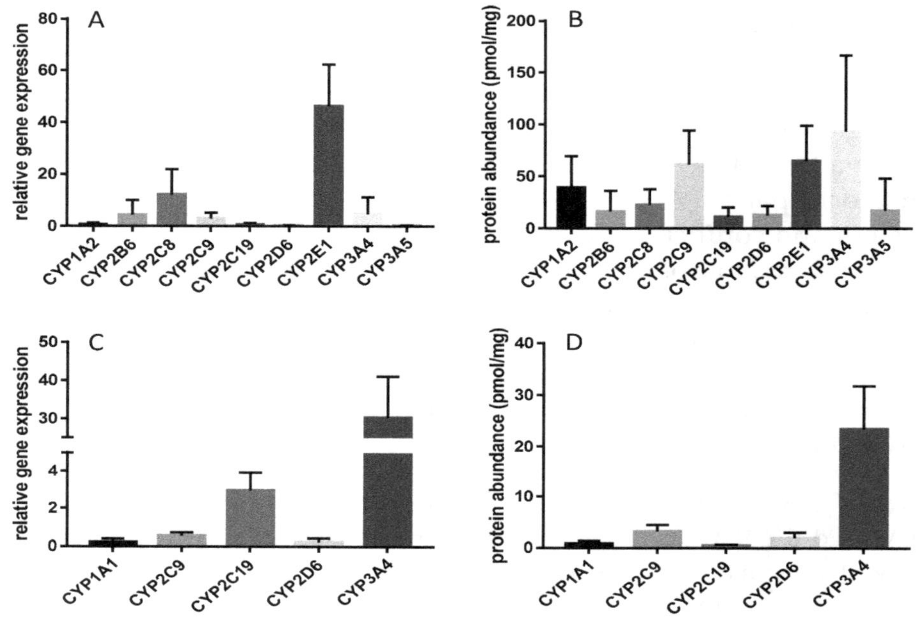

Figure 1. Comparative intestinal and hepatic gene expression and protein abundance of CYP1A1 and CYP1A2 (mean ± SD). Relative gene expression and absolute protein abundance of clinically relevant CYP450 enzymes in the human liver is presented in section (**A**,**B**) (data taken from Drozdzik et al. 2019 (**A**) and Achour et al. 2014 (**B**)). Sections C and D show relative gene expression and absolute protein abundance of clinically relevant CYP450 enzymes in the human small intestine observed in 30 ((**C**), own unpublished data) and 28 human jejunal tissue samples ((**D**), Miyauchi et al. 2016).

In contrast to the mentioned controversies on CYP1A1, CYP1A2 is doubtlessly expressed at considerable levels in the human liver, but not in the intestine (Table 1). A meta-analysis on the expression of 15 hepatic drug-metabolizing enzymes revealed that CYP1A2 contributes about 10% to all CYP enzymes [34]. After CYP3A4, CYP2E1, and CYP2C9, CYP1A2 showed the fourth highest protein abundance of all investigated hepatic CYP enzymes. These data have been confirmed by more recent mass spectrometry-based studies [24,31,35–37]. The mean hepatic microsomal protein abundance ranged from 14 to 35 pmol/mg, as determined by targeted proteomics [18,22,28,31,36,38]. Former data as derived from immunostaining studies determined considerably higher abundance, up to 65 pmol/mg [39,40], which might be interpreted with caution considering the issue of unspecific binding of antibodies. As a general feature of CYP1A1 and CYP1A2 expression, one must consider a substantial inter-subject variability, which seems to be caused by a complex interplay of genetic, epigenetics, and environmental factors [11,41].

3. Regulation

3.1. Transcriptional Regulation

The promoter region of CYP1A1 and CYP1A2 genes contains several Aryl hydrocarbon receptor (AhR) response elements [42,43], which, after binding of respective compounds, initiate coordinated transcription of both genes. Consequently, both genes are highly inducible by AhR ligands such as polycyclic aromatic hydrocarbons (PAHs), dioxins and numerous xenobiotics [44]. Examples for well-established experimental inducers are 2,3,7,8-tetrachlorodibenzo-p-dioxon (TCDD), 3-methlycholanthrene and β-naphthoflavone [45,46]. In addition, omeprazole was shown to be a potent model inducer for CYP1A1 and CYP1A2 [47–49]. There is evidence that the induction of CYP1A1 by AhR is stronger than that of CYP1A2 [44,49,50]. This is also in agreement with the fact that tissues possessing high expression of CYP1A1 (i.e., lung, placenta, intestine, urinary bladder) also show high expression levels of AhR [51]. Table 2 provides an overview of in vitro, in vivo, and ex vivo data on CYP1A1/1A2 induction by clinically relevant drugs. In this regard, albendazole, carbamazepine, omeprazole, lansoprazole, primaquine, and rosiglitazone were shown to be strong inducers of both, expression and metabolic activity of CYP1A1 and CYP1A2 [48–50,52]. As discussed later, these findings do not necessarily translate for all compounds to clinically relevant drug–drug interactions (e.g., for omeprazole). Relevant exogenous sources of AhR activators are charcoal grilled food, tobacco smoking as well as other natural sources including broccoli or fish oil supplementation, which strikingly induce endogenous eicosanoids [11,53,54]. Consequently, some of these environmental factors may contribute to the substantial variability in the expression and function of both CYP1A isoenzymes. Associated with this—tobacco smoking, especially, was shown to have significant effects on the pharmacokinetics and actions of many CYP1A substrates (see paragraph "Drug–Drug Interactions").

Table 2. Impact of clinically relevant drugs, smoking, and diet on the induction of CYP1A1/1A2 mRNA, protein, and activity.

Drug	Object of Investigation	Induction Effect	Reference
Albendazole (5–30 μM)	HepG2 cells	↑CYP1A1 (32-fold) and CYP1A2 mRNA (5.6-fold); ↑EROD-activity (4-fold)	[49,50]
Carbamazepine (7–183 μM)	HepaRG cells	↑CYP1A2 mRNA (10-fold)	[52]
Carbamazepine	Pediatric patients	↑hepatic CYP1A2 activity (CBT, 2.2-fold)	[55]
Lansoprazole (50 μM)	Human hepatocytes	↑CYP1A2 mRNA (26-fold); ↑CYP1A2 protein (32-fold); ↑EROD activity (32-fold)	[48]
Omeprazole (0.03–3 μM)	Human hepatocytes	↑CYP1A1 mRNA (37-fold)	[47]
Omeprazole (50 μM)	Human hepatocytes	↑CYP1A2 mRNA (12-fold); ↑CYP1A2 protein (4.6-fold); ↑EROD activity (39-fold)	[48]
Omeprazole (25 μM)	HepG2 cells	↑CYP1A1 and CYP1A2 mRNA	[49]
Omeprazole (treatment)	Human duodenal biopsies	↑CYP1A1 protein; ↑EROD activity (2.2-fold)	[56]
Omeprazole (20 mg SID, 4 d)	Human liver biopsies	↑CYP1A2 protein (3.4-fold); ↑EROD activity (6-fold)	[57]
Phenobarbital (100–250 μM)	Human hepatocytes	↑EROD activity (1.9-fold)	[46]
Phenobarbital (1 mM)	Human hepatocytes	↑CYP1A2 mRNA (1.5-fold); ↑CYP1A2 protein (1.8-fold); ↑POD activity (3.1-fold)	[58]
Primaquine (10–30 μM)	HepG2 cells	↑CYP1A1 (~7-fold) and CYP1A2 (~3-fold) mRNA; ↑EROD-activity (7.5-fold)	[49,50]

Table 2. *Cont.*

Drug	Object of Investigation	Induction Effect	Reference
Quinine (30 μM)	HepG2 cells	↑CYP1A1 (~9-fold) and CYP1A2 mRNA (2.4-fold); ↑EROD-activity (5.5-fold)	[50]
Rifampicin (10/33 μM)	Human hepatocytes	↑CYP1A1 (2.2-fold) and CYP1A2 mRNA (2.2-fold)	[47,59–61]
Rifampicin (20/50 μM)	Human hepatocytes	↑EROD-activity (2.3-fold)	[46]
Ritonavir (0.1–5 μM)	Human hepatocytes	±CYP1A2 mRNA (0.8-fold); ±CYP1A2 protein (1.0-fold); ↑POD activity (1.6-fold)	[58]
Ritonavir (1–25 μM)	Human hepatocytes	↑CYP1A2 mRNA (4-fold); ↑POD activity (2-fold)	[61]
Rosiglitazone (10 μM)	Human hepatocytes	↑CYP1A2 mRNA (11-fold); ↑CYP1A2 protein (7-fold); ↑EROD activity (37-fold)	[48]
Smoking	Human liver biopsies	↑EROD activity (3.3-fold)	[62]
Smoking (3–30/d), 7d	Human duodenal biopsies	↑EROD activity (4.2-fold)	[56]
Chargrilled meat diet (7 d)	Human duodenal biopsies	↑CYP1A1 protein, ↑hepatic CYP1A2 activity (CBT, 1.9-fold)	[33]

↑, increase; ±, unchanged; CBT, caffeine breath test; EROD, 7-ethoxyresorufin O-deethylase; POD, phenacetin O-deethylation.

As already described for genes regulated by other nuclear receptors (e.g., *ABCB1* by pregnane-X-receptor (PXR)), a partial transactivation of human CYP1A by nuclear receptors other than AhR is possible. In this regard, CYP1A1 and 1A2 were also shown to be induced upon activation of the human constitutive androstane receptor (CAR) [63]. This explains considerable induction of CYP1A enzymes by typical CAR ligands, such as carbamazepine, phenobarbital and phenytoin. On the other side, the relevance of PXR in the regulation of CYP1A seems to be negligible as shown in vitro [47,59,60] and in vivo [64].

3.2. Impact of Gender, Age, and Diseases

In addition to the described transcriptional regulation, also several nongenetic factors seem to influence CYP1A2 expression and function. For example, protein abundance and metabolic CYP1A2 activity for different substrates was shown to be considerably lower in woman than in men [31,65–67]. However, as smoking and the intake of oral contraceptives (inhibitors of CYP1A function) represent substantial confounders of CYP1A2 expression and function, those data have to be interpreted with caution and need further verification. Moreover, in analyzing potential gender differences in the pharmacokinetics of CYP1A substrates, dose-adjustment was shown to be essential as demonstrated for tizanidine [68]. There is also evidence that CYP1A2 activity is significantly higher in younger (<20 years) than in older people (>20–60 years and >60 years) [65].

Disease-related changes have been also reported for CYP1A. Here, CYP1A2 expression in liver dysfunction and cholestasis was found to be decreased [40,69]. Other studies failed to confirm those differences in vivo [53,54] and in human liver tissue at both, mRNA and protein levels [40,70]. More recent mRNA expression data demonstrated that the expression of CYP1A2 was decreased by about 90% in hepatocellular carcinoma livers, 80% in alcoholic cirrhosis, and 65% in severe cirrhosis [71]. In parallel, analysis of liver biopsy samples of patients with chronic hepatitis C revealed significantly lower gene expression levels of CYP1A1 and CYP1A2 [72,73]. These data have been recently confirmed by a targeted proteomic analysis [74]. Likewise, nonalcoholic fatty liver disease (NAFLD) was associated with decreased mRNA, protein amount, and functional activity of microsomal CYP1A2 compared to healthy liver tissue [75].

3.3. Genetics and Epigenetics

The large inter-individual variability in the elimination of drugs undergoing CYP1A2 metabolism has been attributed to genetic and environmental factors [11,76,77]. In this regard, Rasmussen and colleagues demonstrated in a large study in 378 mono- and dizygotic twins for the caffeine metabolic ratio (a surrogate for CYP1A2 activity) a strong overall heritability of 0.72 [78].

Common polymorphisms in the CYP1 gene have been found to be only of limited relevance for human drug metabolism. However, considering the involvement of CYP1A enzymes in bioactivation of procarcinogens, many studies investigated certain single nucleotide polymorphisms in association to various types of cancer [10,11]. The Pharmacogene Variation Consortium website (www.pharmvar.org) lists 15 alleles for CYP1A1 [79]. Of the most frequent variants m1 to m4, only the common non-synonymous variant CYP1A1*2C (rs1048943, 2454A>G, Ile462Val), which has a global minor allele frequency of about 12%, was shown to be associated with substantially modified enzymatic activity, i.e., 6- to 12-fold higher for its substrates 17β-estradiol and estrone [80]. This variant was associated with an increased risk for lung cancer in Chinese and breast, and prostate cancer in Caucasians [10,11].

Several alleles, namely 24, have been also reported for CYP1A2 [79], of which only the most established will be briefly mentioned here. The CYP1A2*6 variant was shown to result in a nonfunctional protein [81]. However, considering the rare occurrence of this and other variants [82], they are expected to be of limited clinical relevance. The CYP1A2*1C was associated with reduced CYP1A2 induction by cigarette smoking in Japanese [83]. On the contrary, the CYP1A2*1F variant (–163C>A) was linked with enhanced enzyme inducibility in Caucasian smokers [53,84] and heavy coffee drinkers [85]. Interestingly, carriers of the combined genotype CYP1A2*1C/*1F were not inducible by the AhR ligand omeprazole [86]. Both variants were described to increase the susceptibility to certain cancers. Despite the described multiplicity of CYP1A2 polymorphisms, clear gene dose relationships by comparing common SNPs to the respective protein abundance or metabolic phenotype could not be demonstrated yet. Thus, so far no single SNP or haplotype in the CYP1A2 gene seems to be predictive [41]. In this regard, a multivariate linear modeling by Klein et al. revealed that genetic polymorphisms contribute about 35% of hepatic CYP1A2 activity variation, whereas some 40% of the variation were explained by nongenetic factors together [40].

However, the clinical impact of genetic variation in terms of susceptibility factors for cancer or pharmacokinetics, efficacy and safety of certain CYP1A substrates is not systematically covered here but was excellently summarized by others [10,11,87–90].

Finally, there is also evidence for an epigenetic regulation of CYP1A2 expression as concluded from the observation that the extent of DNA methylation of a CpG island close to the translation start site was inversely correlated to the hepatic CYP1A2 mRNA expression [53,54]. Recent studies point also to an involvement of certain microRNAs in the expression and induction of CYP1A2 [91,92].

4. Metabolic Function, Substrates, and Inhibitors

4.1. Metabolic Features

Considering that CYP1A2 shares about 80% amino acid sequence identity with CYP1A1, it is not surprising that the substrate specificities of these enzymes often overlap, owing to a CYP1 family–specific distortion of the F helix in the area of the substrate binding cavity, which produces bending of the helix and results in the formation of an enclosed and planar substrate binding site observed in both CYP1A1 and CYP1A2 [93]. It has been demonstrated that commonly used probe drugs for CYP1A2 such as caffeine, theophylline, phenacetin, propranolol, and 7-ethoxyresorufin are metabolized by both CYP1A isoenzymes [94,95]. Despite this considerable similarity, CYP1A1 shows a preference for planar aromatic hydrocarbons (e.g., naphthalene, PAHs), while CYP1A2 prefers aromatic amines and heterocyclic compounds (e.g., 2-naphthylamine, xanthines) (Table 3). The metabolic feature of CYP1A1 in combination with its expression pattern in tissues potentially exposed to high amounts of PAHs (e.g., the lung via tobacco smoke, the intestine via charbroiled food) makes it plausible that increased expression and function of CYP1A1 may result in higher formation rates of potentially carcinogenic metabolites. In this regard, benzo[a]pyrene and other procarcinogens (e.g., arylarenes, nitroarenes, arylamines) are bioactivated by CYP1A1 to reactive and carcinogenic intermediates such as epoxides which may cause DNA damage and in long term malignancies. In the same manner, CYP1A2 is involved in the bioactivation of heterocyclic aromatic amines (HAAs) originating from cook muscle meats such as beef, pork, or fish to carcinogenic hydroxylamines. Thus, it can be assumed that induction of CYP1A1/1A2 in smokers by inhaling frequently high amounts of PAHs may contribute to strikingly increased risk for lung cancer [96]. However, the toxicological impact of both isoenzymes on the bioactivation of carinogenes from environmental compounds is beyond the scope of this article but summarized elsewhere [11,97].

Table 3. Overview for clinically relevant drugs undergoing significant CYP1A2-mediated metabolism (≥25%).

Substrate	Drug Class	Metabolic Reaction	Contribution of CYP1A2 (Other CYPs)	Reference
Aminopyrine	Analgesic drug	N-demethylation	40–50% (CYP2C8/2C19)	[98]
Agomelatine	melatonin receptor agonist (antidepressant)	hydroxylation and demethylation	90% (10% CYP2C9)	[99]
Caffeine	CNS stimulant	N-demethylation	>95%	[94,95]
Clozapine	Atypical antipsychotic drug	N-demethylation and N-oxidation	40–55% (CYP3A4/2C19)	[100]
Dacarbazine	Anticancer drug	N-demethylation	20–40% (CYP1A1/2E1)	[101]
Duloxetine	Antidepressant	4-, 5- and 6-hydroxylation major extent substrate	30–40% (CYP2D6/2C9)	[102]
Flutamide	Non-steroidal antiandrogen	2-Hydroxylation	~25% (CYP3A4/2C19)	[103]
Leflunomide	Disease-modifying anti-inflammatory drug	N-O bond cleavage	40–55%	[104]
Melatonin	Pineal hormone	6-hydroxylation and O-demethylation	40–60% (CYP1A1/1B1)	[105]
Mirtazapine	Antidepressant	8-hydroxylation and N-demethylation	30–50% (CYP3A4/2D6)	[106]
Nabumetone	NSAID	aliphatic hydroxylation	30–40% (CYP2C9)	[107]
Olanzapine	Atypical antipsychotic drug	N-demethylation and 7-hydroxylation	30–40% (CYP2D6)	[108]
Phenacetin	Analgesic drug	O-deethylation and C-hydroxylation	86%	[94]
Promazine	Antipsychotic drug	N-demethylation and 5-sulfoxidation	30–45% (CYP2C19/3A4)	[109]
Propranolol	β-Blocker	N-deisopropylation, and 4- and 5-hydroxylation	30–50% (CYP2D6)	[110]
Ramelteon	Melatonin receptor agonist (hypnotic)	Aliphatic hydroxylation	~50% (CYP2C19/3A4)	[111]
Rasagiline	Antiparkinson drug	N-dealkylation and hydroxylation	>50%	[112]
Riluzole	Antiglutamate agent (treatment of ALS)	N-hydroxylation	~80%	[113]
Ropinirole	Antiparkinson drug	N-depropylation and hydroxylation (major)	30–45%	[114]
Ropivacaine	Local anesthetic drug	3-, 4-hydroxylation	50–65% (CYP3A4)	[115]
Tacrine	cholinesterase inhibitor (Alzheimer's disease)	1-, 2-, 4- and 7-Hydroxylation	50–65%	[116]
Theophylline	Bronchodilator (Asthma/COPD)	N-demethylation	90–95%	[117]
Tizanidine	Muscle relaxant	Hydroxylation	80–95%	[118,119]
Verpamil	Calcium channel blocker	N-demethylation and N-dealkylation	20–30% (CYP2C8/3A4)	[120]
Zolmitriptan	Selective 5-$HT_{1B/1D}$ (treatment of migraine)	N-demethylation and O-demethlyation	30–40%	[121]

5-HT, 5-hydroxy tryptamine; ALS, Amyotrophic lateral sclerosis; CNS, central nervous system; COPD, Chronic obstructive pulmonary disease; NSAID, non-steroidal anti-inflammatory drug.

4.2. Substrates

Under the consideration that CYP1A1 is markedly lower expressed in the human liver than CYP1A2 and is also considered to be of extrahepatic relevance, its impact on the metabolic clearance of drugs was formerly assumed to be negligible [10,11]. In contrast to this conclusion, recent studies have clearly verified CYP1A1 protein abundance in human intestine and liver, which challenges the former paradigm of the pharmacokinetically irrelevant CYP1A1 [18,23,30]. Moreover, 15–20 years ago, several studies convincingly demonstrated high metabolic CYP1A1 activity of intestinal and hepatic microsomal fractions [14,27,122]. Associated to this, riociguat (guanylate cyclase stimulator used for the treatment of pulmonary hypertension) and granisetron (5-HT3 receptor antagonist for the treatment of nausea and vomiting following chemotherapy or radiotherapy) were shown to be highly and specifically biotransformed by CYP1A1 [18,122]. In addition, the tyrosine kinase inhibitors axitinib, erlotinib, gefitinib, and ningetinib as well as the toll-like receptor agonist imiquimod and conivaptan (inhibitor of the antidiuretic hormone) have been reported as substrates of CYP1A1 [18,123,124]. Thus, one has to conclude that CYP1A1 should be considered as an additional potentially relevant clearance pathway for some drugs. However, in the past, the metabolic stability of a drug was in most cases studied by using human liver microsomes or recombinant CYP1A2, but not for both isoforms of CYP1A, as done in very recent studies [18,123]. Consequently, the individual contribution of CYP1A1 to the metabolism of established CYP1A2 substrates as summarized in Table 3 remains uncertain, and asks for additional research efforts. However, even today, these kind of head-to-head comparisons of CYP1A1 and CYP1A2 in drug metabolism are challenging because established manufactures of life science consumables (e.g., Thermo Fisher Scientific and Corning) do not provide microsomal preparations of recombinant CYP1A1, but almost exclusively CYP1A2.

It was estimated by analyzing the metabolic pathways of about 250 frequently used drugs, that CYP1A2 is involved in the biotransformation of about 10% of drugs on the market [10]. CYP1A2-typical biotransformation reactions include N-demethylation of caffeine to 1,7-dimethylxanthine (paraxanthine), N-demethylation of clozapine, O-deethylation of phenacetin, and N-demethylation as well as 8-hydroxylation of theophylline. In particular, caffeine and phenacetin were frequently used as probe compounds in vitro and for phenotype determination in vivo [11,125]. Due to its high abundance in the human liver, CYP1A2 plays an important role in the metabolism of many clinically important drugs, including antipsychotics (clozapine, olanzapine), antidepressants (duloxetine, agomelatine, mirtazapine), cardiovascular drugs (propranolol, verapamil), non-steroidal anti-inflammatory drugs (NSAID) (phenacetin), the Alzheimer's disease drug tacrine, a cholinesterase inhibitor, the muscle relaxant tizanidine, antiparkinson drugs (rasagilin, ropinirol), and the methylxanthines caffeine, and theophylline [10,11]. Over 100 clinically used drugs have been described to be substrates of CYP1A2 [11]. However, many compounds are subjected to complex metabolism by several CYP enzymes so that the allover contribution of CYP1A2 is limited (~5–20%) and dominated by other pathways. Examples for drugs that are frequently and somewhat misleadingly labelled as typical CYP1A2 substrates are acetaminophen, amitriptyline, bupivacaine, carbamazepine, estradiol, fluvoxamine, haloperidol, imipramine, lidocaine, mianserin, naproxen, ondansetrone, triamterene, warfarin, and zolpidem. Although, CYP1A2 contributes to their metabolism, relevant drug-drug interactions (DDIs) cannot be expected as other metabolic pathways take over in the case of CYP1A2 inhibition. Thus, Table 3 summarizes only drugs whose systemic clearance is assumed to be >25% dependent on CYP1A2 metabolism based on the in vitro phenotyping studies and human pharmacokinetic data, as also suggested by the current Food and Drug Administration (FDA) guidance of drug–drug interactions (https://www.fda.gov/regulatory-information/search-fda-guidance-documents/vitro-drug-interaction-studies-cytochrome-p450-enzyme-and-transporter-mediated-drug-interactions). Similar to CYP3A4, CYP1A2 is a rather low affinity but high capacity metabolic enzyme. Thus, only very high concentrations of respective substrates are able to cause competitive inhibition (e.g., by extremely high doses of caffeine).

Endogenous substrates of CYP1A include arachidonic acid, bilirubin, prostaglandins, estrogens, melatonin and retinoic acid [11,126].

4.3. Inhibitors

Established inhibitors of CYP1A function include 7-hydroxyflavone and α-naphthoflavone that have been extensively used in vitro [11,14,18,94]. Ketoconazole, a potent inhibitor of CYP3A4 and P-glycoprotein, was also shown to inhibit CYP1A1 in a significant manner [27]. Again, we must state that there are so far insufficient data on the specific inhibitory properties of established CYP1A2 inhibitors on the function of CYP1A1. Considering the similarity in terms of sequence and function, one may hypothesize again a substantial overlap between both isoenzymes. An exception of this conclusion is furafylline, a methylxanthine, which was demonstrated to inhibit specifically CYP1A2 but not CYP1A1 [94]. Thus, it serves as an in vitro tool to distinguish between the metabolic activites of both isoenzymes in microsomal studies.

Typical inhibitors of CYP1A2 are rather small molecules, which are often heterocyclic or halogenated. Drugs resulting in potent competitive but reversible inhibition of CYP1A2 include fluoroquinolones such as ciprofloxacin and enoxacin, selective serotonin reuptake inhibiting (SSRI) antidepressants fluvoxamine and fluoxetin, the azole antimycotics ketoconazole, and clotrimazole, as well as estrogens (oral contraceptives). Some drugs (e.g., amiodarone, carbamazepine, duloxetine, isoniazid, resveratrol, and rofecoxib) were described to be mechanism-based inhibitors [11], i.e., they cause irreversible inhibition of CYP1A enzymes, which requires de novo synthesis of the respective proteins, which, in turn, results in long-lasting enzyme inhibition. Table 4 provides an overview of clinically used drugs that were identified as potent inhibitors of CYP1A. As it can be seen from the given inhibitory potential of each compound as assessed in vitro (Ki or IC_{50} values), compounds with high inhibition potency, such as ciprofloxacin (Ki, 144 nM for CYP1A2), fluxoxamine (Ki, 11-40 nM for CYP1A2), or ketoconazole (Ki, 40 nM for CYP1A1) are especially expected to cause clinically relevant drug–drug interactions [27,127,128].

Table 4. Overview of clinically relevant drugs with inhibitory properties on CYP1A1/1A2.

Drug	Drug Class	In Vitro System	Inhibitory Effect (Isoenzyme)	Reference
Alosetron [1]	$5HT_3$-receptor antagonist (irritable bowel syndrome)	HLM	IC_{50} = 2 μM (CYP1A2)	[129]
Amiodarone [1]	Antiarrhythmic drug	HLM	IC_{50} = 86 μM	[130]
Artemesinin [1]	Antimalaria drug	HLM	Ki = 0.43 μM (CYP1A2)	[131]
Carbamazepine [2]	Anticonvulsant	HLM	n.d. (CYP1A2)	[132]
Celecoxib [1]	COX-2 inhibitor	HLM	Ki = 25.4 μM (CYP1A2)	[127]
Ciprofloxacin [1]	Antibiotic (fluoroquinolone)	HLM HLM	70.4% (CYP1A2) Ki = 144 nM (CYP1A2)	[133] [127]
Cimetidine [1]	H_2-receptor antagonist	HLM	Ki = 200 μM (CYP1A2)	[134]
Clotrimazole [1]	Antifungal agent	human lymphoblast cells	Ki = 7.9 μM (CYP1A2)	[135]
Desogestrel [1]	Hormone (oral contraceptive)	HLM	Ki = 39.4 μM (CYP1A2)	[127]
Duloxetine [2]	Antidepressant (SSRI)	HLM	n.d. (CYP1A2)	[136]
Enoxacin [1]	Antibiotic (fluoroquinolone)	HLM	74.9% (CYP1A2)	[133]
Ethinyl estradiol [1]	Hormone (oral contraceptive)	HLM	Ki = 10.6 μM (CYP1A2)	[127]
Fluoxetine [1]	Antidepressant (SSRI)	HLM	Ki = 4.4 μM (CYP1A2)	[137]
Fluvoxamine [1]	Antidepressant (SSRI)	HLM	Ki = 33 μM (CYP1A1) Ki = 40 nM (CYP1A2) Ki = 11 nM (CYP1A2)	[128] [128] [127]

Table 4. *Cont.*

Drug	Drug Class	In Vitro System	Inhibitory Effect (Isoenzyme)	Reference
Isoniazid [2]	Antibiotic	HLM	Ki = 285 μM (CYP1A2)	[138]
Ketoconazole [1]	Antifungal agent	HIM HLM	Ki = 40 nM (CYP1A1) IC_{50} = 0.33 μM CYP1A2)	[27] [139]
Miconazole [1]	Antifungal agent	human lymphoblast cells	Ki = 3.2 μM (CYP1A2)	[135]
Nifedipine [1]	Calcium channel blocker	HLM	n.c. (CYP1A1) n.d. (CYP1A2)	[94]
Norfloxacin [1]	Antibiotic (fluoroquinolone)	HLM	55.7% (CYP1A2)	[133]
Paroxetine [1]	Antidepressant (SSRI)	HLM	Ki = 5.5 μM (CYP1A2)	[137]
Propafenone [1]	Antiarrhythmic drug	HLM	IC_{50} = 29 μM	[130]
Propranolol	Beta blocker	HLM	n.c. (CYP1A1) n.d. (CYP1A2)	[94]
Resveratrol [2]	Natural compound	HLM	IC_{50} = 23 μM (CYP1A1) Ki = 2.2 μM (CYP1A2)	[140] [141]
Riluzole [1]	Amyotrophic lateral sclerosis drug	HLM	Ki = 12 1 μM (CYP1A2)	[113]
Rofecoxib [2]	COX-2 inhibitor	HLM	Ki = 6.2 μM (CYP1A2)	[127]
Sertraline [1]	Antidepressant (SSRI)	HLM	Ki = 8.8 μM (CYP1A2)	[137]
Sulconazole	Antifungal agent	human lymphoblast cells	Ki = 0.4 μM (CYP1A2)	[135]
Thiabendazol [2]	Antifungal/antiparasitic agent	HLM	Ki = 1.54 μM (CYP1A2)	[131]
Tioconazole [1]	Antifungal agent	human lymphoblast cells	Ki = 0.4 μM (CYP1A2)	[135]
Tolfenamic acid [1]	NSAID	HLM	Ki= 1.4 μM (CYP1A2)	[127]

[1] Competitive (reversible) inhibitor; [2] mechanism-based (irreversible) inhibitor; 5-HT, 5-hydroxy tryptamine; COX, cyclooxygenase; HLM, human liver microsomes; IC_{50}, half maximal inhibitory concentration; Ki, inhibition constant; NSAID, nonsteroidal anti-inflammatory drug; SSRI, selective serotonin reuptake inhibitor.

5. Drug–Drug Interactions

Under consideration of the high number of frequently prescribed drugs that were described to be substrates (Table 3), inhibitors (Table 4), or inducers (Table 2) of human CYP1A1/A2, several unwanted drug–drug interactions can be assumed in the case of combined administration.

5.1. Inhibition Studies

In this regard, the most pronounced interactions have been described for the combination of CYP1A substrates with potent inhibitors including ciprofloxacin, fluvoxamine, ethinyl estradiol, and rofecoxib. Their combination with established CYP1A substrates resulted in clinically relevant interactions increasing the systemic drug exposure of caffeine, clozapine, mirtazapine, olanzapine and theophylline by 1.5 to 3-fold [106,131,142–144]. For agomelatine, ramelteon, tracrine, and tizanidine much more dramatic increases of serum area under the concentration-time curve (AUC) by 10–190-fold have been observed [118,119,145,146], which is expected to cause drug-related side effects and even toxicity. For example, the elevation of plasma levels of clozapine by ciprofloxacine resulted in rhabdomyolysis, delirium, and death during combination in psychotic patients [147,148].

The reasons for these dramatic interactions might be due to extensive metabolism by CYP1A enzymes and/or a high volume of distribution of the victim drug (e.g., 168 and 349 l for tizanidine and tacrine). In order to estimate the in vivo potential of a certain CYP1A inhibitor (Table 4) of an in vitro function, to cause clinically relevant interactions, focusing on the observed inhibitory potential (Ki, IC_{50} value) alone is not sufficient, but additional pharmacokinetic aspect of the perpetrator compounds must be considered as well. For sufficient inhibitory potential in vivo, a perpetrator drug needs to generate free unbound concentrations (fraction unbound, fu) around or above the observed Ki/IC_{50} value and needs to be present in the systemic circulation for several hours to cause substantial metabolic inhibition as determined by an elimination half-life of several hours. Consequently, fluvoxamine and ciprofloxacin that are characterized by rather low-to-medium protein binding (fu, 0.23 for fluvoxamine and fu, 0.8 for ciprofloxacin), but high serum levels as caused by their comparatively high administered doses (50–100 mg for fluvoxamine, 100–750 mg for ciprofloxacin) and medium to long terminal half-lives (4–7 h for ciprofloxacin, 17–22 h for fluvoxamine), cause that both drugs are strong inhibitors of CYP1A2 in vivo, and cause many clinically relevant drug–drug interactions.

This scenario is not true for other drugs mentioned in Table 4. For example, although the NSAIDs celecoxib and tolfenamic acid demonstrated a considerable inhibition of CYP1A2 in human liver microsomes (HLM) with a Ki values of 25 μM and 1.4 μM [127], they did not show clinically relevant interactions, most likely due to their high protein binding of ~98% and 99.7%, respectively. As a conclusion, drugs undergoing substantial CYP1A1/2 metabolism should be combined with caution together with the perpetrator drugs mentioned in Table 5. If possible, dose escalation combined with therapeutic drug monitoring should be used for CYP1A2 drugs with a narrow therapeutic index such as theophylline, clozapine or tizanidine. Whether the mentioned in vivo inhibitors of CYP1A2 may also cause clinically relevant interactions with CYP1A1 substrates remains uncertain and requires further studies.

Table 5. Overview of clinically relevant interaction as caused by inhibition of CYP1A1/1A2 enzymes.

Substrate (Victim Drug)	Perpetrator (Inhibitor)	PK Change	Reference
Agomelatine	Fluvoxamine	AUC ↑ 60-fold	Product information
Caffeine (137 mg, SD)	Thiabendazol (500 mg, SD)	AUC ↑ 1.6-fold $t_{1/2}$ ↑ 2.4-fold	[131]
Clozapine (50–700 mg)	Fluvoxamine (50–100 mg, SID, MD)	C_{SS} ↑ 5-10-fold	[149]
Clozapine (2.5–3.0 mg/kg)	Fluvoxamine (50 mg, SID, MD)	C_{SS} ↑ 3-fold	[150]
Clozapine (200–350 mg)	Fluvoxamine (50 mg, SID, MD)	C_{SS} ↑ 2.2-fold	[142]
Clozapine (150–400 mg)	Ciprofloxacin (250 mg BID, 7 d)	C_{SS} ↑ 1.3-fold	[151]
Duloxetine (60 mg, SD)	Fluvoxamine (100 mg SID, 16 d)	AUC ↑ 5.6-fold C_{MAX} ↑ 2.4-fold	[102]
Melatonin (5 mg, SD)	Fluvoxamine (50 mg, SD)	AUC ↑ 17-fold C_{MAX} ↑ 12-fold	[105]
Mirtazapin (15–30 mg)	Fluvoxamine (50–100 mg, SID, MD)	C_{SS} ↑ 1.3-fold	[106]
Olanzapine (10 mg, SD)	Fluvoxamine (100 mg, SID, 14 d)	AUC ↑ 1.5-fold C_{MAX} ↑ 1.6-fold	[143]
Propranolol (160 mg, SID)	Fluvoxamine (100 mg)	C_{MAX} ↑ 5-fold	[152]
Ramelteon (16 mg, SD)	Fluvoxamine (100 mg BID, 3 d)	AUC ↑ 190-fold C_{MAX} ↑ 70-fold	Product information [111]
Ropivacaine (0.6 mg/kg, iv)	Ciprofloxacin (500 mg BID, 2.5 d)	CL ↓ 31%	[153]
Tacrine (40 mg, SD)	Fluvoxamine (100 mg SID, 6 d)	AUC ↑ 8.3-fold C_{MAX} ↑ 5.6-fold	[145]
Theophylline (250 mg, SD)	Fluvoxamine (75 mg, SD)	AUC ↑ 2.4-fold $t_{1/2}$ ↑ 2.5-fold	[144]

Table 5. *Cont.*

Substrate (Victim Drug)	Perpetrator (Inhibitor)	PK Change	Reference
Theophylline (3.4 mg/kg, SD)	Ciprofloxacin (500 mg BID, 3 d)	CL ↓ 19% $t_{1/2}$ ↑ 26%	[154]
Tizanidine (4 mg, SD)	Rofecoxib (25 mg SID, 4d)	AUC ↑ 13.6-fold C_{MAX} ^ 6.1-fold	[146]
Tizanidine (4 mg, SD)	Ciprofloxacin (500 mg BID, 3 d)	AUC ↑ 10-fold C_{MAX} ↑ 7-fold	[118]
Tizanidine (4 mg, SD)	Fluvoxamine (100 mg SID, 4d)	AUC ↑ 33-fold C_{MAX} ↑ 12-fold	[119]
Tizanidine (4 mg, SD)	Ethinyl estradiol 20–30 µg, gestodene 75 µg	AUC ↑ 3.9-fold C_{MAX} ↑ 3-fold	[155]
Ropivacaine (0.6 mg/kg, iv)	Ciprofloxacin (500 mg BID, 2.5 d)	CL ↓ 31%	[153]

↑, increase; ↓, decrease; AUC, area under the concentration-time curve; BID, twice daily; CL, clearance; Cmax, maximum serum concentration; Css, trough serum concentrations at steady-state; d, days; MD, multiple doses; PK, pharmacokinetic; SID, once daily; SD, single dose; t1/2, elimination half-life.

5.2. Induction Studies

On the other side, carbamazepine, lansoprazole, omeprazole, phenobarbital, primaquine, and rosiglitazone were reported to be potent inducers of CYP1A1/1A2 by binding to AhR or CAR receptor as briefly described above [44,46–49] (Table 2), while the effects of prototypical PXR activators such as rifampicin, ritonavir and St. John's wort are rather negligible [47,58–60,156]. Of these drugs, omeprazole was one of the most potent and most extensively investigated inducer in vitro and in vivo, resulting in several-fold induction of the gene expression, protein abundance and metabolic function of CYP1A1/2. However, significant effects on the pharmacokinetics and efficacy of CYP1A substrates have not been observed yet. Well-established substrates, including caffeine, phenacetin, theophylline, or propranolol did not show any changes in their pharmacokinetics in the presence of omeprazole [157–160]. Thus, one might conclude that the interaction potential of omeprazole and other proton pump inhibitors for clinically relevant DDIs might be very limited although there are also data from a case report indicating slight increase in CYP1A2 metabolism [161]. An explanation could be found in the relatively low peak concentrations of omeprazole (0.7–4.6 µM) in the systemic circulation compared to the inductive in vitro concentrations (25–50 µM) and its short half-life of 0.5–1 h (Regardh et al. 1990). In contrast to this, treatment with carbamazepine considerably induced clozapine metabolism, leading to significantly lower serum level in schizophrenic patients [149]. Carbamazepine was furthermore shown to induce hepatic caffeine metabolism as well as the systemic clearance of olanzapine and mirtazapine in a significant manner [55,162,163]. Thus, it can be stated that CYP1A2 substrates should not be combined with carbamazepine or dose-adjustment should be taken into account.

However, estimations on potential drug interactions using in vitro data on induction properties alone can be misleading. An example for that phenomenon is ritonavir, a HIV protease inhibitor. Although it showed no (or only weak) induction of CYP1A2 mRNA and activity in human hepatocytes [58,61], the pharmacokinetics of caffeine and olanzapine was significantly affected, i.e., AUC was reduced by 75% and 53% [164,165]. To overcome decreased drug efficacy due to the considerable changes in the pharmacokinetics, Jacobs et al. (2014) proposed that doubling the dose of olanzapine as a successful strategy in the case of co-medication with ritonavir [166]. The same disconnection between in vitro and in vivo effects could be observed for rifampicin, which has not been shown to be an AhR ligand and demonstrated also only a weak induction of CYP1A2 expression and metabolic function in human hepatocytes [46,47,59,61]. Accordingly, rifampicin premedication for 5–15 days reduced serum AUC of caffeine and tizanidine by 50–60% [64,164]. The reasons for this surprising finding might rely on nuclear receptor cross-talk or insensitivity of the respective in vitro on nuclear receptor activation [167]. Table 6 provides an overview about clinically relevant interactions of CYP1A substrates caused by enzyme induction.

Table 6. Overview of clinically relevant interaction as caused by induction of CYP1A1/1A2 enzymes.

Substrate (Victim Drug)	Perpetrator	PK Change	Reference
Antipyrine (20 mg/kg, SD)	Smoking	CL ↑ 46%	[62]
Caffeine (100 mg, SD)	Carbamazepine (400 mg, SID, 14 d)	CL ↑ 27–47%	[163]
Caffeine (2 mg/mg, SD)	Lopinavir (400 mg)/Ritonavir (100 mg), BID, 14 d	MR ↑ 43%	[168]
Caffeine (200 mg, SD)	Rifampicin (400 mg BID, 14 d)	AUC ↓ 60% CL ↑ 214%	[164]
Caffeine (200 mg, SD)	Ritonavir (400 mg BID, 14 d)	AUC ↓ 75% CL ↑ 290%	[164]
Clozapine (150–900 mg)	Smoking (7–>20/d)	C_{SS} ↓ 50% C_{SS} ↓ 40%	[169] [170]
Clozapine (325 mg)	Omeprazole (40–60 mg, MD)	C_{SS} ↓ 42–45%	[161]
Clozapine	Carbamazepine	C_{SS} ↓ 50%	[149]
Duloxetine (86–102 mg, MD)	Smoking	C_{SS} ↓ 53%	[171]
Estradiol (1–2 mg)	Smoking	C_{SS} ↓ 43%	[172]
Mirtazapine (15–30 mg, SID, 7 d)	Carbamazepine (200-400 mg, BID, 21 d)	AUC ↓ 63% C_{max} ↓ 44%	[173]
Mirtazapine (30 mg, SID, 28 d)	Smoking	C_{SS} ↓ 41%	[174]
Olanzapine	Carbamazepine	CL ↑ 46% $t_{1/2}$ ↓ 20%	[162]
Olanzapine (10 mg, SD)	Rifampicin, 600 mg, SID, 7 d	AUC ↓ 48% C_{max} ↓ 11%	[175]
Olanzapine	Ritonavir (300–500 mg BID, 3–5 d)	AUC ↓ 53% C_{MAX} ↓ 40%	[165]
Olanzapine	Smoking (light, 1–4/d) Smoking (medium, >5) Smoking (heavy, 7–>20)	AUC ↓ 45% AUC ↓ 68% C_{SS} ↓ 67%	[176] [176] [169]
Theophylline	Smoking	CL ↑ 58–100% $t_{1/2}$ ↓ 63%	[177]
Tizanidine	Rifampicin, 500 mg, SID, 5 d	AUC ↓ 53%	[64]
Tizanidine	Smoking	AUC ↓ 33%	[68]
Verapamil	Smoking	AUC ↓ 20%	[178]

↑, increase; ↓, decrease; AUC, area under the concentration-time curve; BID, twice daily; CL, clearance; C_{max}, maximum serum concentration; Css, trough serum concentrations at steady-state; d, days; MD, multiple doses; MR, metabolic ratio; PK, pharmacokinetic; SID, once daily; SD, single dose; $t_{1/2}$, elimination half-life.

Although it was shown in vitro experiments that CYP1A1 can be inhibited and induced by several compounds (Tables 2 and 4), there are to the best of our knowledge no clinical drug–drug interactions that can be attributed by specific CYP1A1 inhibition or induction. However, considering the overlap in substrate recognition, inhibitors, and inducers one might speculate similar interactions as described for CYP1A2 substrates (Tables 5 and 6). Accordingly, relevant DDIs have been estimated for CYP1A1 [179]. Nevertheless, given the low expression levels of CYP1A1 in human intestine and liver (if even), the extent of these interactions is expected to be much lower than those caused by inhibition or induction of hepatic CYP1A2.

5.3. Impact of Smoking and Diet

Finally, smoking can have a profound effect on the pharmacokinetics and efficacy of several CYP1A1/2 substrates, which is comparable to potent inducing drugs, as summarized in Table 6. In all summarized examples, the systemic drug exposure of CYP1A substrates was significantly decreased in smokers compared to nonsmokers by 30–70% (Figure 2). Thus, smokers require higher doses than nonsmokers. A questionable benefit might be that smokers show also less adverse drug reactions than nonsmokers [177,180]. However, this is so far only well established in neuropsychopharmacology, i.e., treatment with antipsychotics and antidepressants. Here, individual dose adjustment is routinely performed in dependence on therapeutic drug monitoring [181].

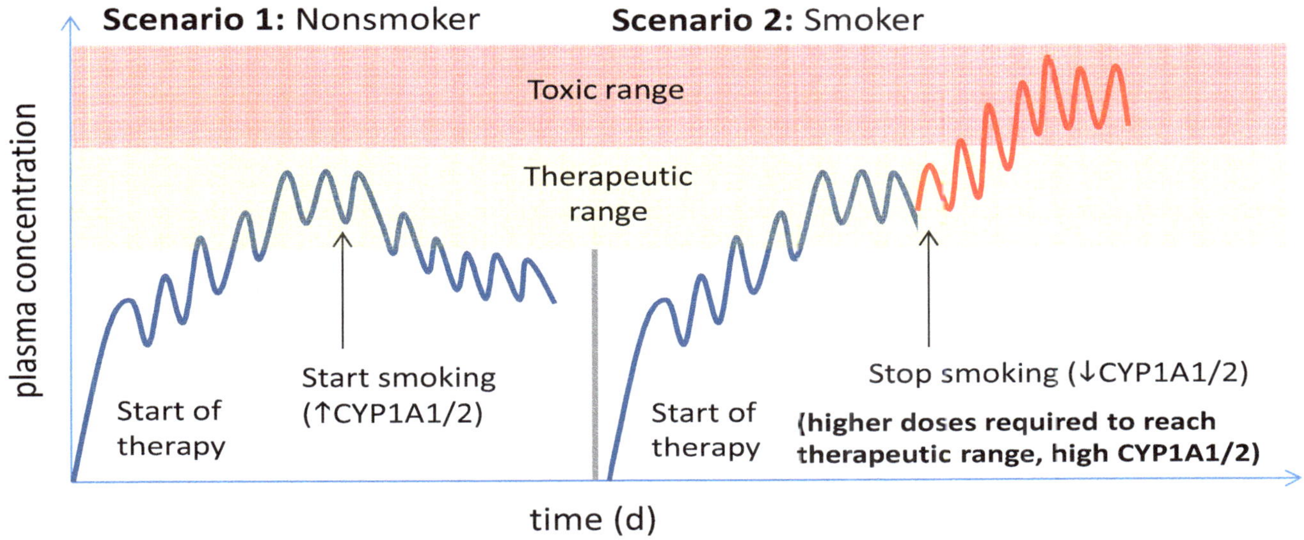

Figure 2. Schematic overview of potential interaction scenarios of tobacco smoking. In scenario 1, a nonsmoker reaches the steady state conditions of a certain CYP1A1/2 substrate after 5–6 half-lives using standard doses. After start smoking, CYP1A enzymes are significantly induced in intestine and liver resulting in increased drug clearance and decreasing plasma levels of the respective drug. In scenario 2, a smoker, who has already substantially higher expression and metabolic activity of CYP1A1/2, requires significantly higher doses to reach the therapeutic range. After stopping smoking, CYP1A1/2 will gradually return to the native expression levels, while the daily drug doses are not adjusted, which results in markedly increased and potentially toxic plasma concentrations.

It was shown that tobacco consumption induces CYP1A2 activity in a dose-dependent manner; smoking of daily 1–5, 6–10 and >10 cigarettes increases CYP1A2 activity 1.2-, 1.5- and 1.7-fold [182]. The maximum induction effect is already reached after smoking about 10 cigarettes daily, which abates after about three days of stopping smoking [182,183]. In particular, the latter effect may cause safety issues in the case of treatment with highly CYP1A-metabolized drugs with serious side effects, such as clozapine, olanzapine, tacrine, theophylline, or tizanidine. In this case, systemic drug exposure will substantially increase due to decreasing metabolic capacity, but unchanged high doses associated with an augmented risk for side effects, or even drug-related toxicity (Figure 2). Associated with this, cases of agranulocytosis and seizures have been reported for clozapine [181,184]. Because nicotine alone does not possess any inductive effects on CYP1A, the same risk is true in case of using e-cigarettes and other ways of nicotine substitution [185]. This should be considered by adjusting the appropriate dose, especially in case of changes in smoking habit (Figure 2).

Although a chargrilled meat diet was shown to significantly induce intestinal CYP1A1 protein as well as the metabolic activity of hepatic CYP1A2, as concluded from the caffeine breath test [33], altered pharmacokinetics of tacrine and caffeine could not be observed in a respective clinical study [186]. Some in vivo findings suggest also a potential in vivo inducing effects of broccoli [187] and another brassica vegetable, kale [188], on CYP1A2 mediated metabolism of caffeine. The brassica vegetable CYP1A2 induction is most probably mediated by 3,3′-diindolylmethane (DIM), a condensation product of indole-3-carbinol being a metabolite of the indole glucosinolate glucobrassicin. DIM has been shown to induce CYP1A2 in cultured human liver slices [189]. However, there is a lack of information about brassica vegetables interaction with clinically relevant drugs.

6. Summary and Conclusions

CYP1A1 and CYP1A2 are expressed in human intestine and liver. However, their inter-subject expression and function is highly variable as most likely caused by genetic, epigenetic, environmental factors (smoking, diet) and diseases. Considering the high number of drugs that have been identified as substrates, inhibitors, or inducers of CYP1A enzymes, many clinically relevant interactions have been reported and can be expected for other substrates. Thus, respective combinations should be avoided or appropriate dose adjustment is recommended in case of victim drugs with a narrow therapeutic index. In general, there is a substantial lack of data regarding CYP1A1 and its distinct role in the pharmacokinetics of drugs. However, from today's perspective, its allover contribution to serious drug–drug interactions seems to be limited considering its low expression levels and the potential functional compensation by CYP1A2. On the other hand, CYP1A2 has to be considered as one of the big five hepatic drug metabolizing enzymes (along with CYP3A4, CYP2C9, CYP2C19, CYP2D6, CYP2E1), which is of high clinical relevance in terms of inter-subject variability of drug efficacy and safety, as well as drug–drug interactions.

Author Contributions: Conceptualization, investigation, writing—original draft preparation, and writing—review and editing, F.K., C.W., M.D., and S.O. All authors have read and agreed to the published version of the manuscript.

References

1. Tanaka, E. Clinically important pharmacokinetic drug-drug interactions: Role of cytochrome P450 enzymes. *J. Clin. Pharm. Ther.* **1998**, *23*, 403–416. [CrossRef] [PubMed]
2. Palleria, C.; Di Paolo, A.; Giofrè, C.; Caglioti, C.; Leuzzi, G.; Siniscalchi, A.; de Sarro, G.; Gallelli, L. Pharmacokinetic drug-drug interaction and their implication in clinical management. *J. Res. Med. Sci.* **2013**, *18*, 601–610. [PubMed]
3. Paine, M.F.; Shen, D.D.; Kunze, K.L.; Perkins, J.D.; Marsh, C.L.; McVicar, J.P.; Barr, D.M.; Gillies, B.S.; Thummel, K.E. First-pass metabolism of midazolam by the human intestine. *Clin. Pharmacol. Ther.* **1996**, *60*, 14–24. [CrossRef]
4. Thummel, K.E.; O'Shea, D.; Paine, M.F.; Shen, D.D.; Kunze, K.L.; Perkins, J.D.; Wilkinson, G.R. Oral first-pass elimination of midazolam involves both gastrointestinal and hepatic CYP3A-mediated metabolism. *Clin. Pharmacol. Ther.* **1996**, *59*, 491–502. [CrossRef]
5. Galetin, A.; Houston, J.B. Intestinal and hepatic metabolic activity of five cytochrome P450 enzymes: Impact on prediction of first-pass metabolism. *J. Pharmacol. Exp. Ther.* **2006**, *318*, 1220–1229. [CrossRef]
6. Eichelbaum, M.; Ingelman-Sundberg, M.; Evans, W.E. Pharmacogenomics and individualized drug therapy. *Annu. Rev. Med.* **2006**, *57*, 119–137. [CrossRef]
7. Evans, W.E.; Relling, M.V. Moving towards individualized medicine with pharmacogenomics. *Nature* **2004**, *429*, 464–468. [CrossRef]
8. Dresser, G.K.; Spence, J.D.; Bailey, D.G. Pharmacokinetic-pharmacodynamic consequences and clinical relevance of cytochrome P450 3A4 inhibition. *Clin. Pharmacokinet.* **2000**, *38*, 41–57. [CrossRef]
9. Bahar, M.A.; Setiawan, D.; Hak, E.; Wilffert, B. Pharmacogenetics of drug-drug interaction and drug-drug-gene interaction: A systematic review on CYP2C9, CYP2C19 and CYP2D6. *Pharmacogenomics* **2017**, *18*, 701–739. [CrossRef]
10. Zanger, U.M.; Schwab, M. Cytochrome P450 enzymes in drug metabolism: Regulation of gene expression, enzyme activities, and impact of genetic variation. *Pharmacol. Ther.* **2013**, *138*, 103–141. [CrossRef]

11. Zhou, S.-F.; Wang, B.; Yang, L.-P.; Liu, J.-P. Structure, function, regulation and polymorphism and the clinical significance of human cytochrome P450 1A2. *Drug Metab. Rev.* **2010**, *42*, 268–354. [CrossRef] [PubMed]
12. Murray, G.I.; Melvin, W.T.; Greenlee, W.F.; Burke, M.D. Regulation, function, and tissue-specific expression of cytochrome P450 CYP1B1. *Annu. Rev. Pharmacol. Toxicol.* **2001**, *41*, 297–316. [CrossRef] [PubMed]
13. Schweikl, H.; Taylor, J.A.; Kitareewan, S.; Linko, P.; Nagorney, D.; Goldstein, J.A. Expression of CYP1A1 and CYP1A2 genes in human liver. *Pharmacogenetics* **1993**, *3*, 239–249. [CrossRef] [PubMed]
14. Stiborová, M.; Martínek, V.; Rýdlová, H.; Koblas, T.; Hodek, P. Expression of cytochrome P450 1A1 and its contribution to oxidation of a potential human carcinogen 1-phenylazo-2-naphthol (Sudan I) in human livers. *Cancer Lett.* **2005**, *220*, 145–154. [CrossRef] [PubMed]
15. Nishimura, M.; Yaguti, H.; Yoshitsugu, H.; Naito, S.; Satoh, T. Tissue distribution of mRNA expression of human cytochrome P450 isoforms assessed by high-sensitivity real-time reverse transcription PCR. *Yakugaku Zasshi* **2003**, *123*, 369–375. [CrossRef] [PubMed]
16. Paine, M.F.; Hart, H.L.; Ludington, S.S.; Haining, R.L.; Rettie, A.E.; Zeldin, D.C. The human intestinal cytochrome P450 "pie". *Drug Metab. Dispos.* **2006**, *34*, 880–886. [CrossRef]
17. Bièche, I.; Narjoz, C.; Asselah, T.; Vacher, S.; Marcellin, P.; Lidereau, R.; Beaune, P.; de Waziers, I. Reverse transcriptase-PCR quantification of mRNA levels from cytochrome (CYP)1, CYP2 and CYP3 families in 22 different human tissues. *Pharmacogenet. Genom.* **2007**, *17*, 731–742. [CrossRef]
18. Lang, D.; Radtke, M.; Bairlein, M. Highly Variable Expression of CYP1A1 in Human Liver and Impact on Pharmacokinetics of Riociguat and Granisetron in Humans. *Chem. Res. Toxicol.* **2019**, *32*, 1115–1122. [CrossRef]
19. Ding, X.; Kaminsky, L.S. Human extrahepatic cytochromes P450: Function in xenobiotic metabolism and tissue-selective chemical toxicity in the respiratory and gastrointestinal tracts. *Annu. Rev. Pharmacol. Toxicol.* **2003**, *43*, 149–173. [CrossRef]
20. Murray, B.P.; Edwards, R.J.; Murray, S.; Singleton, A.M.; Davies, D.S.; Boobis, A.R. Human hepatic CYP1A1 and CYP1A2 content, determined with specific anti-peptide antibodies, correlates with the mutagenic activation of PhIP. *Carcinogenesis* **1993**, *14*, 585–592. [CrossRef]
21. Chang, T.K.H.; Chen, J.; Pillay, V.; Ho, J.-Y.; Bandiera, S.M. Real-time polymerase chain reaction analysis of CYP1B1 gene expression in human liver. *Toxicol. Sci.* **2003**, *71*, 11–19. [CrossRef] [PubMed]
22. Grangeon, A.; Clermont, V.; Barama, A.; Gaudette, F.; Turgeon, J.; Michaud, V. Development and validation of an absolute protein assay for the simultaneous quantification of fourteen CYP450s in human microsomes by HPLC-MS/MS-based targeted proteomics. *J. Pharm. Biomed. Anal.* **2019**, *173*, 96–107. [CrossRef] [PubMed]
23. Shrivas, K.; Mindaye, S.T.; Getie-Kebtie, M.; Alterman, M.A. Mass spectrometry-based proteomic analysis of human liver cytochrome(s) P450. *Toxicol. Appl. Pharmacol.* **2013**, *267*, 125–136. [CrossRef] [PubMed]
24. Drozdzik, M.; Busch, D.; Lapczuk, J.; Müller, J.; Ostrowski, M.; Kurzawski, M.; Oswald, S. Protein Abundance of Clinically Relevant Drug-Metabolizing Enzymes in the Human Liver and Intestine: A Comparative Analysis in Paired Tissue Specimens. *Clin. Pharmacol. Ther.* **2018**, *104*, 515–524. [CrossRef]
25. Drahushuk, A.T.; McGarrigle, B.P.; Larsen, K.E.; Stegeman, J.J.; Olson, J.R. Detection of CYP1A1 protein in human liver and induction by TCDD in precision-cut liver slices incubated in dynamic organ culture. *Carcinogenesis* **1998**, *19*, 1361–1368. [CrossRef]
26. Zhang, Q.Y.; Dunbar, D.; Ostrowska, A.; Zeisloft, S.; Yang, J.; Kaminsky, L.S. Characterization of human small intestinal cytochromes P-450. *Drug Metab. Dispos.* **1999**, *27*, 804–809.
27. Paine, M.F.; Schmiedlin-Ren, P.; Watkins, P.B. Cytochrome P-450 1A1 expression in human small bowel: Interindividual variation and inhibition by ketoconazole. *Drug Metab. Dispos.* **1999**, *27*, 360–364.
28. Ohtsuki, S.; Schaefer, O.; Kawakami, H.; Inoue, T.; Liehner, S.; Saito, A.; Ishiguro, N.; Kishimoto, W.; Ludwig-Schwellinger, E.; Ebner, T.; et al. Simultaneous absolute protein quantification of transporters, cytochromes P450, and UDP-glucuronosyltransferases as a novel approach for the characterization of individual human liver: Comparison with mRNA levels and activities. *Drug Metab. Dispos.* **2012**, *40*, 83–92. [CrossRef]
29. Nakamura, K.; Hirayama-Kurogi, M.; Ito, S.; Kuno, T.; Yoneyama, T.; Obuchi, W.; Terasaki, T.; Ohtsuki, S. Large-scale multiplex absolute protein quantification of drug-metabolizing enzymes and transporters in human intestine, liver, and kidney microsomes by SWATH-MS: Comparison with MRM/SRM and HR-MRM/PRM. *Proteomics* **2016**, *16*, 2106–2117. [CrossRef]

30. Miyauchi, E.; Tachikawa, M.; Declèves, X.; Uchida, Y.; Bouillot, J.-L.; Poitou, C.; Oppert, J.-M.; Mouly, S.; Bergmann, J.-F.; Terasaki, T.; et al. Quantitative Atlas of Cytochrome P450, UDP-Glucuronosyltransferase, and Transporter Proteins in Jejunum of Morbidly Obese Subjects. *Mol. Pharm.* **2016**, *13*, 2631–2640. [CrossRef]
31. Couto, N.; Al-Majdoub, Z.M.; Achour, B.; Wright, P.C.; Rostami-Hodjegan, A.; Barber, J. Quantification of Proteins Involved in Drug Metabolism and Disposition in the Human Liver Using Label-Free Global Proteomics. *Mol. Pharm.* **2019**, *16*, 632–647. [CrossRef] [PubMed]
32. Clermont, V.; Grangeon, A.; Barama, A.; Turgeon, J.; Lallier, M.; Malaise, J.; Michaud, V. Activity and mRNA expression levels of selected cytochromes P450 in various sections of the human small intestine. *Br. J. Clin. Pharmacol.* **2019**, *85*, 1367–1377. [CrossRef]
33. Fontana, R.J.; Lown, K.S.; Paine, M.F.; Fortlage, L.; Santella, R.M.; Felton, J.S.; Knize, M.G.; Greenberg, A.; Watkins, P.B. Effects of a chargrilled meat diet on expression of CYP3A, CYP1A, and P-glycoprotein levels in healthy volunteers. *Gastroenterology* **1999**, *117*, 89–98. [CrossRef]
34. Achour, B.; Barber, J.; Rostami-Hodjegan, A. Expression of hepatic drug-metabolizing cytochrome p450 enzymes and their intercorrelations: A meta-analysis. *Drug Metab. Dispos.* **2014**, *42*, 1349–1356. [CrossRef] [PubMed]
35. Vildhede, A.; Wiśniewski, J.R.; Norén, A.; Karlgren, M.; Artursson, P. Comparative Proteomic Analysis of Human Liver Tissue and Isolated Hepatocytes with a Focus on Proteins Determining Drug Exposure. *J. Proteome Res.* **2015**, *14*, 3305–3314. [CrossRef]
36. Achour, B.; Al Feteisi, H.; Lanucara, F.; Rostami-Hodjegan, A.; Barber, J. Global Proteomic Analysis of Human Liver Microsomes: Rapid Characterization and Quantification of Hepatic Drug-Metabolizing Enzymes. *Drug Metab. Dispos.* **2017**, *45*, 666–675. [CrossRef]
37. Achour, B.; Russell, M.R.; Barber, J.; Rostami-Hodjegan, A. Simultaneous quantification of the abundance of several cytochrome P450 and uridine 5′-diphospho-glucuronosyltransferase enzymes in human liver microsomes using multiplexed targeted proteomics. *Drug Metab. Dispos.* **2014**, *42*, 500–510. [CrossRef]
38. Kawakami, H.; Ohtsuki, S.; Kamiie, J.; Suzuki, T.; Abe, T.; Terasaki, T. Simultaneous absolute quantification of 11 cytochrome P450 isoforms in human liver microsomes by liquid chromatography tandem mass spectrometry with in silico target peptide selection. *J. Pharm. Sci.* **2011**, *100*, 341–352. [CrossRef]
39. Shimada, T.; Yamazaki, H.; Mimura, M.; Inui, Y.; Guengerich, F.P. Interindividual variations in human liver cytochrome P-450 enzymes involved in the oxidation of drugs, carcinogens and toxic chemicals: Studies with liver microsomes of 30 Japanese and 30 Caucasians. *J. Pharmacol. Exp. Ther.* **1994**, *270*, 414–423.
40. Klein, K.; Winter, S.; Turpeinen, M.; Schwab, M.; Zanger, U.M. Pathway-Targeted Pharmacogenomics of CYP1A2 in Human Liver. *Front. Pharmacol.* **2010**, *1*, 129. [CrossRef]
41. Jiang, Z.; Dragin, N.; Jorge-Nebert, L.F.; Martin, M.V.; Guengerich, F.P.; Aklillu, E.; Ingelman-Sundberg, M.; Hammons, G.J.; Lyn-Cook, B.D.; Kadlubar, F.F.; et al. Search for an association between the human CYP1A2 genotype and CYP1A2 metabolic phenotype. *Pharmacogenet. Genom.* **2006**, *16*, 359–367. [CrossRef]
42. Ueda, R.; Iketaki, H.; Nagata, K.; Kimura, S.; Gonzalez, F.J.; Kusano, K.; Yoshimura, T.; Yamazoe, Y. A common regulatory region functions bidirectionally in transcriptional activation of the human CYP1A1 and CYP1A2 genes. *Mol. Pharmacol.* **2006**, *69*, 1924–1930. [CrossRef]
43. Jorge-Nebert, L.F.; Jiang, Z.; Chakraborty, R.; Watson, J.; Jin, L.; McGarvey, S.T.; Deka, R.; Nebert, D.W. Analysis of human CYP1A1 and CYP1A2 genes and their shared bidirectional promoter in eight world populations. *Hum. Mutat.* **2010**, *31*, 27–40. [CrossRef] [PubMed]
44. Nebert, D.W.; Dalton, T.P.; Okey, A.B.; Gonzalez, F.J. Role of aryl hydrocarbon receptor-mediated induction of the CYP1 enzymes in environmental toxicity and cancer. *J. Biol. Chem.* **2004**, *279*, 23847–23850. [CrossRef] [PubMed]
45. Edwards, R.J.; Price, R.J.; Watts, P.S.; Renwick, A.B.; Tredger, J.M.; Boobis, A.R.; Lake, B.G. Induction of cytochrome P450 enzymes in cultured precision-cut human liver slices. *Drug Metab. Dispos.* **2003**, *31*, 282–288. [CrossRef] [PubMed]
46. Madan, A.; Graham, R.A.; Carroll, K.M.; Mudra, D.R.; Burton, L.A.; Krueger, L.A.; Downey, A.D.; Czerwinski, M.; Forster, J.; Ribadeneira, M.D.; et al. Effects of prototypical microsomal enzyme inducers on cytochrome P450 expression in cultured human hepatocytes. *Drug Metab. Dispos.* **2003**, *31*, 421–431. [CrossRef] [PubMed]

47. Moscovitz, J.E.; Kalgutkar, A.S.; Nulick, K.; Johnson, N.; Lin, Z.; Goosen, T.C.; Weng, Y. Establishing Transcriptional Signatures to Differentiate PXR-, CAR-, and AhR-Mediated Regulation of Drug Metabolism and Transport Genes in Cryopreserved Human Hepatocytes. *J. Pharmacol. Exp. Ther.* **2018**, *365*, 262–271. [CrossRef]
48. Roymans, D.; van Looveren, C.; Leone, A.; Parker, J.B.; McMillian, M.; Johnson, M.D.; Koganti, A.; Gilissen, R.; Silber, P.; Mannens, G.; et al. Determination of cytochrome P450 1A2 and cytochrome P450 3A4 induction in cryopreserved human hepatocytes. *Biochem. Pharmacol.* **2004**, *67*, 427–437. [CrossRef]
49. Yoshinari, K.; Ueda, R.; Kusano, K.; Yoshimura, T.; Nagata, K.; Yamazoe, Y. Omeprazole transactivates human CYP1A1 and CYP1A2 expression through the common regulatory region containing multiple xenobiotic-responsive elements. *Biochem. Pharmacol.* **2008**, *76*, 139–145. [CrossRef]
50. Bapiro, T.E.; Andersson, T.B.; Otter, C.; Hasler, J.A.; Masimirembwa, C.M. Cytochrome P450 1A1/2 induction by antiparasitic drugs: Dose-dependent increase in ethoxyresorufin O-deethylase activity and mRNA caused by quinine, primaquine and albendazole in HepG2 cells. *Eur. J. Clin. Pharmacol.* **2002**, *58*, 537–542. [CrossRef]
51. Dolwick, K.M.; Swanson, H.I.; Bradfield, C.A. In vitro analysis of Ah receptor domains involved in ligand-activated DNA recognition. *Proc. Natl. Acad. Sci. USA* **1993**, *90*, 8566–8570. [CrossRef] [PubMed]
52. Sugiyama, I.; Murayama, N.; Kuroki, A.; Kota, J.; Iwano, S.; Yamazaki, H.; Hirota, T. Evaluation of cytochrome P450 inductions by anti-epileptic drug oxcarbazepine, 10-hydroxyoxcarbazepine, and carbamazepine using human hepatocytes and HepaRG cells. *Xenobiotica* **2016**, *46*, 765–774. [CrossRef]
53. Ghotbi, R.; Christensen, M.; Roh, H.-K.; Ingelman-Sundberg, M.; Aklillu, E.; Bertilsson, L. Comparisons of CYP1A2 genetic polymorphisms, enzyme activity and the genotype-phenotype relationship in Swedes and Koreans. *Eur. J. Clin. Pharmacol.* **2007**, *63*, 537–546. [CrossRef] [PubMed]
54. Dobrinas, M.; Cornuz, J.; Oneda, B.; Kohler Serra, M.; Puhl, M.; Eap, C.B. Impact of smoking, smoking cessation, and genetic polymorphisms on CYP1A2 activity and inducibility. *Clin. Pharmacol. Ther.* **2011**, *90*, 117–125. [CrossRef] [PubMed]
55. Yoshinari, K.; Yoda, N.; Toriyabe, T.; Yamazoe, Y. Constitutive androstane receptor transcriptionally activates human CYP1A1 and CYP1A2 genes through a common regulatory element in the 5′-flanking region. *Biochem. Pharmacol.* **2010**, *79*, 261–269. [CrossRef] [PubMed]
56. Feidt, D.M.; Klein, K.; Hofmann, U.; Riedmaier, S.; Knobeloch, D.; Thasler, W.E.; Weiss, T.S.; Schwab, M.; Zanger, U.M. Profiling induction of cytochrome p450 enzyme activity by statins using a new liquid chromatography-tandem mass spectrometry cocktail assay in human hepatocytes. *Drug Metab. Dispos.* **2010**, *38*, 1589–1597. [CrossRef] [PubMed]
57. Rae, J.M.; Johnson, M.D.; Lippman, M.E.; Flockhart, D.A. Rifampin is a selective, pleiotropic inducer of drug metabolism genes in human hepatocytes: Studies with cDNA and oligonucleotide expression arrays. *J. Pharmacol. Exp. Ther.* **2001**, *299*, 849–857. [PubMed]
58. Backman, J.T.; Granfors, M.T.; Neuvonen, P.J. Rifampicin is only a weak inducer of CYP1A2-mediated presystemic and systemic metabolism: Studies with tizanidine and caffeine. *Eur. J. Clin. Pharmacol.* **2006**, *62*, 451–461. [CrossRef] [PubMed]
59. Parkinson, A.; Mudra, D.R.; Johnson, C.; Dwyer, A.; Carroll, K.M. The effects of gender, age, ethnicity, and liver cirrhosis on cytochrome P450 enzyme activity in human liver microsomes and inducibility in cultured human hepatocytes. *Toxicol. Appl. Pharmacol.* **2004**, *199*, 193–209. [CrossRef] [PubMed]
60. Relling, M.V.; Lin, J.S.; Ayers, G.D.; Evans, W.E. Racial and gender differences in N-acetyltransferase, xanthine oxidase, and CYP1A2 activities. *Clin. Pharmacol. Ther.* **1992**, *52*, 643–658. [CrossRef]
61. Ou-Yang, D.S.; Huang, S.L.; Wang, W.; Xie, H.G.; Xu, Z.H.; Shu, Y.; Zhou, H.H. Phenotypic polymorphism and gender-related differences of CYP1A2 activity in a Chinese population. *Br. J. Clin. Pharmacol.* **2000**, *49*, 145–151. [CrossRef] [PubMed]
62. Backman, J.T.; Schröder, M.T.; Neuvonen, P.J. Effects of gender and moderate smoking on the pharmacokinetics and effects of the CYP1A2 substrate tizanidine. *Eur. J. Clin. Pharmacol.* **2008**, *64*, 17–24. [CrossRef] [PubMed]
63. Orlando, R.; Padrini, R.; Perazzi, M.; de Martin, S.; Piccoli, P.; Palatini, P. Liver dysfunction markedly decreases the inhibition of cytochrome P450 1A2-mediated theophylline metabolism by fluvoxamine. *Clin. Pharmacol. Ther.* **2006**, *79*, 489–499. [CrossRef] [PubMed]
64. Zhang, Y.; Klein, K.; Sugathan, A.; Nassery, N.; Dombkowski, A.; Zanger, U.M.; Waxman, D.J. Transcriptional profiling of human liver identifies sex-biased genes associated with polygenic dyslipidemia and coronary artery disease. *PLoS ONE* **2011**, *6*, e23506. [CrossRef] [PubMed]

65. Chen, H.; Shen, Z.-Y.; Xu, W.; Fan, T.-Y.; Li, J.; Lu, Y.-F.; Cheng, M.-L.; Liu, J. Expression of P450 and nuclear receptors in normal and end-stage Chinese livers. *World J. Gastroenterol.* **2014**, *20*, 8681–8690. [CrossRef] [PubMed]
66. Nakai, K.; Tanaka, H.; Hanada, K.; Ogata, H.; Suzuki, F.; Kumada, H.; Miyajima, A.; Ishida, S.; Sunouchi, M.; Habano, W.; et al. Decreased expression of cytochromes P450 1A2, 2E1, and 3A4 and drug transporters Na+-taurocholate-cotransporting polypeptide, organic cation transporter 1, and organic anion-transporting peptide-C correlates with the progression of liver fibrosis in chronic hepatitis C patients. *Drug Metab. Dispos.* **2008**, *36*, 1786–1793. [CrossRef] [PubMed]
67. Hanada, K.; Nakai, K.; Tanaka, H.; Suzuki, F.; Kumada, H.; Ohno, Y.; Ozawa, S.; Ogata, H. Effect of nuclear receptor downregulation on hepatic expression of cytochrome P450 and transporters in chronic hepatitis C in association with fibrosis development. *Drug Metab. Pharmacokinet.* **2012**, *27*, 301–306. [CrossRef]
68. Prasad, B.; Bhatt, D.K.; Johnson, K.; Chapa, R.; Chu, X.; Salphati, L.; Xiao, G.; Lee, C.; Hop, C.E.C.A.; Mathias, A.; et al. Abundance of Phase 1 and 2 Drug-Metabolizing Enzymes in Alcoholic and Hepatitis C Cirrhotic Livers: A Quantitative Targeted Proteomics Study. *Drug Metab. Dispos.* **2018**, *46*, 943–952. [CrossRef]
69. Fisher, C.D.; Lickteig, A.J.; Augustine, L.M.; Ranger-Moore, J.; Jackson, J.P.; Ferguson, S.S.; Cherrington, N.J. Hepatic cytochrome P450 enzyme alterations in humans with progressive stages of nonalcoholic fatty liver disease. *Drug Metab. Dispos.* **2009**, *37*, 2087–2094. [CrossRef]
70. Parker, A.C.; Pritchard, P.; Preston, T.; Choonara, I. Induction of CYP1A2 activity by carbamazepine in children using the caffeine breath test. *Br. J. Clin. Pharmacol.* **1998**, *45*, 176–178. [CrossRef]
71. Buchthal, J.; Grund, K.E.; Buchmann, A.; Schrenk, D.; Beaune, P.; Bock, K.W. Induction of cytochrome P4501A by smoking or omeprazole in comparison with UDP-glucuronosyltransferase in biopsies of human duodenal mucosa. *Eur. J. Clin. Pharmacol.* **1995**, *47*, 431–435. [CrossRef]
72. Diaz, D.; Fabrev, I.; Daujat, M.; Aubert, B.S.; Bories, P.; Michel, H.; Maurel, P. Omeprazole is an aryl hydrocarbon-like inducer of human hepatic cytochrome P450. *Gastroenterology* **1990**, *99*, 737–747. [CrossRef]
73. Halladay, J.S.; Wong, S.; Khojasteh, S.C.; Grepper, S. An 'all-inclusive' 96-well cytochrome P450 induction method: Measuring enzyme activity, mRNA levels, protein levels, and cytotoxicity from one well using cryopreserved human hepatocytes. *J. Pharmacol. Toxicol. Methods* **2012**, *66*, 270–275. [CrossRef] [PubMed]
74. Dixit, V.; Hariparsad, N.; Li, F.; Desai, P.; Thummel, K.E.; Unadkat, J.D. Cytochrome P450 enzymes and transporters induced by anti-human immunodeficiency virus protease inhibitors in human hepatocytes: Implications for predicting clinical drug interactions. *Drug Metab. Dispos.* **2007**, *35*, 1853–1859. [CrossRef] [PubMed]
75. Pelkonen, O.; Pasanen, M.; Kuha, H.; Gachalyi, B.; Kairaluoma, M.; Sotaniemi, E.A.; Park, S.S.; Friedman, F.K.; Gelboin, H.V. The effect of cigarette smoking on 7-ethoxyresorufin O-deethylase and other monooxygenase activities in human liver: Analyses with monoclonal antibodies. *Br. J. Clin. Pharmacol.* **1986**, *22*, 125–134. [CrossRef] [PubMed]
76. Gunes, A.; Dahl, M.-L. Variation in CYP1A2 activity and its clinical implications: Influence of environmental factors and genetic polymorphisms. *Pharmacogenomics* **2008**, *9*, 625–637. [CrossRef] [PubMed]
77. Ingelman-Sundberg, M.; Sim, S.C.; Gomez, A.; Rodriguez-Antona, C. Influence of cytochrome P450 polymorphisms on drug therapies: Pharmacogenetic, pharmacoepigenetic and clinical aspects. *Pharmacol. Ther.* **2007**, *116*, 496–526. [CrossRef] [PubMed]
78. Rasmussen, B.B.; Brix, T.H.; Kyvik, K.O.; Brøsen, K. The interindividual differences in the 3-demthylation of caffeine alias CYP1A2 is determined by both genetic and environmental factors. *Pharmacogenetics* **2002**, *12*, 473–478. [CrossRef]
79. Zanger, U.M.; Klein, K.; Thomas, M.; Rieger, J.K.; Tremmel, R.; Kandel, B.A.; Klein, M.; Magdy, T. Genetics, epigenetics, and regulation of drug-metabolizing cytochrome p450 enzymes. *Clin. Pharmacol. Ther.* **2014**, *95*, 258–261. [CrossRef]
80. Kisselev, P.; Schunck, W.-H.; Roots, I.; Schwarz, D. Association of CYP1A1 polymorphisms with differential metabolic activation of 17beta-estradiol and estrone. *Cancer Res.* **2005**, *65*, 2972–2978. [CrossRef]
81. Zhou, H.; Josephy, P.D.; Kim, D.; Guengerich, F.P. Functional characterization of four allelic variants of human cytochrome P450 1A2. *Arch. Biochem. Biophys.* **2004**, *422*, 23–30. [CrossRef] [PubMed]

82. Palma, B.B.; Silva E Sousa, M.; Vosmeer, C.R.; Lastdrager, J.; Rueff, J.; Vermeulen, N.P.E.; Kranendonk, M. Functional characterization of eight human cytochrome P450 1A2 gene variants by recombinant protein expression. *Pharm. J.* **2010**, *10*, 478–488. [CrossRef] [PubMed]
83. Nakajima, M.; Yokoi, T.; Mizutani, M.; Kinoshita, M.; Funayama, M.; Kamataki, T. Genetic polymorphism in the 5′-flanking region of human CYP1A2 gene: Effect on the CYP1A2 inducibility in humans. *J. Biochem.* **1999**, *125*, 803–808. [CrossRef] [PubMed]
84. Sachse, C.; Brockmöller, J.; Bauer, S.; Roots, I. Functional significance of a C–A polymorphism in intron 1 of the cytochrome P450 CYP1A2 gene tested with caffeine. *Br. J. Clin. Pharmacol.* **1999**, *47*, 445–449. [CrossRef] [PubMed]
85. Djordjevic, N.; Ghotbi, R.; Jankovic, S.; Aklillu, E. Induction of CYP1A2 by heavy coffee consumption is associated with the CYP1A2 -163CA polymorphism. *Eur. J. Clin. Pharmacol.* **2010**, *66*, 697–703. [CrossRef]
86. Han, X.-M.; Ouyang, D.-S.; Chen, X.-P.; Shu, Y.; Jiang, C.-H.; Tan, Z.-R.; Zhou, H.-H. Inducibility of CYP1A2 by omeprazole in vivo related to the genetic polymorphism of CYP1A2. *Br. J. Clin. Pharmacol.* **2002**, *54*, 540–543. [CrossRef]
87. Sergentanis, T.N.; Economopoulos, K.P. Four polymorphisms in cytochrome P450 1A1 (CYP1A1) gene and breast cancer risk: A meta-analysis. *Breast Cancer Res. Treat.* **2010**, *122*, 459–469. [CrossRef]
88. Yao, L.; Yu, X.; Yu, L. Lack of significant association between CYP1A1 T3801C polymorphism and breast cancer risk: A meta-analysis involving 25,087 subjects. *Breast Cancer Res. Treat.* **2010**, *122*, 503–507. [CrossRef]
89. Cui, X.; Lu, X.; Hiura, M.; Omori, H.; Miyazaki, W.; Katoh, T. Association of genotypes of carcinogen-metabolizing enzymes and smoking status with bladder cancer in a Japanese population. *Environ. Health Prev. Med.* **2013**, *18*, 136–142. [CrossRef]
90. Wang, H.; Zhang, Z.; Han, S.; Lu, Y.; Feng, F.; Yuan, J. CYP1A2 rs762551 polymorphism contributes to cancer susceptibility: A meta-analysis from 19 case-control studies. *BMC Cancer* **2012**, *12*, 528. [CrossRef]
91. Chen, Y.; Zeng, L.; Wang, Y.; Tolleson, W.H.; Knox, B.; Chen, S.; Ren, Z.; Guo, L.; Mei, N.; Qian, F.; et al. The expression, induction and pharmacological activity of CYP1A2 are post-transcriptionally regulated by microRNA hsa-miR-132-5p. *Biochem. Pharmacol.* **2017**, *145*, 178–191. [CrossRef] [PubMed]
92. Gill, P.; Bhattacharyya, S.; McCullough, S.; Letzig, L.; Mishra, P.J.; Luo, C.; Dweep, H.; James, L. MicroRNA regulation of CYP 1A2, CYP3A4 and CYP2E1 expression in acetaminophen toxicity. *Sci. Rep.* **2017**, *7*, 12331. [CrossRef] [PubMed]
93. Sansen, S.; Yano, J.K.; Reynald, R.L.; Schoch, G.A.; Griffin, K.J.; Stout, C.D.; Johnson, E.F. Adaptations for the oxidation of polycyclic aromatic hydrocarbons exhibited by the structure of human P450 1A2. *J. Biol. Chem.* **2007**, *282*, 14348–14355. [CrossRef] [PubMed]
94. Tassaneeyakul, W.; Birkett, D.J.; Veronese, M.E.; McManus, M.E.; Tukey, R.H.; Quattrochi, L.C.; Gelboin, H.V.; Miners, J.O. Specificity of substrate and inhibitor probes for human cytochromes P450 1A1 and 1A2. *J. Pharmacol. Exp. Ther.* **1993**, *265*, 401–407. [PubMed]
95. Tassaneeyakul, W.; Mohamed, Z.; Birkett, D.J.; McManus, M.E.; Veronese, M.E.; Tukey, R.H.; Quattrochi, L.C.; Gonzalez, F.J.; Miners, J.O. Caffeine as a probe for human cytochromes P450: Validation using cDNA-expression, immunoinhibition and microsomal kinetic and inhibitor techniques. *Pharmacogenetics* **1992**, *2*, 173–183. [CrossRef] [PubMed]
96. Ma, Q.; Lu, A.Y.H. CYP1A induction and human risk assessment: An evolving tale of in vitro and in vivo studies. *Drug Metab. Dispos.* **2007**, *35*, 1009–1016. [CrossRef]
97. Androutsopoulos, V.P.; Tsatsakis, A.M.; Spandidos, D.A. Cytochrome P450 CYP1A1: Wider roles in cancer progression and prevention. *BMC Cancer* **2009**, *9*, 187. [CrossRef]
98. Nakamura, H.; Ariyoshi, N.; Okada, K.; Nakasa, H.; Nakazawa, K.; Kitada, M. CYP1A1 is a major enzyme responsible for the metabolism of granisetron in human liver microsomes. *Curr. Drug Metab.* **2005**, *6*, 469–480. [CrossRef]
99. Mescher, M.; Tigges, J.; Rolfes, K.M.; Shen, A.L.; Yee, J.S.; Vogeley, C.; Krutmann, J.; Bradfield, C.A.; Lang, D.; Haarmann-Stemmann, T. The Toll-like receptor agonist imiquimod is metabolized by aryl hydrocarbon receptor-regulated cytochrome P450 enzymes in human keratinocytes and mouse liver. *Arch. Toxicol.* **2019**, *93*, 1917–1926. [CrossRef]
100. Liu, L.; Wang, Q.; Xie, C.; Xi, N.; Guo, Z.; Li, M.; Hou, X.; Xie, N.; Sun, M.; Li, J.; et al. Drug interaction of ningetinib and gefitinib involving CYP1A1 and efflux transporters in non-small cell lung cancer patients. *Br. J. Clin. Pharmacol.* **2020**. [CrossRef]

101. Niwa, T.; Sato, R.; Yabusaki, Y.; Ishibashi, F.; Katagiri, M. Contribution of human hepatic cytochrome P450s and steroidogenic CYP17 to the N-demethylation of aminopyrine. *Xenobiotica* **1999**, *29*, 187–193 [CrossRef] [PubMed]
102. Norman, T.R.; Olver, J.S. Agomelatine for depression: Expanding the horizons? *Expert Opin. Pharmacother.* **2019**, *20*, 647–656. [CrossRef] [PubMed]
103. Bertilsson, L.; Carrillo, J.A.; Dahl, M.L.; Llerena, A.; Alm, C.; Bondesson, U.; Lindström, L.; La Rodriguez de Rubia, I.; Ramos, S.; BENITEZ, J. Clozapine disposition covaries with CYP1A2 activity determined by a caffeine test. *Br. J. Clin. Pharmacol.* **1994**, *38*, 471–473. [CrossRef] [PubMed]
104. Long, L.; Dolan, M.E. Role of cytochrome P450 isoenzymes in metabolism of O(6)-benzylguanine: Implications for dacarbazine activation. *Clin. Cancer Res.* **2001**, *7*, 4239–4244.
105. Lobo, E.D.; Bergstrom, R.F.; Reddy, S.; Quinlan, T.; Chappell, J.; Hong, Q.; Ring, B.; Knadler, M.P. In vitro and in vivo evaluations of cytochrome P450 1A2 interactions with duloxetine. *Clin. Pharmacokinet.* **2008**, *47*, 191–202. [CrossRef] [PubMed]
106. Shet, M.S.; McPhaul, M.; Fisher, C.W.; Stallings, N.R.; Estabrook, R.W. Metabolism of the antiandrogenic drug (Flutamide) by human CYP1A2. *Drug Metab. Dispos.* **1997**, *25*, 1298–1303.
107. Kalgutkar, A.S.; Nguyen, H.T.; Vaz, A.D.N.; Doan, A.; Dalvie, D.K.; McLeod, D.G.; Murray, J.C. In vitro metabolism studies on the isoxazole ring scission in the anti-inflammatory agent lefluonomide to its active alpha-cyanoenol metabolite A771726: Mechanistic similarities with the cytochrome P450-catalyzed dehydration of aldoximes. *Drug Metab. Dispos.* **2003**, *31*, 1240–1250. [CrossRef]
108. Härtter, S.; Grözinger, M.; Weigmann, H.; Röschke, J.; Hiemke, C. Increased bioavailability of oral melatonin after fluvoxamine coadministration. *Clin. Pharmacol. Ther.* **2000**, *67*, 1–6. [CrossRef]
109. Anttila, A.K.; Rasanen, L.; Leinonen, E.V. Fluvoxamine augmentation increases serum mirtazapine concentrations three- to fourfold. *Ann. Pharmacother.* **2001**, *35*, 1221–1223. [CrossRef]
110. Turpeinen, M.; Hofmann, U.; Klein, K.; Mürdter, T.; Schwab, M.; Zanger, U.M. A predominate role of CYP1A2 for the metabolism of nabumetone to the active metabolite, 6-methoxy-2-naphthylacetic acid, in human liver microsomes. *Drug Metab. Dispos.* **2009**, *37*, 1017–1024. [CrossRef]
111. Ring, B.J.; Catlow, J.; Lindsay, T.J.; Gillespie, T.; Roskos, L.K.; Cerimele, B.J.; Swanson, S.P.; Hamman, M.A.; Wrighton, S.A. Identification of the human cytochromes P450 responsible for the in vitro formation of the major oxidative metabolites of the antipsychotic agent olanzapine. *J. Pharmacol. Exp. Ther.* **1996**, *276*, 658–666. [PubMed]
112. Wójcikowski, J.; Pichard-Garcia, L.; Maurel, P.; Daniel, W.A. Contribution of human cytochrome p-450 isoforms to the metabolism of the simplest phenothiazine neuroleptic promazine. *Br. J. Pharmacol.* **2003**, *138*, 1465–1474. [CrossRef]
113. Masubuchi, Y.; Hosokawa, S.; Horie, T.; Suzuki, T.; Ohmori, S.; Kitada, M.; Narimatsu, S. Cytochrome P450 isozymes involved in propranolol metabolism in human liver microsomes. The role of CYP2D6 as ring-hydroxylase and CYP1A2 as N-desisopropylase. *Drug Metab. Dispos.* **1994**, *22*, 909–915. [PubMed]
114. Obach, R.S.; Ryder, T.F. Metabolism of ramelteon in human liver microsomes and correlation with the effect of fluvoxamine on ramelteon pharmacokinetics. *Drug Metab. Dispos.* **2010**, *38*, 1381–1391. [CrossRef] [PubMed]
115. Guay, D.R.P. Rasagiline (TVP-1012): A new selective monoamine oxidase inhibitor for Parkinson's disease. *Am. J. Geriatr. Pharmacother.* **2006**, *4*, 330–346. [CrossRef] [PubMed]
116. Sanderink, G.J.; Bournique, B.; Stevens, J.; Petry, M.; Martinet, M. Involvement of human CYP1A isoenzymes in the metabolism and drug interactions of riluzole in vitro. *J. Pharmacol. Exp. Ther.* **1997**, *282*, 1465–1472.
117. Kaye, C.M.; Nicholls, B. Clinical pharmacokinetics of ropinirole. *Clin. Pharmacokinet.* **2000**, *39*, 243–254. [CrossRef]
118. Oda, Y.; Furuichi, K.; Tanaka, K.; Hiroi, T.; Imaoka, S.; Asada, A.; Fujimori, M.; Funae, Y. Metabolism of a new local anesthetic, ropivacaine, by human hepatic cytochrome P450. *Anesthesiology* **1995**, *82*, 214–220. [CrossRef] [PubMed]
119. Spaldin, V.; Madden, S.; Pool, W.F.; Woolf, T.F.; Park, B.K. The effect of enzyme inhibition on the metabolism and activation of tacrine by human liver microsomes. *Br. J. Clin. Pharmacol.* **1994**, *38*, 15–22. [CrossRef] [PubMed]
120. Ha, H.R.; Chen, J.; Freiburghaus, A.U.; Follath, F. Metabolism of theophylline by cDNA-expressed human cytochromes P-450. *Br. J. Clin. Pharmacol.* **1995**, *39*, 321–326. [CrossRef] [PubMed]
121. Granfors, M.T.; Backman, J.T.; Neuvonen, M.; Neuvonen, P.J. Ciprofloxacin greatly increases concentrations and hypotensive effect of tizanidine by inhibiting its cytochrome P450 1A2-mediated presystemic metabolism. *Clin. Pharmacol. Ther.* **2004**, *76*, 598–606. [CrossRef] [PubMed]

122. Granfors, M.T.; Backman, J.T.; Neuvonen, M.; Ahonen, J.; Neuvonen, P.J. Fluvoxamine drastically increases concentrations and effects of tizanidine: A potentially hazardous interaction. *Clin. Pharmacol. Ther.* **2004**, *75*, 331–341. [CrossRef] [PubMed]
123. Kroemer, H.K.; Gautier, J.C.; Beaune, P.; Henderson, C.; Wolf, C.R.; Eichelbaum, M. Identification of P450 enzymes involved in metabolism of verapamil in humans. *Naunyn Schmiedebergs Arch. Pharmacol.* **1993**, *348*, 332–337. [CrossRef] [PubMed]
124. Wild, M.J.; McKillop, D.; Butters, C.J. Determination of the human cytochrome P450 isoforms involved in the metabolism of zolmitriptan. *Xenobiotica* **1999**, *29*, 847–857. [CrossRef]
125. Fuhr, U.; Jetter, A.; Kirchheiner, J. Appropriate phenotyping procedures for drug metabolizing enzymes and transporters in humans and their simultaneous use in the "cocktail" approach. *Clin. Pharmacol. Ther.* **2007**, *81*, 270–283. [CrossRef]
126. Nebert, D.W.; Dalton, T.P. The role of cytochrome P450 enzymes in endogenous signalling pathways and environmental carcinogenesis. *Nat. Reviews Cancer* **2006**, *6*, 947–960. [CrossRef]
127. Karjalainen, M.J.; Neuvonen, P.J.; Backman, J.T. In vitro inhibition of CYP1A2 by model inhibitors, anti-inflammatory analgesics and female sex steroids: Predictability of in vivo interactions. *Basic Clin. Pharmacol. Toxicol.* **2008**, *103*, 157–165. [CrossRef]
128. Pastrakuljic, A.; Tang, B.K.; Roberts, E.A.; Kalow, W. Distinction of CYP1A1 and CYP1A2 activity by selective inhibition using fluvoxamine and isosafrole. *Biochem. Pharmacol.* **1997**, *53*, 531–538. [CrossRef]
129. Somers, G.I.; Harris, A.J.; Bayliss, M.K.; Houston, J.B. The metabolism of the 5HT3 antagonists ondansetron, alosetron and GR87442 I: A comparison of in vitro and in vivo metabolism and in vitro enzyme kinetics in rat, dog and human hepatocytes, microsomes and recombinant human enzymes. *Xenobiotica* **2007**, *37*, 832–854. [CrossRef]
130. Kobayashi, K.; Nakajima, M.; Chiba, K.; Yamamoto, T.; Tani, M.; Ishizaki, T.; Kuroiwa, Y. Inhibitory effects of antiarrhythmic drugs on phenacetin O-deethylation catalysed by human CYP1A2. *Br. J. Clin. Pharmacol.* **1998**, *45*, 361–368. [CrossRef]
131. Bapiro, T.E.; Sayi, J.; Hasler, J.A.; Jande, M.; Rimoy, G.; Masselle, A.; Masimirembwa, C.M. Artemisinin and thiabendazole are potent inhibitors of cytochrome P450 1A2 (CYP1A2) activity in humans. *Eur. J. Clin. Pharmacol.* **2005**, *61*, 755–761. [CrossRef] [PubMed]
132. Masubuchi, Y.; Nakano, T.; Ose, A.; Horie, T. Differential selectivity in carbamazepine-induced inactivation of cytochrome P450 enzymes in rat and human liver. *Arch. Toxicol.* **2001**, *75*, 538–543. [CrossRef] [PubMed]
133. Fuhr, U.; Anders, E.M.; Mahr, G.; Sörgel, F.; Staib, A.H. Inhibitory potency of quinolone antibacterial agents against cytochrome P450IA2 activity in vivo and in vitro. *Antimicrob. Agents Chemother.* **1992**, *36*, 942–948. [CrossRef] [PubMed]
134. Martinez, C.; Albet, C.; Agundez, J.; Herrero, E.; Carrillo, J.; Marquez, M.; Benitez, J.; Ortiz, J. Comparative in vitro and in vivo inhibition of cytochrome P450 CYP1A2, CYP2D6, and CYP3A by H -receptor antagonists. *Clin. Pharmacol. Ther.* **1999**, *65*, 369–376. [CrossRef]
135. Zhang, W.; Ramamoorthy, Y.; Kilicarslan, T.; Nolte, H.; Tyndale, R.F.; Sellers, E.M. Inhibition of cytochromes P450 by antifungal imidazole derivatives. *Drug Metab. Dispos.* **2002**, *30*, 314–318. [CrossRef] [PubMed]
136. Paris, B.L.; Ogilvie, B.W.; Scheinkoenig, J.A.; Ndikum-Moffor, F.; Gibson, R.; Parkinson, A. In vitro inhibition and induction of human liver cytochrome p450 enzymes by milnacipran. *Drug Metab. Dispos.* **2009**, *37*, 2045–2054. [CrossRef] [PubMed]
137. von Moltke, L.L.; Greenblatt, D.J.; Schmider, J.; Duan, S.X.; Wright, C.E.; Harmatz, J.S.; Shader, R.I. Midazolam hydroxylation by human liver microsomes in vitro: Inhibition by fluoxetine, norfluoxetine, and by azole antifungal agents. *J. Clin. Pharmacol.* **1996**, *36*, 783–791. [CrossRef]
138. Wen, X.; Wang, J.-S.; Neuvonen, P.J.; Backman, J.T. Isoniazid is a mechanism-based inhibitor of cytochrome P450 1A2, 2A6, 2C19 and 3A4 isoforms in human liver microsomes. *Eur. J. Clin. Pharmacol.* **2002**, *57*, 799–804. [CrossRef]
139. Sai, Y.; Dai, R.; Yang, T.J.; Krausz, K.W.; Gonzalez, F.J.; Gelboin, H.V.; Shou, M. Assessment of specificity of eight chemical inhibitors using cDNA-expressed cytochromes P450. *Xenobiotica* **2000**, *30*, 327–343. [CrossRef]
140. Chun, Y.J.; Kim, M.Y.; Guengerich, F.P. Resveratrol is a selective human cytochrome P450 1A1 inhibitor. *Biochem. Biophys. Res. Commun.* **1999**, *262*, 20–24. [CrossRef]

141. Chang, T.K.; Chen, J.; Lee, W.B. Differential inhibition and inactivation of human CYP1 enzymes by trans-resveratrol: Evidence for mechanism-based inactivation of CYP1A2. *J. Pharmacol. Exp. Ther.* **2001**, *299*, 874–882. [PubMed]
142. Augustin, M.; Schoretsanitis, G.; Pfeifer, P.; Gründer, G.; Liebe, C.; Paulzen, M. Effect of fluvoxamine augmentation and smoking on clozapine serum concentrations. *Schizophr. Res.* **2019**, *210*, 143–148. [CrossRef] [PubMed]
143. Chiu, C.-C.; Lane, H.-Y.; Huang, M.-C.; Liu, H.-C.; Jann, M.W.; Hon, Y.-Y.; Chang, W.-H.; Lu, M.-L. Dose-dependent alternations in the pharmacokinetics of olanzapine during coadministration of fluvoxamine in patients with schizophrenia. *J. Clin. Pharmacol.* **2004**, *44*, 1385–1390. [CrossRef] [PubMed]
144. Yao, C.; Kunze, K.L.; Kharasch, E.D.; Wang, Y.; Trager, W.F.; Ragueneau, I.; Levy, R.H. Fluvoxamine-theophylline interaction: Gap between in vitro and in vivo inhibition constants toward cytochrome P4501A2. *Clin. Pharmacol. Ther.* **2001**, *70*, 415–424. [CrossRef]
145. Becquemont, L.; Ragueneau, I.; Le Bot, M.A.; Riche, C.; Funck-Brentano, C.; Jaillon, P. Influence of the CYP1A2 inhibitor fluvoxamine on tacrine pharmacokinetics in humans. *Clin. Pharmacol. Ther.* **1997**, *61*, 619–627. [CrossRef]
146. Backman, J.T.; Karjalainen, M.J.; Neuvonen, M.; Laitila, J.; Neuvonen, P.J. Rofecoxib is a potent inhibitor of cytochrome P450 1A2: Studies with tizanidine and caffeine in healthy subjects. *Br. J. Clin. Pharmacol.* **2006**, *62*, 345–357. [CrossRef]
147. Meyer, J.M.; Proctor, G.; Cummings, M.A.; Dardashti, L.J.; Stahl, S.M. Ciprofloxacin and Clozapine: A Potentially Fatal but Underappreciated Interaction. *Case Rep. Psychiatry* **2016**, *2016*, 5606098. [CrossRef]
148. Brouwers, E.E.M.; Söhne, M.; Kuipers, S.; van Gorp, E.C.M.; Schellens, J.H.M.; Koks, C.H.W.; Beijnen, J.H.; Huitema, A.D.R. Ciprofloxacin strongly inhibits clozapine metabolism: Two case reports. *Clin. Drug Investig.* **2009**, *29*, 59–63. [CrossRef]
149. Jerling, M.; Lindström, L.; Bondesson, U.; Bertilsson, L. Fluvoxamine inhibition and carbamazepine induction of the metabolism of clozapine: Evidence from a therapeutic drug monitoring service. *Ther. Drug Monit.* **1994**, *16*, 368–374. [CrossRef]
150. Wetzel, H.; Anghelescu, I.; Szegedi, A.; Wiesner, J.; Weigmann, H.; Härter, S.; Hiemke, C. Pharmacokinetic interactions of clozapine with selective serotonin reuptake inhibitors: Differential effects of fluvoxamine and paroxetine in a prospective study. *J. Clin. Psychopharmacol.* **1998**, *18*, 2–9. [CrossRef]
151. Raaska, K.; Neuvonen, P.J. Ciprofloxacin increases serum clozapine and N-desmethylclozapine: A study in patients with schizophrenia. *Eur. J. Clin. Pharmacol.* **2000**, *56*, 585–589. [CrossRef] [PubMed]
152. Perucca, E.; Gatti, G.; Spina, E. Clinical pharmacokinetics of fluvoxamine. *Clin. Pharmacokinet.* **1994**, *27*, 175–190. [CrossRef] [PubMed]
153. Jokinen, M.J.; Olkkola, K.T.; Ahonen, J.; Neuvonen, P.J. Effect of ciprofloxacin on the pharmacokinetics of ropivacaine. *Eur. J. Clin. Pharmacol.* **2003**, *58*, 653–657. [CrossRef] [PubMed]
154. Batty, K.T.; Davis, T.M.; Ilett, K.F.; Dusci, L.J.; Langton, S.R. The effect of ciprofloxacin on theophylline pharmacokinetics in healthy subjects. *Br. J. Clin. Pharmacol.* **1995**, *39*, 305–311. [CrossRef]
155. Granfors, M.T.; Backman, J.T.; Laitila, J.; Neuvonen, P.J. Oral contraceptives containing ethinyl estradiol and gestodene markedly increase plasma concentrations and effects of tizanidine by inhibiting cytochrome P450 1A2. *Clin. Pharmacol. Ther.* **2005**, *78*, 400–411. [CrossRef]
156. Komoroski, B.J.; Zhang, S.; Cai, H.; Hutzler, J.M.; Frye, R.; Tracy, T.S.; Strom, S.C.; Lehmann, T.; Ang, C.Y.W.; Cui, Y.Y.; et al. Induction and inhibition of cytochromes P450 by the St. John's wort constituent hyperforin in human hepatocyte cultures. *Drug Metab. Dispos.* **2004**, *32*, 512–518. [CrossRef]
157. Andersson, T.; Bergstrand, R.; Cederberg, C.; Eriksson, S.; Lagerström, P.-O.; Skånberg, I. Omeprazole treatment does not affect the metabolism of caffeine. *Gastroenterology* **1991**, *101*, 943–947. [CrossRef]
158. Rizzo, N.; Padoin, C.; Palombo, S.; Scherrmann, J.M.; Girre, C. Omeprazole and lansoprazole are not inducers of cytochrome P4501A2 under conventional therapeutic conditions. *Eur. J. Clin. Pharmacol.* **1996**, *49*, 491–495. [CrossRef]
159. Dilger, K.; Zheng, Z.; Klotz, U. Lack of drug interaction between omeprazole, lansoprazole, pantoprazole and theophylline. *Br. J. Clin. Pharmacol.* **1999**, *48*, 438–444. [CrossRef]
160. Henry, D.; Brent, P.; Whyte, I.; Mihaly, G.; Devenish-Meares, S. Propranolol steady-state pharmacokinetics are unaltered by omeprazole. *Eur. J. Clin. Pharmacol.* **1987**, *33*, 369–373. [CrossRef]

161. Frick, A.; Kopitz, J.; Bergemann, N. Omeprazole reduces clozapine plasma concentrations. A case report. *Pharmacopsychiatry* **2003**, *36*, 121–123. [CrossRef] [PubMed]
162. Lucas, R.A.; Gilfillan, D.J.; Bergstrom, R.F. A pharmacokinetic interaction between carbamazepine and olanzapine: Observations on possible mechanism. *Eur. J. Clin. Pharmacol.* **1998**, *54*, 639–643. [CrossRef] [PubMed]
163. Magnusson, M.O.; Dahl, M.-L.; Cederberg, J.; Karlsson, M.O.; Sandström, R. Pharmacodynamics of carbamazepine-mediated induction of CYP3A4, CYP1A2, and Pgp as assessed by probe substrates midazolam, caffeine, and digoxin. *Clin. Pharmacol. Ther.* **2008**, *84*, 52–62. [CrossRef] [PubMed]
164. Kirby, B.J.; Collier, A.C.; Kharasch, E.D.; Dixit, V.; Desai, P.; Whittington, D.; Thummel, K.E.; Unadkat, J.D. Complex drug interactions of HIV protease inhibitors 2: In vivo induction and in vitro to in vivo correlation of induction of cytochrome P450 1A2, 2B6, and 2C9 by ritonavir or nelfinavir. *Drug Metab. Dispos.* **2011**, *39*, 2329–2337. [CrossRef] [PubMed]
165. Penzak, S.R.; Hon, Y.Y.; Lawhorn, W.D.; Shirley, K.L.; Spratlin, V.; Jann, M.W. Influence of ritonavir on olanzapine pharmacokinetics in healthy volunteers. *J. Clin. Psychopharmacol.* **2002**, *22*, 366–370. [CrossRef] [PubMed]
166. Jacobs, B.S.; Colbers, A.P.H.; Velthoven-Graafland, K.; Schouwenberg, B.J.J.W.; Burger, D.M. Effect of fosamprenavir/ritonavir on the pharmacokinetics of single-dose olanzapine in healthy volunteers. *Int. J. Antimicrob. Agents* **2014**, *44*, 173–177. [CrossRef]
167. Pascussi, J.-M.; Gerbal-Chaloin, S.; Duret, C.; Daujat-Chavanieu, M.; Vilarem, M.-J.; Maurel, P. The tangle of nuclear receptors that controls xenobiotic metabolism and transport: Crosstalk and consequences. *Annu. Rev. Pharmacol. Toxicol.* **2008**, *48*, 1–32. [CrossRef]
168. Yeh, R.F.; Gaver, V.E.; Patterson, K.B.; Rezk, N.L.; Baxter-Meheux, F.; Blake, M.J.; Eron, J.J.; Klein, C.E.; Rublein, J.C.; Kashuba, A.D.M. Lopinavir/ritonavir induces the hepatic activity of cytochrome P450 enzymes CYP2C9, CYP2C19, and CYP1A2 but inhibits the hepatic and intestinal activity of CYP3A as measured by a phenotyping drug cocktail in healthy volunteers. *J. Acquir. Immune Defic. Syndr.* **2006**, *42*, 52–60. [CrossRef]
169. Haslemo, T.; Eikeseth, P.H.; Tanum, L.; Molden, E.; Refsum, H. The effect of variable cigarette consumption on the interaction with clozapine and olanzapine. *Eur. J. Clin. Pharmacol.* **2006**, *62*, 1049–1053. [CrossRef]
170. Seppälä, N.H.; Leinonen, E.V.; Lehtonen, M.L.; Kivistö, K.T. Clozapine serum concentrations are lower in smoking than in non-smoking schizophrenic patients. *Pharmacol. Toxicol.* **1999**, *85*, 244–246. [CrossRef]
171. Fric, M.; Pfuhlmann, B.; Laux, G.; Riederer, P.; Distler, G.; Artmann, S.; Wohlschläger, M.; Liebmann, M.; Deckert, J. The influence of smoking on the serum level of duloxetine. *Pharmacopsychiatry* **2008**, *41*, 151–155. [CrossRef] [PubMed]
172. Cassidenti, D.L.; Vijod, A.G.; Vijod, M.A.; Stanczyk, F.Z.; Lobo, R.A. Short-term effects of smoking on the pharmacokinetic profiles of micronized estradiol in postmenopausal women. *Am. J. Obstet. Gynecol.* **1990**, *163*, 1953–1960. [CrossRef]
173. Sitsen, J.; Maris, F.; Timmer, C. Drug-drug interaction studies with mirtazapine and carbamazepine in healthy male subjects. *Eur. J. Drug Metab. Pharmacokinet.* **2001**, *26*, 109–121. [CrossRef] [PubMed]
174. Lind, A.-B.; Reis, M.; Bengtsson, F.; Jonzier-Perey, M.; Powell Golay, K.; Ahlner, J.; Baumann, P.; Dahl, M.-L. Steady-state concentrations of mirtazapine, N-desmethylmirtazapine, 8-hydroxymirtazapine and their enantiomers in relation to cytochrome P450 2D6 genotype, age and smoking behaviour. *Clin. Pharmacokinet.* **2009**, *48*, 63–70. [CrossRef] [PubMed]
175. Sun, L.; McDonnell, D.; Yu, M.; Kumar, V.; Moltke, L. von. A Phase I Open-Label Study to Evaluate the Effects of Rifampin on the Pharmacokinetics of Olanzapine and Samidorphan Administered in Combination in Healthy Human Subjects. *Clin. Drug Investig.* **2019**, *39*, 477–484. [CrossRef]
176. Wu, T.-H.; Chiu, C.-C.; Shen, W.W.; Lin, F.-W.; Wang, L.-H.; Chen, H.-Y.; Lu, M.-L. Pharmacokinetics of olanzapine in Chinese male schizophrenic patients with various smoking behaviors. *Prog. Neuropsychopharmacol. Biol. Psychiatry* **2008**, *32*, 1889–1893. [CrossRef] [PubMed]
177. Zevin, S.; Benowitz, N.L. Drug interactions with tobacco smoking. An update. *Clin. Pharmacokinet.* **1999**, *36*, 425–438. [CrossRef]
178. Fuhr, U.; Woodcock, B.G.; Siewert, M. Verapamil and drug metabolism by the cytochrome P450 isoform CYP1A2. *Eur. J. Clin. Pharmacol.* **1992**, *42*, 463–464. [CrossRef]

179. Jungmann, N.A.; Lang, D.; Saleh, S.; van der Mey, D.; Gerisch, M. In vitro-in vivo correlation of the drug-drug interaction potential of antiretroviral HIV treatment regimens on CYP1A1 substrate riociguat. *Expert Opin. Drug Metab. Toxicol.* **2019**, *15*, 975–984. [CrossRef]
180. Kroon, L.A. Drug interactions with smoking. *Am. J. Health Syst. Pharm.* **2007**, *64*, 1917–1921. [CrossRef]
181. Hiemke, C.; Bergemann, N.; Clement, H.W.; Conca, A.; Deckert, J.; Domschke, K.; Eckermann, G.; Egberts, K.; Gerlach, M.; Greiner, C.; et al. Consensus Guidelines for Therapeutic Drug Monitoring in Neuropsychopharmacology: Update 2017. *Pharmacopsychiatry* **2018**, *51*, 9–62. [CrossRef] [PubMed]
182. Faber, M.S.; Fuhr, U. Time response of cytochrome P450 1A2 activity on cessation of heavy smoking *Clin. Pharmacol. Ther.* **2004**, *76*, 178–184. [CrossRef] [PubMed]
183. Faber, M.S.; Jetter, A.; Fuhr, U. Assessment of CYP1A2 activity in clinical practice: Why, how, and when? *Basic Clin. Pharmacol. Toxicol.* **2005**, *97*, 125–134. [CrossRef]
184. Chochol, M.D.; Kataria, L.; O'Rourke, M.C.; Lamotte, G. Clozapine-Associated Myoclonus and Stuttering Secondary to Smoking Cessation and Drug Interaction: A Case Report. *J. Clin. Psychopharmacol.* **2019**, *39*, 275–277. [CrossRef] [PubMed]
185. Kocar, T.; Freudenmann, R.W.; Spitzer, M.; Graf, H. Switching From Tobacco Smoking to Electronic Cigarettes and the Impact on Clozapine Levels. *J. Clin. Psychopharmacol.* **2018**, *38*, 528–529. [CrossRef]
186. Larsen, J.T.; Brøsen, K. Consumption of charcoal-broiled meat as an experimental tool for discerning CYP1A2-mediated drug metabolism in vivo. *Basic Clin. Pharmacol. Toxicol.* **2005**, *97*, 141–148 [CrossRef] [PubMed]
187. Hakooz, N.; Hamdan, I. Effects of dietary broccoli on human in vivo caffeine metabolism: A pilot study on a group of Jordanian volunteers. *Curr. Drug Metab.* **2007**, *8*, 9–15. [CrossRef]
188. Charron, C.S.; Novotny, J.A.; Jeffery, E.H.; Kramer, M.; Ross, S.A.; Seifried, H.E. Consumption of baby kale increased cytochrome P450 1A2 (CYP1A2) activity and influenced bilirubin metabolism in a randomized clinical trial. *J. Funct. Foods* **2020**, *64*, 103624. [CrossRef]
189. Lake, B.G.; Tredger, J.M.; Renwick, A.B.; Barton, P.T.; Price, R.J. 3,3′-Diindolylmethane induces CYP1A2 in cultured precision-cut human liver slices. *Xenobiotica* **1998**, *28*, 803–811. [CrossRef]

14

Prevalence of Potential Drug–Drug Interaction Risk among Chronic Kidney Disease Patients in a Spanish Hospital

Gracia Santos-Díaz [1], Ana María Pérez-Pico [2], Miguel Ángel Suárez-Santisteban [1,3], Vanesa García-Bernalt [3], Raquel Mayordomo [4] and Pedro Dorado [1,*]

1 Biosanitary Research Institute of Extremadura (INUBE), University of Extremadura, 06006 Badajoz, Spain; grsantosd@unex.es (G.S.-D.); miguelangel.suarez@salud-juntaex.es (M.Á.S.-S.)
2 Department of Nursing, University of Extremadura, 10600 Plasencia, Spain; aperpic@unex.es
3 Nephrology Department, Virgen del Puerto Hospital, Servicio Extremeño de Salud, 10600 Plasencia, Spain; vanesa.garcia@salud-juntaex.es
4 Department of Anatomy, Cellular Biology and Zoology, University of Extremadura, 10600 Plasencia, Spain; rmayordo@unex.es
* Correspondence: pdorado@unex.es

Abstract: Chronic kidney disease (CKD) is a major health problem worldwide and, in Spain, it is present in 15.1% of individuals. CKD is frequently associated with some comorbidities and patients need to be prescribed multiple medications. Polypharmacy increases the risk of adverse drug reactions (ADRs). There are no published studies evaluating the prevalence of potential drug–drug interactions (pDDIs) among CKD patients in any European country. This study was aimed to determine the prevalence, pattern, and factors associated with pDDIs among CKD patients using a drug interactions program. An observational cross-sectional study was carried out at Plasencia Hospital, located in Spain. Data were collected among patients with CKD diagnoses and pDDIs were assessed by the Lexicomp® Drug Interactions platform. Data were obtained from 112 CKD patients. A total number of 957 prescribed medications were acknowledged, and 928 pDDIs were identified in 91% of patients. Age and concomitant drugs were significantly associated with the number of pDDIs ($p < 0.05$). According to the results, the use of programs for the determination of pDDIs (such as Lexicomp®) is recommended in the clinical practice of CKD patients in order to avoid serious adverse effects, as is paying attention to contraindicated drug combinations.

Keywords: chronic kidney disease; drug–drug interactions; polypharmacy; adverse drug reactions; Lexicomp

---

1. Introduction

As specified by the Kidney Disease Improving Global Outcomes (NKF KDIGO) guidelines [1], chronic kidney disease (CKD) is defined as abnormalities of kidney structure or function, present for more than three months, with implications for health. CKD is a general term for various heterogeneous disorders affecting kidney structure and function with variable clinical presentations; in part, related to the cause, severity, and rate of progression. The glomerular filtration rate (GFR) is generally accepted as the best overall index of kidney function, and is classified into different stages (G1, G2, G3a, G3b, G4, and G5). The diagnostic criteria of CKD are those denominated as kidney damage markers or a threshold of GFR < 60 mL/min/1.73 m^2 (GFR categories G3a–G5), or both, for more than three months.

CKD is a major health problem worldwide; in 2017, 1.2 million people died from CKD. Furthermore, between 1990 and 2017, the global all-age mortality rate from CKD increased by 41.5% [2]. In Spain,

CKD is present in 15.1% of individuals and this prevalence is more than three times higher in men than in women (23.1% vs. 7.3%) and increases with age [3]. Diabetes and hypertension are the main causes of CKD in all high-income and middle-income countries and in many low-income countries [4]. Among other reasons, the prevalence of CKD is increasing worldwide due to the fact that the prevalence of both hypertension and diabetes is also rising. Diabetes is expected to increase by 69% in high-income countries and 20% in low-income and middle-income countries from 2010 to 2030 [5]. Regarding hypertension, it is predicted to increase by 60% from 2000 to 2025 [6]. Additionally, CKD is also associated with other comorbidities such as dyslipidemia, hyperuricemia, or cardiovascular disease [7], and patients need to be prescribed multiple medications.

Polypharmacy is usually defined as the concomitant prescription of five or more medications [8] and it is a major risk factor of drug–drug interactions, which increases with the number of prescribed drugs leading to 100% with eight or more medications [9]. The elderly are at risk for polypharmacy, and this fact increases the risk of adverse drug reactions (ADRs) from 13 to 58% with two and five medications, respectively. Seven or more medications increase the risk of ADRs to 82% [9].

Previous studies have evaluated the prevalence and severity of potential drug–drug interactions (pDDIs) using different drug–drug interaction programs among CKD patients from Brazil [10,11], India [12,13], Pakistan [14], Palestine [15], and Nigeria [16–19]; however, there are no published studies evaluating the prevalence of pDDIs among CKD patients in any European country.

Lexicomp® (Wolters Kluwer Clinical Drug Information) is considered one of the best performing drug–drug interaction programs and it was reported to be highly sensitive and specific (around 90–100%). It focuses on the depth and duplication of information and it is a resource of choices for locating the mechanism of a drug–drug interaction [20–22].

This study was aimed to determine the prevalence, pattern, and factors associated with potential drug–drug interaction among CKD patients attending a hospital nephrology department using the drug interaction program Lexicomp®.

2. Materials and Methods

2.1. Subjects

An observational cross-sectional study was carried out at Virgen del Puerto Hospital in Plasencia (Cáceres, Spain). All participants were patients attended by the nephrology department, and were invited to participate in the study. The inclusion criteria were: patients with CKD diagnosis, over the age of 18, and having signed an informed consent form. Data were collected during 2019 and included: age, gender, list of medications at the time of last clinic visit, comorbidities, and serum creatinine.

The study was performed in accordance with the principles of the Declaration of Helsinki of 1975, revised in 2013, and approved by the Clinical Research Ethics Committee, Cáceres (reference: MASR/2016), and the Bioethics and Biosecurity Committee, University of Extremadura (reference: 64/2016).

The serum creatinine value was used to calculate eGFR (estimated glomerular filtration rate in mL/min/1.73 m^2) and patients were classified following the criteria of the KDIGO Guideline 1 into different CKD stages: G1, eGFR $\geq$ 90; G2, eGFR 60–89; G3a, eGFR 45–59; G3b, eGFR 30–44; G4, eGFR 15–29; G5, eGFR < 15.

2.2. Methods

The electronic drug–drug interactions (DDIs) checking platform Lexicomp® was used to evaluate patient medication regimens for pDDIs. The Lexicomp® (Wolters Kluwer Health Inc. Riverwoods, IL, USA) database system provides accurate information about the risk, type, mechanism, and pattern of distribution of pDDIs. It also gives recommendations on how to prevent and manage DDIs if they occur. This software identifies and classifies pDDIs into five types according to the degree of clinical significance. Type A: no known interaction, Type B: minor or mild interaction, Type C:

moderate or significant interaction, Type D: major or serious interaction, and Type X: contraindication or avoid combination.

2.3. Statistical Analysis

Descriptive statistics were used, and results were presented as percentages and frequencies. ANOVA Kruskal–Wallis test or Mann–Whitney t-test analyses were performed to evaluate the effect of covariates on the incidence of pDDIs. A *p*-value of less than 0.05 was considered statistically significant. All statistical analyses were performed using IBM SPSS v.22 (SPSS Inc., Chicago, IL, USA).

3. Results

3.1. Clinical and Demographic and Characteristics of Patients

Data were obtained from 112 CKD patients, 69 (61.6%) females and 43 (38.4%) males. The mean age of this study population was 77.1 ± 10.4 years: 11 patients (10.0%) were between 30 and 60 years, 8 (7.1%) were between 61 and 70 years, 44 (39.3%) were between 71 and 80 years, and 49 (43.7%) were older than 80 years (Table 1).

Table 1. Characteristics of the study population (n = 112).

Characteristics	N (%) or Mean ± SD
Female	69 (61.6)
Male	43 (38.4)
Mean age (years)	77.1 ± 10.4
Age group (years)	
30–60	11 (10.0)
61–70	8 (7.1)
71–80	44 (39.3)
>80	49 (43.7)
CKD stage	
1	10 (8.9)
2	15 (13.4)
3a	34 (30.3)
3b	33 (29.5)
4	15 (13.4)
5	5 (4.5)
Comorbidities	91 (81.2)
Hypertension	52 (46.4)
Diabetes mellitus	25 (22.3)
Dyslipidemia/hypercholesterolemia	33 (29.5)
Anemia	13 (11.6)
Hyperuricemia	11 (9.8)
Mean prescribed drugs per patient	8.6 ± 3.4
Number of prescribed drugs	
≤5	22 (19.6)
6–10	59 (53.2)
11–15	29 (25.9)
≥16	2 (1.8)

The most common comorbid conditions (Table 1) were hypertension in 52 patients (46.4%), diabetes mellitus in 25 (22.3%), dyslipidemia in 33 (29.5%), anemia in 13 (11.6%), and hyperuricemia in 11 (9.8%).

3.2. Prevalence and Pattern of Potential Drug–Drug Interactions

A total number of 957 prescribed medications were identified. The minimum number of prescribed medications per patient was 1, the maximum was 17, and the mean number was

8.6 ± 3.4 medications. Only one patient was not taking any medication. The most commonly prescribed medications were omeprazole (30.6%), acetaminophen (30.6%), salicylic acid (26.1%), bisoprolol (25.2%), furosemide (22.5%), and allopurinol (21.6%).

Among 111 individuals 928 pDDIs were identified, and 67 (60.3%) patients showed 1–10 pDDIs, while 34 (30.6%) presented more than 10. Only 10 patients (9%) did not have any interaction (Table 2)

Table 2. Frequency of potential drug–drug interactions (pDDIs) per patient (n = 111 *).

Number of pDDIs	N	%
None	10	9.0
1–5	40	36.0
6–10	27	24.3
11–15	15	13.5
16–20	11	9.9
21–25	4	3.6
>25	4	3.6

* One patient had not taken any drugs.

According to the Lexicomp® severity classification, 11 (1.2%) pDDIs were Type A (no known interaction), 84 (9.1%) were Type B (mild severity), 717 (77.3%) were Type C (moderate severity), 106 (11.4%) were Type D (major severity), and 10 (1.1%) were Type X (avoid drug combination) (Table 3)

Table 3. Severity of potential drug–drug interactions (pDDIs; n = 928) among studied chronic kidney disease (CKD) patients.

Severity of pDDIs	N	%
Type A (No known interaction)	11	1.2
Type B (mild severity)	84	9.1
Type C (moderate severity)	717	77.3
Type D (major severity)	106	11.4
Type X (avoid drug combination)	10	1.1

Table 4 shows the most frequent pDDIs by severity group: levothyroxine + omeprazole with 9 cases in the Type B group (10.7%), acenocoumarol + omeprazole with 11 cases in Type C (1.5%), and acenocoumarol + allopurinol with 8 cases in Type D (7.5%).

Table 4. Most frequent potential drug–drug interactions (pDDIs) by severity group.

Severity of pDDI	N	PDDIs	Frequency (%)
Type B (mild severity)	84	Levothyroxine + Omeprazole	10.7
		Levothyroxine + Furosemide	9.5
		Acenocoumarol + Spironolactone	7.1
Type C (moderate severity)	717	Acenocoumarol + Omeprazole	1.5
		Ferrous Sulfate + Omeprazole	1.3
		Metformin + Acetylsalicylic Acid	1.3
Type D (major severity)	106	Acenocoumarol + Allopurinol	7.5
		Levothyroxine + Ferrous Sulfate	4.7
		Tramadol + Trazodone	3.8

In addition, Type X (avoid drug combination) pDDIs were found in 10 CKD patients (Table 5).

Table 5. Potential drug–drug interactions Type X (avoid drug combination) found in the studied CKD patients.

Drug–Drug Interaction	Potential Adverse Effects	Severity	Reliability Rating
Amitriptyline + Aclidinium	Aclidinium may enhance the anticholinergic effect of Anticholinergic Agents	Major	Fair
Doxazosin + Dutasteride and Tamsulosin	Alpha1-Blockers may enhance the antihypertensive effect of other Alpha1-Blockers	Major	Fair
Dutasteride And Tamsulosin + Tamsulosin	Alpha1-Blockers may enhance the antihypertensive effect of other Alpha1-Blockers	Major	Fair
Levosulpiride + Solifenacin	Anticholinergic Agents may diminish the therapeutic effect of Levosulpiride	Major	Fair
Aclidinium and Formoterol + Propranolol	Beta-Blockers (Nonselective) may diminish the bronchodilatory effect of Beta2-Agonists	Major	Fair
Metamizole + Dexketoprofen	Dexketoprofen may enhance the adverse/toxic effect of Nonsteroidal Anti-Inflammatory Agents	Major	Fair
Tramadol and Acetaminophen + Buprenorphine	Opioids (Mixed Agonist/Antagonist) may diminish the analgesic effect of Opioid Agonists	Major	Good
Atenolol + Rivastigmine	Rivastigmine may enhance the bradycardic effect of Beta-Blockers	Moderate	Fair
Bisoprolol + Rivastigmine	Rivastigmine may enhance the bradycardic effect of Beta-Blockers	Moderate	Fair
Dexketoprofen + Acetylsalicylic Acid	Salicylates may enhance the adverse/toxic effect of Dexketoprofen. Dexketoprofen may diminish the therapeutic effect of Salicylates. Salicylates may decrease the serum concentration of Dexketoprofen	Major	Fair

It was also observed that some drugs were present in a large number of pDDIs such as hydrochlorothiazide (15%), acetylsalicylic acid (10%), or furosemide (9%). The most frequent drugs present in pDDIs in the study group are shown in Figure 1.

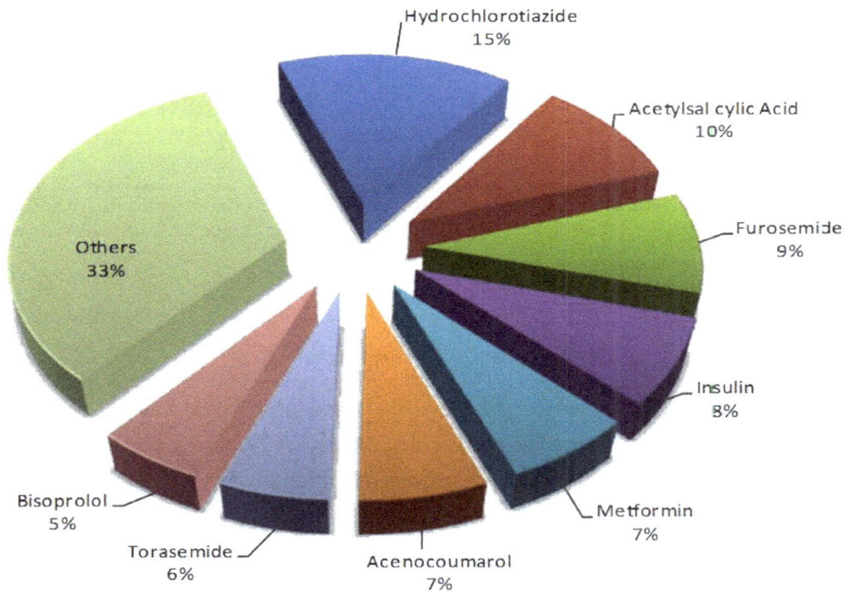

Figure 1. Frequency of main drugs with potential drug–drug interactions (n = 928).

3.3. Factors Associated with Potential Drug–Drug Interactions on CKD Patients

Age and concomitant drugs were significantly associated with the number of pDDIs ($p < 0.05$; Table 6). In contrast, demographic and clinical variables, such as gender, CKD stage, or the number of chronic comorbid diseases were not significantly associated with the number of pDDIs (Table 6).

Table 6. Potential drug–drug interactions (pDDIs) among 111 * CKD patients according to demographic and clinical variables groups.

Variable	Number	Median (25%–75% Percentile)	*p*–Value [1]
Gender			0.5768 [2]
Female	68	7 (2–12.7)	
Male	43	7 (2–11)	
Age			0.0191
30–60	11	2 (0–5)	
61–70	8	3.5 (0.5–7.7)	
71–80	44	8 (3.2–16)	
>80	48	8 (3–11)	
CKD stage **			0.4930
G1	10	3.5 (0.7–12.7)	
G2	15	8 (3–12)	
G3a	34	5 (1–9.2)	
G3b	33	8 (3–13)	
G4	14	4 (3–13)	
G5	5	11 (4–17.5)	
Concomitant drugs			<0.0001
≤5	21	1 (0–2)	
6–10	59	6 (4–9)	
11–15	29	16 (11–20)	
>15	2	26 (16–36)	
Chronic comorbid disease			0.0611
0	20	6.5 (3.2–11)	
1	21	7 (2–12.5)	
2	20	6.5 (3–10.7)	
3	10	12 (7.2–20.5)	
4	17	7 (1–17.5)	
≥5	23	4 (1–7)	

* One patient had not taken any drugs; ** according to the classification of chronic kidney disease from Kidney Disease: Improving Global Outcomes (KDIGO); [1] ANOVA Kruskal–Wallis test; [2] Mann–Whitney *t*-test.

4. Discussion

4.1. Frequency and Severity of Potential Drug–Drug Interactions

Table 8 shows previous reports in which the prevalence and severity of pDDIs has been evaluated on CKD patients. It is remarkable that there are two studies published in 2017 that were carried out in different hospitals in Nigeria, with different numbers of individuals, but their results are practically identical despite using different analysis tools [17,18].

Table 7. Previous studies in which prevalence and severity of potential drug–drug interactions has been evaluated on CKD patients.

Study	Number of Patients (% Female)	Years (Mean ± SD)	Country	CKD Patients on Stage 5 or Hemodialysis (%)	Software for Potential DDI	Number of Drugs per Patient (Mean ± SD)	Most Frequent Drug Combinations with Potential DDIs (%)	Number of Patients with Potential DDIs Contraindicated (%)
Rama et al. [12].	205 (25.8%)	48.6 ± 16.2	India	68.5%	Micromedex	12.1 ± 6.3	Ascorbid Acid + Cyanocobalamine (12.4%) Clonidine + Metoprolol (3.8%) Amlodipine + Metoprolol (3.4%) Insulin + Metoprolol (2.9%)	0 (0.0%)
Marquito et al. [10].	558 (45.3%)	n.s.	Brazil	6.6%	Micromedex	5.6 ± 3.2	Furosemide + Aspirin (7.8%) Enalapril + Furosemide (5.9%) Captopril + Furosemide (5.1%) Enalapril + Losartan (3.7%)	5 (0.9%)
Sgnaolin et al. [11].	65 (50.8%)	59.1±14.7	Brazil	100%	Micromedex	6.3 ± 3.1	Calcium Carbonate + Atenolol (8.0%) Calcium Carbonate + Ferrous Sulfate (8.0%) Calcium Carbonate + Ticlopidine (6.3%) Enalapril + Eritropoietin (4.5%)	2 (3.1%)
Hegde et al. [13].	120 (45%)	58.5 ± 8.4	India	n.s.	Medscape Drug interaction checker	9.4 ± 3.9	Sodium Bicarbonate + Ferrous Sulfate (8.9%) Calcium Carbonate + Ferrous Sulfate (5.5%) Aspirin + Carvedilol (5.5%) Sodium Bicarbonate + Allopurinol (5.5%)	0 (0.0%)
Al-Ramahi et al. [15].	275 (45.1%)	50.7 ± 15.9	Palestina	100%	LexiComp	7.9 ± 2.4	Calcium Carbonate + Amlodipine (12.3%) Calcium Carbonate + Aspirin (8.2%) Aspirin + Furosemide (7.9%) Aspirin + Enoxaparin (4.3%)	2 (0.7%)
Olumuyiwa et al. [18].	123 (33.3%)	53.8 ± 16.0	Nigeria	69.9%	Lexi-Interact database	10.1 ± 4.0	Calcium Carbonate + Ferrous Sulfate (8.4%) Folic Acid + Furosemide (3.4%) Calcium Carbonate + Calcidol (3.2%) Vitamin E + Ferrous Sulfate (3.0%)	1 (0.8%)
Fasipe et al. [17].	123 (48.8%)	53.8 ± 16.0	Nigeria	69.9%	Medscape Drug interaction checker	10.3 ± 3.9	Calcium Carbonate + Ferrous Sulfate (9.9%) Folic Acid + Furosemide (3.4%) Calcium Carbonate + Calcidol (3.2%) Vitamin E + Ferrous Sulfate (3.0%)	1 (0.8%)

Table 8. Previous studies in which prevalence and severity of potential drug–drug interactions has been evaluated on CKD patients.

Study	Number of Patients (% Female)	Years (Mean ± SD)	Country	CKD Patients on Stage 5 or Hemodialysis (%)	Software for Potential DDI	Number of Drugs per Patient (Mean ± SD)	Most Frequent Drug Combinations with Potential DDIs (%)	Number of Patients with Potential DDIs Contraindicated (%)
Saleem et al. [14].	209 (39.2%)	38.3 ± 16.8	Pakistan	74.2%	Micromedex Drug-Reax	n.s.	Ferrous Sulfate + Omeprazole (5.8%) Calcium/Vitamin D + Ciprofloxacin (4.8%) Captopril + Furosemide (4.1%) Calcium Gluconate + Ceftriaxone (3.6%)	28 (13.4)
Adibe et al. [16].	169 (52.1%)	51.0 ± 14.9	Nigeria	28.4%	Medscape Drug interaction checker	6.1 ± 2.0	Lisinopril + Furosemide (9.1%) Furosemide + Calcium Carbonate (7.2%) Calcium Carbonate + Lisinipril (6.1%) Aspirin + Furosemide (4.6%)	0 (0.0%)
Okoro and Farate [19].	201 (66%)	49.5 ± 14.5	Nigeria	69.2%	Omnio drug interaction checker	5.8 ± 1.5	Calcium Carbonate + Ferrous Sulfate (45.8%) Lisinopril + Furosemide (7.7%) Captopril + Furosemide (6.6%) Captopril + Spironolactone (6.6%)	5 (2.5%)
Present study	111 (61.3%)	77.1 ± 10.4	Spain	4.5%	LexiComp	8.6 ± 3.4	Acenocoumarol + Omeprazole (1.1%) Ferrous Sulfate + Omeprazole (1.0%) Metformin + Aspirin (1.0%) Levothyroxine + Omeprazole (1.0%)	10 (9.0%)

n.s.: not studied.

As mentioned, most of the pDDIs were Type C (moderate severity), and 12.5% were Type D (major severity) and Type X (avoid drug combination). These data are similar to those observed in a previous study in Palestinian patients [15]. Other studies highlighted differences in the frequency of pDDIs types (Table 8). Among other causes, the variability in the reported pDDIs could also be a consequence of using different screening platforms to analyze potential drug interactions. In our case, we used Lexicomp®, which classifies pDDIs in different levels of severity. However, other software (Micromedex Drug-Reax, Medscape Drug interaction checker, etc.) for similar drug combinations perform dissimilar categorizations, or find different pDDIs.

Even though the majority of pDDIs reported in this study were Type C, it is necessary to closely monitor patients in order to identify adverse events. Moreover, major severity drug interactions and avoided drug combinations present a high risk to the health of patients and, consequently, physicians or clinical pharmacists must analyze, detect, and early prevent pDDIs.

In the present study, the majority of the patients were in CKD stage 3, and only 4.5% of the total were in CKD stage 5 or hemodialysis. This result is comparable with another study from Brazil [10] in which patients in CKD stage 5 represented 6.6% of the total sample. However, in the remaining previous studies, most of the patients were in stage 5 or hemodialysis (Table 8). This could affect the number and type of prescribed treatment and, therefore, the pDDI. The present study did not only focus on patients on hemodialysis, but on all patients with CKD.

4.2. Factors Associated with Potential Drug–Drug Interactions

Regarding comorbid conditions, these appeared in 91 patients (81.2%), and the most frequent were hypertension (44.6%), dyslipidemia/hypercholesterolemia (28.6%), and diabetes mellitus (22.3%).

The prevalence of hypertension and diabetes in previous studies [10,13–15] were higher than those found in the present study. In addition, each country could have implemented different clinical guidelines for similar disease conditions, which results in the prescription of different drugs and thereby other pDDIs. The selected hospital is a reference hospital with a nephrology unit similar and representative of most hospitals in the country. The percentage of patients with chronic kidney disease is also similar to those other nephrology units in Spain.

In the present study, the mean age of patients was higher (77.1 ± 10.4 years) than in the rest of the studies, which reported mean age data from 38.3 ± 16.8 to 59.1 ± 14.7 years (Table 8). Polypharmacy prevalence increases with advancing age [23], and hence also pDDIs. Furthermore, people aged 80 and over are still much more likely to have DDIs [24]. Therefore, the main reasons for the differences found in the present study, comparing to most of the previous studies, could be the different CKD stages, age, or the country of patients. These factors could affect the number and type of prescribed drug treatment and, therefore, the number and severity of pDDIs. On the other hand, the use of different software to evaluate the pDDIs in the reported studies (Table 8) could lead to differences of the severity of pDDIs. Furthermore, many of the analyzed drugs that appear in Lexicomp® do not appear in some other databases.

This could be one of the reasons for variability in the pattern of frequency and severity of pDDIs observed in the present study compared to previous studies.

5. Conclusions

The frequency and severity of pDDIs could be affected by the type and number of drugs per patient, which, at the same time, could be influenced by comorbidities and age. On the other hand, the advancement of CKD increases the risk of a major cardiac event and the possibility of hospitalization, which increases the number of medications [25,26].

It should be noted that in CKD patients, the association of medications is sometimes inevitable, and according to the present results, the use of programs for determination of pDDIs (such as Lexicomp®) are recommended in clinical practice for CKD patients in order to avoid serious adverse effects, paying attention to the contraindicated drug combinations. Therefore, as a way to classify and identify pDDIs according to interaction risk, severity, and reliability, it would be convenient to consider and evaluate pDDIs in clinical practice in order to avoid or prevent some avoidable adverse effects.

Author Contributions: Conceptualization, G.S.-D., P.D., M.Á.S.-S.; methodology, G.S.-D. and P.D.; software, G.S.-D. and P.D.; investigation, G.S.-D., A.M.P.-P., M.Á.S.-S., V.G.-B., R.M. and P.D.; writing—original draft preparation, G.S.-D. and P.D.; writing—review and editing, G.S.-D., A.M.P.-P., M.Á.S.-S., V.G.-B., R.M. and P.D.; supervision, P.D.; project administration, P.D. All authors have read and agreed to the published version of the manuscript.

Acknowledgments: The authors thank all patients who kindly participated in the study, as well as the clinical assistance of Laura Piquero Calleja and Anika Tyszkiewiez. This work was supported.

References

1. Kidney Disease: Improving Global Outcomes (KDIGO) CKD Work Group. KDIGO clinical practice guideline for the evaluation and management of chronic kidney disease. *Kidney Int. Suppl.* **2013**, *3*, 1–150.
2. GBD Chronic Kidney Disease Collaboration. Global, regional, and national burden of chronic kidney disease, 1990-2017: A systematic analysis for the Global Burden of Disease Study 2017. *Lancet* **2020**, *395*, 709–733. [CrossRef]
3. Gorostidi, M.; Sánchez-Martínez, M.; Ruilope, L.M.; Graciani, A.; de la Cruz, J.J.; Santamaría, R.; del Pino, M.; Guallar-Castillón, P.; de Álvaro, F.; Rodríguez-Artalejo, F.; et al. Prevalencia de enfermedad renal crónica en España: Impacto de la acumulación de factores de riesgo cardiovascular. *Nefrologia* **2018**, *38*, 606–615. [CrossRef]
4. Webster, A.; Nagler, E.; Morton, R.; Masson, P. Chronic Kidney Disease. *Lancet* **2017**, *389*, 1238–1252. [CrossRef]
5. Shaw, J.E.; Sicree, R.A.; Zimmet, P.Z. Global estimates of the prevalence of diabetes for 2010 and 2030. *Diabetes Res. Clin. Pract.* **2010**, *87*, 4–14. [CrossRef]
6. Kearney, P.; Whelton, M.; Reynolds, K.; Muntner, P.; Whelton, P.; He, J. Global burden of hypertension: Analysis of worldwide data. *Lancet* **2005**, *365*, 217–223. [CrossRef]
7. Major, R.; Cheng, M.; Grant, R.; Shantikumar, S.; Xu, G.; Oozeerally, I.; Brunskill, N.; Gray, L. Cardiovascular disease risk factors in chronic kidney disease: A systematic review and meta-analysis. *PLoS ONE* **2018**, *13*, e0192895. [CrossRef] [PubMed]
8. Masnoon, N.; Shakib, S.; Kalisch-Ellett, L.; Caughey, G. What is polypharmacy? A systematic review of definitions. *BMC Geriatr.* **2017**, *17*, 230. [CrossRef] [PubMed]
9. Shah, B.; Hajjar, E. Polypharmacy, Adverse Drug Reactions, and Geriatric Syndromes. *Clin. Geriatr. Med.* **2012**, *28*, 173–186. [CrossRef] [PubMed]
10. Marquito, A.; Fernandes, N.; Colugnati, F.; Paula, R. Identifying potential drug interactions in chronic kidney disease patients. *J. Bras. Nefrol.* **2014**, *36*, 26–34. [CrossRef]
11. Sgnaolin, V.; Sgnaolin, V.; Engroff, P.; De Carli, G.; Prado Lima Figueiredo, A. Avaliação dos medicamentos utilizados e possíveis interações medicamentosas em doentes renais crônicos. *Sci. Med. (Porto Alegre)* **2014**, *24*, 329–335. [CrossRef]
12. Rama, M.; Viswanathan, G.; Acharya, L.; Attur, R.; Reddy, P.; Raghavan, S. Assessment of drug-drug interactions among renal failure patients of nephrology ward in a south Indian tertiary care hospital. *Indian J. Pharm. Sci.* **2012**, *74*, 63–68. [PubMed]
13. Hegde, S.; Udaykumar, P.; Manjuprasad, M.S. Potential drug interactions in chronic kidney disease patients-A cross sectional study. *Int. J. Recent Trends Sci. Technol.* **2015**, *16*, 56–60.
14. Saleem, A.; Masood, I.; Khan, T. Clinical relevancy and determinants of potential drug-drug interactions in chronic kidney disease patients: Results from a retrospective analysis. *Integr. Pharm. Res. Pract.* **2017**, *6*, 71–77. [CrossRef] [PubMed]
15. Al-Ramahi, R.; Raddad, A.; Rashed, A.; Bsharat, A.; Abu-Ghazaleh, D.; Yasin, E.; Shehab, O. Evaluation of potential drug-drug interactions among Palestinian hemodialysis patients. *BMC Nephrol.* **2016**, *17*, 96. [CrossRef] [PubMed]
16. Adibe, M.O.; Ewelum, P.C.; Amorha, K.C. Evaluation of drug-drug interactions among patients with chronic kidney disease in a South-Eastern Nigeria tertiary hospital: A retrospective study. *Pan Afr. Med. J.* **2017**, *28*, 199. [CrossRef]

17. Fasipe, O.J.; Akhideno, P.E.; Nwaiwu, O.; Adelosoye, A.A. Assessment of prescribed medications and pattern of distribution for potential drug–drug interactions among chronic kidney disease patients attending the Nephrology Clinic of Lagos University Teaching Hospital in Sub-Saharan West Africa. *Clin. Pharmacol.* **2017**, *9*, 125–132. [CrossRef] [PubMed]
18. Olumuyiwa, J.F.; Akinwumi, A.A.; Ademola, O.A.; Oluwole, B.A.; Ibiene, E.O. Prevalence and pattern of potential drug-drug interactions among chronic kidney disease patients in south-western Nigeria. *Niger. Postgrad. Med. J.* **2017**, *24*, 88–92.
19. Okoro, R.; Farate, V. Evaluation of potential drug–drug interactions among patients with chronic kidney disease in northeastern Nigeria. *Afr. J. Nephrol.* **2019**, *22*, 77–81.
20. Roblek, T.; Vaupotic, T.; Mrhar, A.; Lainscak, M. Drug-drug interaction software in clinical practice: A systematic review. *Eur. J. Clin. Pharmacol.* **2015**, *1*, 131–142. [CrossRef]
21. Kheshti, R.; Aalipour, M.; Namazi, S. A comparison of five common drug-drug interaction software programs regarding accuracy and comprehensiveness. *J. Res. Pharm. Pract.* **2016**, *5*, 257–263. [PubMed]
22. Patel, R.I.; Beckett, R.D. Evaluation of resources for analyzing drug interactions. *J. Med. Libr. Assoc.* **2016**, *104*, 290–295. [CrossRef] [PubMed]
23. Fulton, M.; Allen, E. Polypharmacy in the elderly: A literature review. *J. Am. Acad. Nurse Pract.* **2005**, *17*, 123–132. [CrossRef] [PubMed]
24. Guthrie, B.; Makubate, B.; Hernandez-Santiago, V.; Dreischulte, T. The rising tide of polypharmacy and drug-drug interactions: Population database analysis 1995–2010. *BMC Med.* **2015**, *13*, 74. [CrossRef] [PubMed]
25. Go, A.S.; Chertow, G.M.; Fan, D.; McCulloch, C.E.; Hsu, C.Y. Chronic kidney disease and the risks of death, cardiovascular events, and hospitalization. *N. Engl. J. Med.* **2004**, *351*, 1296–1305. [CrossRef] [PubMed]
26. Parikh, N.I.; Hwang, S.J.; Larson, M.G.; Levy, D.; Fox, C.S. Chronic kidney disease as a predictor of cardiovascular disease (from the Framingham Heart Study). *Am. J. Cardiol.* **2008**, *102*, 47–53. [CrossRef]

15

Role of OATP1B1 and OATP1B3 in Drug-Drug Interactions Mediated by Tyrosine Kinase Inhibitors

Dominique A. Garrison †, Zahra Talebi †, Eric D. Eisenmann, Alex Sparreboom * and Sharyn D. Baker *

Division of Pharmaceutics and Pharmacology, College of Pharmacy, The Ohio State University, Columbus, OH 43210, USA; garrison.220@osu.edu (D.A.G.); talebi.9@osu.edu (Z.T.); eisenmann.11@osu.edu (E.D.E.)
* Correspondence: sparreboom.1@osu.edu (A.S.); baker.2480@osu.edu (S.D.B.)

† These authors contributed equally to this work.

Abstract: Failure to recognize important features of a drug's pharmacokinetic characteristics is a key cause of inappropriate dose and schedule selection, and can lead to reduced efficacy and increased rate of adverse drug reactions requiring medical intervention. As oral chemotherapeutic agents, tyrosine kinase inhibitors (TKIs) are particularly prone to cause drug-drug interactions as many drugs in this class are known or suspected to potently inhibit the hepatic uptake transporters OATP1B1 and OATP1B3. In this article, we provide a comprehensive overview of the published literature and publicly-available regulatory documents in this rapidly emerging field. Our findings indicate that, while many TKIs can potentially inhibit the function of OATP1B1 and/or OATP1B3 and cause clinically-relevant drug-drug interactions, there are many inconsistencies between regulatory documents and the published literature. Potential explanations for these discrepant observations are provided in order to assist prescribing clinicians in designing safe and effective polypharmacy regimens, and to provide researchers with insights into refining experimental strategies to further predict and define the translational significance of TKI-mediated drug-drug interactions.

Keywords: OATP1B1; OATP1B3; tyrosine kinase inhibitors; drug-drug interactions

1. Introduction

The economic burden of drug-related morbidity and mortality as a result of non-optimized medication therapy is estimated to be more than 16% of total US health care annual expenditures [1] Overlooking major pharmacokinetic characteristics of a drug is one of the key players in inappropriate pharmaceutical dosing, which can lead to reduced efficacy and an increased rate of adverse drug reactions (ADRs) requiring medical intervention [2]. Pharmacokinetic drug-drug interactions (DDIs) can be responsible for about half of all DDIs depending on the patient group [3,4]. Furthermore, these DDIs have the potential to cause very pronounced (several hundred-fold) and abrupt changes in concentration and effect of the victim drug, depending on the start and stop of the causative (perpetrator) comedication and on fluctuations of its concentration during therapy [2,5,6].

Different components in absorption, distribution, metabolism and excretion can affect the overall pharmacokinetic profile of drugs. For agents that primarily undergo hepatic elimination, transport-mediated mechanisms of hepatocellular uptake can have a particularly significant clinical impact on pharmacotherapy; thus, this field of research has gained increased attention in recent years [7]. The organic anion transporting polypeptides OATP1B1 and OATP1B3 are examples of such transporters that can facilitate the uptake of a diverse array of xenobiotics, including many anticancer drugs, into the liver in advance of metabolism, and that are sensitive to inhibition by other medicines given concurrently.

Two of the most commonly acknowledged risk factors of DDIs are polypharmacy and advanced age [2,8–10]. Consistent with this notion, cancer patients are particularly at high risk for the occurrence of potentially harmful DDIs, since they often take a large number of medications concomitantly, which tends to increase as their disease progresses, and because the majority of cancer diagnoses happens in older ages [10,11]. Indeed, prior investigations have demonstrated that as many as 30% of cancer patients receiving chemotherapeutic treatment are at a risk for DDIs [12,13]. As the number of new treatment options in oncology continues to grow, DDIs are increasingly recognized as significant health hazards that can negatively influence treatment outcomes. These issues are particularly concerning given the increasing use orally-administered chemotherapeutic agents. While such drugs offer advantages in terms of patient preference, the convenience of use, reduced healthcare resource utilization, the possibility to achieve sustained drug exposure associated with the need for chronic use without requiring prolonged drug infusions, and may improve the overall quality of life, recent studies have suggested that the use of such agents increases the risk of potentially serious DDIs with commonly used outpatient medications [14]. In addition, unsupervised administration of other medications as well as their possibly prolonged use has been advanced as concerns with oral chemotherapy drugs, which could potentiate DDIs that may remain unanticipated. Although recent studies have suggested that the prevalence of DDIs with oral chemotherapy drugs is as high as 50% with nearly 20% potentially increasing toxicity, the clinical impact of DDIs involving oral chemotherapy remains largely unstudied [10].

In this article, we provide an overview of this field of research in relation to tyrosine kinase inhibitors (TKIs), a rapidly expanding group of orally-administered drugs commonly used in the treatment of solid tumors and hematological malignancies, with particular emphasis on OATP1B1- and OATP1B3-related mechanisms. In addition to reviewing existing published data, we aimed to identify potential knowledge gaps that could help improve our understanding of the clinical impact of DDIs mediated through this mechanism.

2. Tyrosine Kinase Inhibitors (TKIs)

Since the US Food and Drug Administration (FDA) approval of the first TKI, imatinib, in 2001 for the treatment of chronic myeloid leukemia (CML), almost 50 additional TKIs have been approved for the treatment of various cancers, and many more are currently being developed and evaluated [15,16]. Protein tyrosine kinases (PTKs) are enzymes that catalyze the transfer of a gamma phosphate group from adenosine triphosphate (ATP) to a tyrosine residue on a protein. The phosphorylation of PTKs leads to the downstream activation of signal transduction pathways that are important in the regulation of cell growth, differentiation, and a series of other physiological and biochemical processes involved in cell survival and migration. Dysregulation of PTK function results in proliferation disorders, with those most notably being cancers [17–19]. Because of their importance in signal transduction, many PTKs have been the target of therapeutic intervention with the use of small-molecule TKIs. As a result, TKIs function by competing with ATP for the ATP-binding pocket of PTKs, thus reducing the downstream signaling cascade and provide useful targeted strategies in oncogenic treatment [20,21].

While TKIs have revolutionized anticancer therapy, some challenges have also risen in the use of these agents. Unlike conventional cytotoxic agents that are given intravenously, TKIs are administered orally and daily for prolonged periods [22]. As mentioned before, while this is more convenient, this also increases their susceptibility to unpredictable patterns of oral absorption and causes both wide inter-individual pharmacokinetic variability and potential for DDIs with co-administered agents [23–25]. Most TKIs are highly prone to cause DDIs [26], as patients receiving these agents are often subsequently treated for concomitant diseases, and because polypharmacy is highly prevalent [25]. Comorbid conditions such as hypertension, chronic obstructive pulmonary disease, diabetes, cardiovascular disease, congestive heart failure, and peripheral vascular disease are frequently reported in the population of cancer patients [27], and this further increases the risk for potential DDIs. Indeed, a recent study indicated that 97.1% of patients receiving treatment with TKIs were using at least one other drug simultaneously, with a median of 4 concurrent medications, and 47.4% experienced at least one potential TKI-mediated DDI [28]. In another study, 44.7% of the potential DDIs identified involving TKIs were considered severe [29]. Interestingly, most available data in this field have investigated TKIs as victims in DDIs [30–33], and conclusive information on their role as perpetrators in DDIs is generally lacking.

3. Organic Anion Transporting Polypeptides (OATPs)

The vast majority of orally-administered TKIs are eliminated from the body by enzyme-mediated metabolism, which occurs predominantly in the liver, followed by biliary or urinary excretion of the metabolites. These processes require drugs to cross the selectively permeable biological membrane of hepatocytes and are dependent, at least in part, on interaction with membrane transporters. These include the organic anion transporting polypeptides (OATPs), a family of influx transporters expressed in various tissues, including the liver [34–36]. Experimental studies with TKIs have predominantly evaluated transport by the liver-specific transporters OATP1B1 and OATP1B3, which are encoded by the *SLCO1B1* and *SLCO1B3* genes [37], respectively. Moreover, it has also been shown that some TKIs can additionally act as inhibitors of the transporters for which they are substrates [38]. Inhibition of OATPs can lead to defective elimination, result in sudden increases in plasma concentration and area under the curve (AUC) for drugs that are substrates of these transporters [36], and ultimately increase the risk of therapy-related side effects. Known substrates of OATP1B1 and OATP1B3 include statins, repaglinide, olmesartan, enalapril, valsartan, several xenobiotic glucuronide metabolites, as well as a host of cytotoxic chemotherapeutic agents, including the taxanes paclitaxel and docetaxel, the platinum-based drug cisplatin, and methotrexate. As hypertension and diabetes are among the prevalent comorbidities in cancer patients, many xenobiotic OATP1B1 and OATP1B3 substrate drugs are likely to be co-administrated with OATP-inhibitory TKIs, and therefore, clinically significant toxicities such as rhabdomyolysis, hyperkalemia, and hypoglycemia can be anticipated [39–41].

4. Regulatory Guidance Documents

As more and more DDIs involving uptake transporters have been reported in recent years, so have regulatory agencies such as the FDA and the European Medicines Agency (EMA) put increasing emphasis on investigating each new drug entity for their potential to induce/inhibit such transporters. It should be noted that both the "EMA Guideline on the Investigation of Drug Interactions" and "FDA guidance for In Vitro Drug Interaction Studies—Cytochrome P450 Enzyme- and Transporter-Mediated Drug Interactions" recognize the fact that the field of transporter interaction assessments is still rapidly evolving and therefore the recommendations offered are relatively flexible and advocate the use of a variety of methods. However, some specifications have been proposed as a means to ensure that the in vitro models have optimal prediction potential for transporter-mediated interactions:

- Both the FDA and EMA documents suggest that the sponsor should conduct in vitro studies to evaluate whether an investigational drug is an inhibitor of OATP1B1 and/or OATP1B3.
- Both documents recommend using an appropriate, predictive in vitro models, such as human hepatocytes or mammalian cells engineered to overexpress transporters of interest (e.g., CHO, HEK293, MDCK) to explore potential transporter interactions.
- Different concentrations of the investigational drug on the transport of a specific substrate should be investigated, such that at least 3 and 4 concentrations should be tested, according to EMA and FDA guidance documents, respectively, and values for the inhibition constant (Ki) should be obtained, with known inhibitors present as controls.
- According to EMA, Ki values that are lower than a concentration representing 25-fold the unbound hepatic inlet concentration after oral administration warrant the conduct of an in vivo DDI study with the use of a prototypical probe substrate. The most recent FDA guidance, which aligns with the EMA, uses unbound concentrations of the investigational drug, not the total drug, for the

calculation of R values with the formula $R = 1 + ((fu,p \times Iin,max)/ IC_{50})$ where fu,p is the unbound fraction in plasma, IC_{50} is the half-maximal inhibitory concentration and Iin, max is the estimated maximum plasma inhibitor concentration at the inlet to the liver. An R-value ≥ 1.1 suggests that the drug has the potential to inhibit OATP1B1 and/or OATP1B3 in vivo.

- The 2017 version of the FDA guidance on in vitro assessment of DDIs requires a strategy employing a 30-min preincubation with the inhibitor before the addition of substrate. Although this design is recommended as it may lead to changes in the observed IC_{50} values, the latest version of the guidance does not specify an exact duration of the preincubation conditions.
- The FDA guidance also mentions that the observed degree of inhibition by a particular agent can be dependent on the substrate used in the experiment, and therefore it has been suggested that substrates more likely to be used in clinical studies, or substrates that usually generate lower IC_{50} values for known inhibitors should be chosen in in vitro investigations to avoid underestimation of effects in vivo.

5. Identification and Retrieval of Relevant Data

Acquisition of the data for this article was compiled independently up to and including June 2020 by various members of the Division of Pharmaceutics and Pharmacology at the Ohio State University with specific expertise in drug transporters (D.A.G.), pharmacy (Z.T.), and cancer pharmacology (E.D.E.), and subsequently reviewed by members with expertise in pharmacokinetics (A.S.) and TKIs (S.D.B.). Data on FDA-approved TKIs was extracted from the full prescribing information as provided by the respective drug manufacturers. A search was subsequently conducted using publicly-available, unpublished databases from the FDA and EMA guidance documents for industry to further collect information on OATP1B1 and OATP1B3 inhibition studies previously conducted for each of the TKIs (Figure 1). It should be noted that although published studies have indicated that certain TKIs such as erlotinib are inhibitors of 2B1 and can cause DDIs, this was considered beyond the scope of the present article since regulatory guidance documents lack information on this transporter [42].

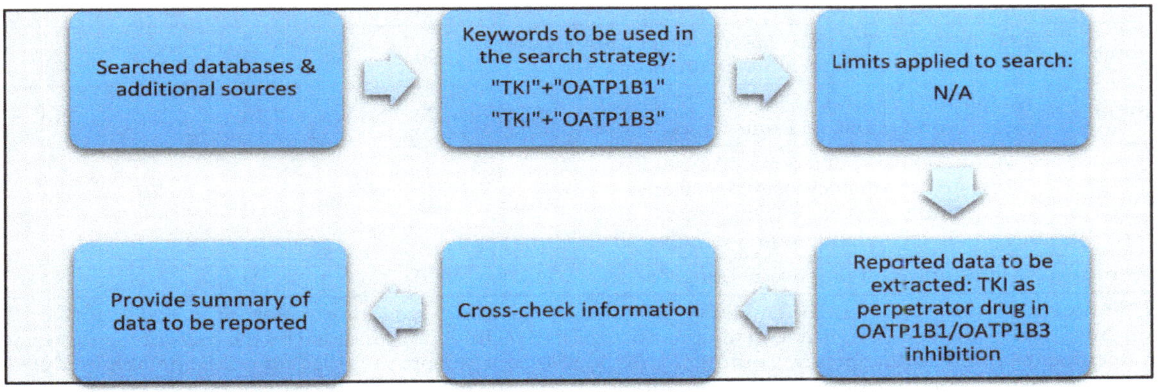

Figure 1. Applied methods for the acquisition of relevant data on TKI-related interactions with OATP1B1 and OATP1B3.

All DDI data included for consideration focused exclusively on the TKIs as inhibitors of the transporter (the perpetrator) of interest. The selection of relevant literature articles for inclusion was performed based on predefined inclusion/exclusion criteria, where eligible articles included either peer-reviewed publications, meeting abstracts, and previously published reviews. As a primary search module, PubMed (National Library of Medicine) was utilized to identify potentially relevant publications using the following MeSH terms in the search strategy: ["TKI of interest"] AND [OATP1B1] or ["TKI of interest"] AND [OATP1B3]. Google Scholar was consecutively consulted to ensure no published article of relevance to this literature review was omitted. Three authors (D.A.G., Z.T., and E.D.E.) independently reviewed the collected data for eligibility and accuracy. In our analysis, concordant outcomes were defined as those for which the prescribing information, documentation from the FDA and/or EMA, and all the retrieved published literature on a specific TKI were in agreement that the TKI was either an inhibitor or not an inhibitor of OATP1B1 and/or OATP1B3. Outcomes were considered discordant outcomes if the identified reports on a particular TKI regarding its inhibitory properties towards OATP1B1 and/or OATP1B3 were conflicting. All data of relevance was tabulated to highlight such discrepancies (see below).

6. Effects of TKIs on the Function of OATP1B1 and OATP1B3

A descriptive summary of the main findings resulting from surveying the available prescribing information (PIs), and FDA and EMA guidance documents are shown in Table 1. The PIs showed that of the 48 FDA-approved TKIs evaluated, 7 (15%) are claimed to be inhibitors of OATP1B1 and 5 (10%) are inhibitors of OATP1B3. In addition, it is reported that of those 48 TKIs, 22 (48%) and 21 (44%) are reported in the PIs to not be inhibitors of OATP1B1 or OATP1B3, respectively. However, it is of note that the PIs for 19 (40%) of the TKIs do not mention whether or not drug interactions with OATP1B1 are of concern, and 22 (46%) do not mention that information for OATP1B3. As shown in Table 1, some inconsistencies were observed for some TKIs between what is reported in the regulatory guidance. Many of the differences can be accounted for by differences in cutoff for IC_{50} values (shown in Supplementary Materials Tables S1–S9).

Table 1. Comparison of regulatory guidance documents on OATP1B inhibition by FDA-approved TKIs.

TKI	Disease Indication	Kinase Target	OATP1B1			OATP1B3		
			PI	FDA	EMA	PI	FDA	EMA
Bacritinib	Rheumatoid Arthritis	JAK	No	No	No	Yes	Yes	No
Ceritinib	Metastatic Non-Small Cell Lung Cancer	ALK	No	Yes	No	No	Yes	No
Crizotinib	Metastatic Non-Small Cell Lung Cancer	ALK, ROS1	No	Yes	-	No	Yes	-
Laroctrectinib	Solid Tumors	NTKR	No	No	Yes	No	No	No
Lenvatinib	Differentiated Thyroid Cancer, Renal Cell Carcinoma, Hepatocellular Carcinoma	VEGFR	No	Yes	Yes	No	No	No
Lorlatinib	Anaplastic Lymphoma Positive Metastatic Non-Small Cell Lung Cancer	ALK	No	No	Yes	No	No	Yes
Midostaurin	Acute Myeloid Leukemia, Aggressive Systemic Mastocytosis, Associated Hematological Neoplasm, Mast Cell Leukemia	FLT3	Yes	Yes	Yes	-	Yes	No
Osimertinib	Metastatic Non-Small Cell Lung Cancer	EGFR	No	No	Yes	No	No	Yes

"Yes" indicates a TKI as an OATP1B1/3 inhibitor provided by the prescribing information, FDA documents, or EMA documents. "No" indicates a TKI is not an inhibitor of OATP1B1/3 inhibitor provided by the prescribing information, FDA documents, or EMA documents. Sources: PI, FDA, EMA documents provided on public databases, details of the links can be found in the Supplementary Materials. Access date: May 2020.

Next, we conducted a literature search on published data addressing OATP1B1 or OATP1B3 inhibition by different TKIs. In vitro, in vivo, and clinical data were extracted. The details of the articles were inserted into tables (shown in Supplementary Materials Tables S1–S9) [43–47] For alectinib, avapritinib, baracitinib, binimetinib, brigatinib, cobimetinib, dacomitinib, encorafenib, erdafitnib, fedratinib, gilteritinib, ibrutinib, laroctrectinib, lorlatinib, midostaurin, pexidartinib, ponatinib, trametinib, and zanbrutinib no published reports were found. In data collected for 17 TKIs, the results of the published data were largely inconsistent in that some of the published results for a given TKI identified the TKI as an inhibitor of OATP1B1 or OATP1B3, while other sources identified it expressly as a non-inhibitor. It should be noted that different transfected cell lines (Flp-In T-Rex293, HEK293, MDCK-II, CHO, SF9, or HepaRG) and different substrates were used in the various studies. The latter included estradiol-17b-D-glucuronide (E2G), 8-(2-(fluoresceinyl)-aminoethylthio)-adenosine-3′,5′-cyclic monophosphate (8FcA), fluorescein (FL), 2′,7′-dichlorofluorescein (DCF), valsartan, atorvastatin, SN-38, Na-Fluo, fluvastatin, estrone-3-sulfate (E1S) for OATP1B1 and taurocholic acid (TCA), cholecystokinin octapeptide (CCK-8) for OATP1B3. Furthermore, the preincubation time, the method of detection, the data analysis metric (percent inhibition or IC_{50}), and even the concentration of the TKI were found to vary among the published reports. The details of these methodological differences are summarized in Table 2.

Data from clinical and in vivo studies were also collected and reviewed for this article, the results of which can be seen in the supplements. Very few studies have directly investigated the role of OATPs in TKI pharmacokinetics with different methodologies, however the results from available studies seem to be consistent with regulatory data. Since the main scope of this review is to focus on discrepancies between published data and FDA and EMA guidelines, their results were not further explored here. Moreover, as OATP1B1 and OATP1B3 substrates used in the retrieved data have complex pharmacokinetic profiles involving drug-metabolizing enzymes and other transporters, the results of such case reports should be carefully analyzed to decide on the importance of each part of the pathway [48–59].

6.1. *Omissions*

In numerous studies, TKIs have been indicated as victims in DDIs while considerably less is known about their role as perpetrators via transporter inhibition [32,60–64]. In this context, it is noteworthy that transporter inhibition studies are not required by regulatory agencies for approval, but rather recommended to evaluate DDI potential [38].

Currently, there are 20 FDA approved TKIs for which the PI does not contain any information on their inhibitory effects on OATP1B1 and/or OATP1B3, and this is the case for both agents approved long ago as well as those that were approved more recently. The transport interactions of some of these omitted drugs have been examined by academic investigators as reported in the published literature, and it seems prudent that this information is captured and included in the future in individual PIs and regulatory databases alike. Interestingly, we found that some of the PIs address DDIs that are plausibly attributable to OATPs but this is not always consistently acknowledged due to inconclusive mechanistic insights. For example, dasatinib can dramatically increase plasma levels of the dual OATP1B1 and CYP3A4 substrate, simvastatin, and the individual contribution of each one of these pharmacokinetic components to the DDI is not clearly defined. On the other hand, for many TKIs, no data were found in the published literature on their potential to inhibit OATP1B1 and/or OATP1B3.

6.2. *Discrepancies*

The discrepancies observed during our evaluation can be categorized into two groups: discrepancies between the information provided by EMA and FDA, and discrepancies between different published articles. Table 1 summarizes the cases where data provided by FDA and EMA data were not congruent in terms of reported OATP-inhibitory properties of TKIs. Specific discrepancies of interest are highlighted below. Authors do acknowledge that reporting an IC_{50}, even when it is relatively low, does not guarantee a significant clinical impact, unless special formulas are implemented, therefore the inconsistencies reported here, address instances where the guidance is not followed and the reported IC_{50} is not further explored:

- The PI and FDA guidance documents for baricitinib report the agent as an OATP1B3 inhibitor, whereas the EMA documents claim that it is not an inhibitor of this transporter. The existence of this discrepancy is not explained or discussed in any of the regulatory materials.
- For ceritinib, the PI and EMA state that based on in vitro data, the TKI is unlikely to inhibit OATP1B1 and OATP1B3 at clinically-relevant concentrations. However, the FDA guidance document for ceritinib reports that ceritinib inhibits OATP1B1 and OATP1B3 by 31.8% and 24.1%, respectively, and that because the R-value is <1.25, an in vivo study was considered unnecessary.

However, the FDA guidance on DDI potential states that a drug has the potential to inhibit OATP1B1 or OATP1B3 in vivo if the R-value is >1.1

- The PI for crizotinib reports the TKI as not an inhibitor of OATP1B1 or OATP1B3, but the FDA guidance reports that crizotinib demonstrated a weak, concentration-dependent inhibitory effect on pravastatin, an OATP1B1 substrate, and rosuvastatin, an OATP1B3 substrate uptake, with IC_{50} values of 48 μM and 44 μM, respectively.
- The PI and FDA documents state that OATP1B1 and OATP1B3 are not inhibited by laroctrectinib, although the EMA materials state that there are inhibitory effects of laroctrectinib on OATP1B1 with an IC_{50} of 48 μM.
- For lenvatinib, the PI states that there is no potential to inhibit OATP1B1 *in vivo*, whereas in the FDA guidance it is concluded that lenvatinib inhibited OATP1B1 with an IC_{50} of 7.29 μM.
- The PI and FDA report that lorlatinib does not inhibit OATP1B1 and OATP1B3, while the EMA claims that this TKI has the potential to inhibit these transporters at clinically-relevant concentrations.
- For osimertinib, the PI and FDA information state that is no observed inhibition of OATP1B1 and OATP1B3, whereas the EMA claims that osimertinib inhibits transport by OATP1B1 and OATP1B3 albeit at concentrations that are unlikely to result in a clinically-significant DDI.

Some of the potential explanations for these discrepancies are similar to those responsible for the apparent discrepant data between different published articles and are discussed in more detail below. However, some interesting points might explain the inconsistencies in regulatory data, such as the equations used to establish whether a clinical evaluation is indeed necessary for the drug or not. While EMA suggests calculating ($R = 1 + Iu,in,max/Ki$ or $IC_{50}) \geq 1.04$, FDA uses a different equation and different cutoff criteria ($R = 1 + Iu,in,max/Ki$ or $IC_{50}) \geq 1.1$). This latter equation has been suggested in the latest FDA draft guidance, although prior versions of this document have proposed alternative criteria for consideration. It has also been suggested recently that, while most of the proposed equations and criteria hold merit, they are different in terms of their potential to ultimately arrive at false positive and false negative predictions. In particular, it has been suggested that the equation applied in the EMA guidance has a lower positive predictive value than the one proposed in the current FDA guidance, which offers arguably more dependable predictions [65]. When comparing data from these two regulatory agencies, this aspect should be taken into consideration, along with different manners of data reporting (either with or without calculation of the R-value), and variation in reported IC_{50} values that could be due to differences in the applied methods.

The results of our comparative literature survey also show that there are instances of substantial inconsistency between reports in the published literature as well as between published studies and publicly-available data reported by manufacturers. Since all this collective work is ultimately aimed at improving clinical decision making, it is pertinent to establish an unequivocal, dependable approach to data interpretation. The following are some of the elements that can potentially contribute to the reported inconsistencies:

- Inhibitor concentration: A large number of the published articles have relied on the use of a single concentration of TKI, although regulatory guidance documents specifically recommend the need to perform experiments with at least 3–4 different concentrations, in order to more rigorously evaluate potential inhibitory properties. This is exemplified by a recent study involving the TKIs afatinib, nintedanib, lenvatinib, and ceritinib in which diverse degrees of inhibition were observed depending on the concentration (up to 30 μM), and where some concentrations would even increase transport function [66]. As TKIs tend to get concentrated in the liver and can potentially increase intracellular levels that are much higher than concurrent levels in plasma [2], the selection of relevant concentration ranges to be used in in vitro uptake studies requires careful consideration.

- Data reporting: Several studies have only reported results as percent inhibition relative to control, while more quantitative measures (IC_{50} or inhibition constant) might be more informative and offer increased predictive value. According to regulatory guidance documents, certain equations could be utilized to predict if the observed degree of inhibition has potential clinical relevance. However, such strategies are rarely implemented and reported studies often fail to include positive and negative control inhibitors into the experimental design, which is recommended in the regulatory guidance documents. These issues complicate the interpretation of data and can result in discrepant views on extrapolating from in vitro studies to the clinical situation, as reported for ruxolitinib or crizotinib, where experimental data would suggest statistically significant but not clinically relevant degrees of inhibition [67–69].
- Substrate selection: Since substrate-dependent inhibition by xenobiotics, including TKIs, has been well documented and is acknowledged expressly in the FDA guidance document, the degree to which findings obtained with one particular substrate can be extrapolated to other conditions is uncertain, and potentially accounts for several reported inconsistencies. Substrate-dependent inhibition has been previously reported when comparing inhibitory properties in OATP1B1-overexpressed models comparing the substrates fluorescein (FL), 2′,7′-dichlorofluorescein (DCF), atorvastatin, SN-38, and valsartan, as well as in a recent study comparing E2G and 8Fc-A [66], where some TKIs such as lapatinib, pazopanib, and nintedanib show inhibitory effects with some but not all test substrates. The difference between the results for different substrates is occasionally quite substantial; for example, ceritinib can cause 50% inhibition of OATP1B1 function when using FL, DCF, atorvastatin, or SN-38 as test substrates, but causes an apparent increase (by 50%) in OATP1B1-mediated transport of valsartan. Similar results have been reported for nintedanib, which stimulated the OATP1B1-mediated uptake of FL and valsartan, while inhibiting that of DCF and SN-38 (by 70%). One strategy recommended by the FDA to prevent the creation of such apparent, internally conflicting results is to advocate the use of test substrates in the in vitro model system that is predicted to generate the lowest IC_{50} value, or alternatively, to use the most clinically-relevant substrate. While this is a generally useful approach, several published examples highlight the limitations associated with this strategy. For example, Koide et al., have demonstrated that the use of DCF as a model substrate generates the lowest IC_{50} values for most but not necessarily all substrate-inhibitor combinations [66,68] and that TKIs with known OATP1B1-inhibitory properties, such as pazopanib, fail to affect transport function when using the clinically relevant substrates atorvastatin and valsartan [70–73]. The reported differences in inhibitory properties of TKIs toward the function of transporters such as OATP1B1 as a function of the test substrate used in in vitro studies can directly impact calculated R-values, and influence the reliability of DDI predictions and the clinical decision-making process, especially for weak-to-moderate inhibitors [74].
- Incubation conditions: Several studies have demonstrated that the mechanism by which TKIs inhibit the function of OATP1B1 and/or OATP1B1 can be time-dependent [75], for example in the case of pazopanib, where preincubation times are inversely correlated with the degree of transport inhibition such as that longer preincubation times result in lower IC_{50} estimates [72]. The FDA guidance recommends the inclusion of a preincubation condition, in addition to simultaneous incubation of inhibitor and substrate, to ensure that optimal prediction values can be derived from in vitro experiments. Despite this recommendation, most of the published literature fails to provide specific detail on the design of the reported experiments where the preincubation condition is either not considered or not defined. Although the original FDA guidance recommendation was to include preincubation times of up to 30 min in the experimental study design, recent studies have demonstrated that more prolonged times, for example, one hour in the case of dasatinib or even up to three hours for other compounds, may be required to obtained reliable results [45,76]. Proper consideration of this aspect is especially relevant for a class of agents such as TKIs as they are generally administrated daily for prolonged periods, and may cause transporter inhibition

predominantly through an indirect, kinase-mediated mechanism involving post-translational events that affect tyrosine phosphorylation. This suggests that a comprehensive evaluation of TKI-transporter inhibition studies require careful consideration and optimization of preincubation times in order to derive translationally useful DDI predictions.

- Cell line selection: Although regulatory guidance documents do not currently expressly specify any particular cell-based model system for standardized use in in vitro transporter studies, prior findings have supported the notion that the choice of cell lines used for transfection can influence conclusions about inhibitory properties of xenobiotics. Indeed, McFeely et al. have argued that the selection of cell lines as one of the most important factors contributing to variability in observed OATP-mediated transport inhibition when using in vitro models [75]. In addition to intrinsic differences between commonly used cell lines that may be linked with differential baseline expression of other transport mechanisms of putative relevance and artificial compensatory dysregulation of other transporters in overexpressed models, factors such cell origin (e.g., mammalian vs amphibian), cell passage number, cell culture conditions, and maintenance procedures, seeding density, media composition (e.g., presence of binding proteins), and duration of time that cells are in culture (e.g., expression drifting), which are often not clearly documented, could further affect the outcome of each study [77].
- Other contributing variables: In addition to the considerations outlined above as well as in Table 2 and Supplementary Materials Tables S1–S9, several other factors can contribute to variation in the reported transport inhibition data. These include the use of non-standardized software when calculating kinetic parameters such as IC_{50} or Ki, and the implementation of varying methods in quantifying levels of substrate drugs used in the transport assays [77,78]. An example of the latter would the use of an LC-MS/MS-based method to measure the intracellular levels of unchanged substrate drugs, whereas more commonly studies would employ the use of fluorescent substrates of radiolabeled substrates that would be analyzed for total fluorescence or total radioactivity, respectively, and thus would simultaneously measure the total of the parent drug and metabolite(s) formed intracellularly. This is an important methodological difference as certain compounds can undergo rapid enzyme-mediated metabolism once inside cells to form metabolites that may easily escape detection and result in underestimating the actual extent of uptake. Furthermore, even the use of identical protocols in different locales can influence the outcome of particular experimental studies as a result of uncontrollable factors such as interlaboratory differences, as has been documented extensively before for P-glycoprotein IC_{50} determinations [77]. It should also be pointed out that inconsistencies, as reported here for inhibition of OATP1B1- and OATP1B3-mediated transport, are relatively common and have previously been documented for models involving several other drug-metabolizing enzymes and transporters with a putative relevance in predicting clinically relevant DDIs [77,79,80].

Table 2. Inconsistencies in reporting OATP1B inhibition by TKIs in published literature.

TKI	1B1 Inhibitor	Reported Values	1B3 Inhibitor	Reported Values	Model	Pre-Incubation (mins)	Substrate	References
Bosutinib	Yes	>60% inhibition at 10 μM			Flp-In T-Rex293/OATP1B1*1A	15	0.1 mM (3H) (E2G)	FDA: No [68,70,81]
	No	121 ± 6% function remaining after incubation with 10 μM	No	109 ± 5% function remaining after incubation with 10 μM	HEK293/OATP1B1 or 3	UNK	300 nM E3S (1B1) or 2 nM CCK-8 (1B3)	
	Yes	>25% 10 μM on E2G, >50% on 8Fc-A			HEK293/OATP1B1	15	E2G 8Fc-A	

Table 2. *Cont.*

TKI	1B1 Inhibitor	Reported Values	1B3 Inhibitor	Reported Values	Model	Pre-Incubation (mins)	Substrate	References
Cabozantinib	No	>15 µM	No	>10 µM	MDCK-II cell monolayers	UNK	OATP1B1: 2 µM; E2G OATP1B3: 2 µM CCK	EMA: No [66,82]
	Yes	59% inhibition at 30 µM			HEK/OATP1B1		3 µM FL	
	Yes	61% inhibition at 30 µM			HEK/OATP1B1		1 µM DCF	
	Yes	74% inhibition at 30 µM			HEK/OATP1B1		1 µM Valsartan	
Ceritinib	Yes	50% inhibition at 30 µM			HEK/OATP1B1	10	3 µM FL	FDA: Yes, PI: No [66]
	Yes	50% inhibition at 30 µM			HEK/OATP1B1	10	1 µM DCF	
	Yes	50% inhibition at 30 µM			HEK/OATP1B1	10	0.5 µM atorvastatin	
	Yes	50% inhibition at 30 µM			HEK/OATP1B1	10	1 µM SN-38	
	No	150% stimulation at 30 µM			HEK/OATP1B1	10	1 µM valsartan	
Crizotinib	No		No		HEK/OATP1B1 or 1B3		11nM (3H]E3S [1B1) 50nM (3H)TCA (1B3) 0.5 µM fluvastatin (1B1) 2 µM fluvastatin (; 1B1)	FDA: Yes, PI: No [67,68]
	Yes	>25% inhibition at 10 µM			HEK293/OATP1B1	15	E2G 8Fc-A	
Erlotinib	No		No		CHO/OATP-1B1 and -1B3	UNK	0.25 µCi/mL (3H)ES (for OATP-1B1) or (3H)CCK-8 (for OATP-1B3)	NI [68,70,81,83]
	Yes	>60% decrease at 10 µM			Flp-In T-Rex293/OATP1B1*1A	15	0.1 mM (3H) (E2G)	
	No	104 ± 5% function remaining after incubation with 10 µM	Yes	50% inhibition at 1.19 µM	HEK293/OATP1B1 or 3	UNK	300 nM E3S (1B1) or 2 nM CCK-8 (1B3)	
	Yes	>25% inhibtion at 10 µM on E2G, >50% inhibition on 8Fc-A			HEK293/OATP1B1	15	E2G 8Fc-A	
Gefitinib	Yes	>70% decrease with 10 µM			Flp-In T-Rex293/OATP1B1*1A	15	0.1 mM (3H) E2G	NI [67,68,70,81]
	Yes	50% inhibition at 17.2 ± 1.47 µM,	Yes	18.8 ± 2.74 mM	HEK293/OATP1B1, OATP1B3,		fluvastatin	
			Inducer	EC50 value of 14.1 ± 4.6 mM	HEK293/ OATP1B1, OATP1B3,		(3H)TCA	
	No	105 ± 3% function remaining after incubation with 10 µM	No	78 ± 3% function remaining after incubation with 10 µM	HEK293/OATP1B1 or 3	UNK	300 nM E3S (1B1) or 2 nM CCK-8 (1B3)	
	Yes	>25% inhibition at 10 µM on E2G, >75% inhibition on 8Fc-A			HEK293/OATP1B1	15	E2G 8Fc-A	
Imatinib	Yes	~20% inhibition at 10 µM			Flp-In T-Rex29/OATP1B1	15	0.1 mM (3H) E2G	NI [47,68,70]
	No				Sf9 /OATP1b1	5	1 µM Na-Fluo	
	Yes	>25% inhibition at 10 µM on both			HEK293/OATP1B1	15	E2G 8Fc-A	

Table 2. *Cont.*

TKI	1B1 Inhibitor	Reported Values	1B3 Inhibitor	Reported Values	Model	Pre-Incubation (mins)	Substrate	References
Lapatinib	Yes	>70% inhibition at 10 μM			HEK293/OATP1B1	15	E2G8Fc-A	YES [68,70,81,84,85]
	Yes	>70% inhibition at 10 μM			Flp-In T-Rex29/ OATP1B1	15	0.1 mM (3H) E2G	
	No		Yes, slight inhibition		CHO/ OATP-1B1 or -1B3	UNK	fluro-methotrexate	
	Yes	50% inhibition at 4.0 μM (Sd:2.1)			CHO-OATP1B1	15–30	(3H) E2G	
	No	123 ± 13% function remaining after incubation with 10 μM	No	98 ± 16% function remaining after incubation with 10 μM	HEK293/OATP1B1 or 3	UNK	300 nM E3S (1B1) or 2 nM CCK-8 (1B3)	
Neratinib	No				HEK/OATP1B1	10	3 μM FL	EMA:No [66,81]
	No				HEK/OATP1B1	10	1 μM DCF	
	No				HEK/OATP1B1	10	0.5 μM atorvastatin	
	Yes	30% inhibition at 30 μM			HEK/OATP1B1	10	1 μM SN-38	
	No				HEK/OATP1B1	10	1 μM valsartan	
	No	123 ± 13% function remaining after incubation with 10 μM	Yes	50% inhibition at 18.13 ± 1.21	HEK293/OATP1B1 or 3	UNK	300 nM E3S (1B1) or 2nM CCK-8 (1B3)	
Nilotinib	No				HEK/OATP1B1	10	3 μM FL	NI [66,68,70,83,86,87]
	Yes	~50% inhibition at 30 μM			HEK/OATP1B1	10	1 μM DCF	
	Yes	~50% inhibition at 30 μM			HEK/OATP1B1	10	0.5 μM atorvastatin	
	Yes	~50% inhibition at 30 μM			HEK/OATP1B1	10	1 μM SN-38	
	Yes	~50% inhibition at 30 μM			HEK/OATP1B1	10	1 μM valsartan	
	Yes	>95% inhibition at 10 μM			Flp-In T-Rex29/ OATP1B1	10	0.1 mM (3H) E2G	
	No	110 ± 7% stimulation at 10 μM	No	100 ± 3% function remaining after incubation with 10 μM	HEK293/OATP1B1 or 3	UNK	300 nM E3S (1B1) or 2nM CCK-8 (1B3)	
	Yes	>80% inhibition at 0–20 μM			HEK/OATP1B1		5–40 μM 8Fc-A or 2 μM E2G	
	Yes	50% inhibition at 1.3 μM	Yes		HEK293/OATP1B1 or 3		E2G or 8FcA	
	Yes	>50% at 10 μM, IC_{50}: ~1 μM			HEK293/OATP1B1	15	E2G or 8FcA	
	Yes	50% inhibition at 2.78 ± 1.13 μM	No		CHO/ OATP-1B1 or -1B3		0.25 μCi/mL (3H)ES (for OATP-1B1) or (3H)CCK-8 (for OATP-1B3)	
Nintedanib	No	312% stimulation at 30 μM			HEK/OATP1B1		3 μM FL	No [66]
	Yes	74% inhibition at 30 μM			HEK/OATP1B1		1 μM DCF	
	No	133% stimulation at 30 μM			HEK/OATP1B1		1 μM Valsartan	
	Yes	78% inhibition at 30 μM			HEK/OATP1B1		1 μM SN-38	

Table 2. *Cont.*

TKI	1B1 Inhibitor	Reported Values	1B3 Inhibitor	Reported Values	Model	Pre-Incubation (mins)	Substrate	References
Pazopanib	No	120% stimulation at 30 μM			HEK/OATP1B1	10	3 μM FL	Yes [66,68,70–73,83]
	No				HEK/OATP1B1	10	1 μM DCF	
	No				HEK/OATP1B1	10	0.5 μM atorvastatin	
	No				HEK/OATP1B1	10	1 μM SN-38	
	No				HEK/OATP1B1	10	1 μM valsartan	
	Yes	50% inhibition 3.89 ± 1.21 μM	No		CHO/ OATP-1B1 or -1B3		0.25 μCi/mL of (3H)ES (for OATP-1B1) or (3H)CCK-8 (for OATP-1B3)	
	Yes	>50% inhibition with 8Fc-A, >90% inhibition with E2G			HEK293/OATP1B1	15	E2G or (1B1),8FcA (1B1, 1B3)	
	Yes	50% inhibition at 0.79 μM			CHO-OATP1B1	15–30	(3H)-EG	
	No				HEK293/OATP1B1		SN-38	
	Yes	>95% inhibition at 10 μM			Flp-In T-Rex29/OATP1B1	15	0.1 μM (3H) E2G	
	Yes	IC_{50} E1S: 1.42 ± 0.23, IC_{50} E2G: 13.5 ± 6.0			HEK293/OATP1B1	0	(3H) E1S and (3H) E2G	
	Yes	IC_{50} E1S:0.594 ± 0.030 IC_{50} E2G: 7.25 ± 0.53			HEK293/OATP1B2	1	(3H) (E1S) and (3H) E2G	
	Yes	IC_{50} E1S: 0.374 ± 0.074, IC_{50} E2G: 2.58 ± 0.77			HEK293/OATP1B4	30	(3H) E1S and (3H) E2G	
	Yes	IC_{50} E1S: 0.530 ± 0.022, IC_{50} E2G:2.03 ± 0.71			HEK293/OATP1B5	60	(3H) E1S and (3H) E2G	
Regorafenib	No	30% stimulation			HEK293/OATP1B6	10	0.5 μM Atorvastatin	FDA: No [66,68,70,88]
	Yes	50% inhibition at ~10 μM	No		HEK293/OATP1B1/1B3	2	estrone-3-sulfate (1B1)/taurocholic acid (1B3)	
	Yes	>50% inhibition at 10 μM			Flp-In T-Rex29/ OATP1B1	15	0.1mM (3H) E2G	
	Yes	>50% inhibition			HEK293/OATP1B1	15	E2G, 8FcA	
Ruxolitinib	Yes	>25% inhibition at 10 μM on 8Fc-A			HEK293/OATP1B1	15	E2G, 8FcA	No [68–70]
	No				HepaRG		4 nM E3S	
	Yes	~20% inhibition at 10 μM			Flp-In T-Rex29/ OATP1B1	15	0.1mM (3H) E2G	
Sorafenib	Yes	>75% at 10 μM on both			HEK293/OATP1B1	15	E2G, 8FcA	NI [66,70,81]
	Yes	>90% inhibition at 10 μM			Flp-In T-Rex293/OATP1B1*1A	15	(3H) E2G 0.1 mM	
	Yes	50% inhibition at 69.6 μM			Flp-In T-Rex293/ OATP1B1*1A	15	0.1 mM (3H) docetaxel	
	No				HEK/OATP1B1	10	3 μM FL	
	No				HEK/OATP1B1	10	1 μM DCF	
	No				HEK/OATP1B1	10	0.5 μM atorvastatin	
	No				HEK/OATP1B1	10	1 μM SN-38	
	No				HEK/OATP1B1	10	1 μM valsartan	
	No	96 ± 7% function remaining after incubation with 10 μM	Yes	68 ± 0.5% function remaining after incubation with 10 μM	HEK293/OATP1B1 or 3	UNK	300nM E3S (1B1) or 2nM CCK-8 (1B3)	

Table 2. *Cont.*

TKI	1B1 Inhibitor	Reported Values	1B3 Inhibitor	Reported Values	Model	Pre-Incubation (mins)	Substrate	References
Sunitinib	Yes	>25% decrease at 10 μM			Flp-In T-Rex293/OATP1B1*1A	15	0.1 mM (3H) E2G	NI [68,70,84]
	No	109 ± 10% function remaining after incubation with 10 μM	No	101 ± 10% function remaining after incubation with 10 μM	HEK293/OATP1B1 or 3	UNK	300nM E3S (1B1) or 2nM CCK-8 (1B3)	
	Yes	>25% inhibition			HEK293/OATP1B1	15	E2G, 8FcA	
Vandetanib	Yes	>25% inhibition at 10 μM			Flp-In T-Rex293/ OATP1B1*1A	15	0.1 mM (3H) E2G	NI [53,68,70,83,84]
	No		Yes	50% inhibition at 18.13 ± 1.21	CHO/ OATP-1B1 or -1B3		0.25 μCi/mL of (3H)ES (for OATP-1B1) or (3H)CCK-8 (for OATP-1B3)	
	No	110 ± 6% function remaining after incubation with 10 μM	Yes	71± 5% function remaining after incubation with 10 μM	HEK293/OATP1B1 or 3	UNK	300nM E3S (1B1) or 2nM CCK-8 (1B3)	
	Yes	>25% inhibition at 10 μM			HEK293/OATP1B1	15	E2G, 8FcA	

UNK indicates not mentioned in the study/Unknown. NI is not indicated

7. Conclusions

The development and use of TKIs as molecular targeted therapies for the treatment of a diverse array of malignant diseases continues to rapidly increase, and 50 of such agents have now been approved for human use. However, polypharmacy regimens commonly applied in oncology with these TKIs creates a high risk for the occurrence of clinically-relevant DDIs. Although the extent to which such DDIs are influenced by the ability of many TKIs to impact the function of transporter-mediated uptake mechanisms in hepatocytes remains relatively poorly studied, data have accumulated in recent years highlighting that TKIs can act as perpetrators in DDIs by inhibiting OATP1B1 and/or OATP1B3 Many of these recent observations have been made with the use of transfected cell-based in vitro models, and a summary of this available evidence has identified substantial methodological differences between various studies and has highlighted several important limitations in the chosen approaches that have generated incongruent reports. Given that these in vitro studies are the most frequently employed nonclinical tool in aiding decision making for patient care, it is pertinent that regulatory guidance documents and available published literature provide consistent and corresponding results To further improve consistency in the outcome of transporter-mediated DDI studies involving TKIs, specific recommendations are offered that may assist investigators in the design of future studies in order to provide unequivocal data pertaining to the inhibitory potential of both established as well as investigational TKIs that could be rationally used to further refine the predictive ability of DDIs and ultimately optimize the outcome of treatment in patients with cancer.

Supplementary Materials:
Table S1: Prescribing Information, Table S2. FDA guidance for TKI interactions with OATP1B1 and OATP1B3, Table S3. EMA guidance for TKI interactions with OATP1B1 and OATP1B3, Table S4. Comparison of PI, FDA, and EMA regulatory documents, Table S5. In vitro studies for TKIs as perpetrators in OATP-mediated DDIs, Table S6. In vivo studies for TKIs as perpetrators in OATP-mediated DDIs Table S7. Literature on clinical studies focused on TKIs in potential DDIs Table S8. Comparison of the PI, FDA, and EMA guidance documents to the literature for OATP1B1 inhibition and OATP1B3 inhibition, Table S9. TKIs for which no relevant literature was found for OATP-mediated inhibition by TKIs.

Author Contributions: Each of the authors have read and approved this version of the manuscript and agrees to be held accountable for the accuracy and integrity of all included content. Each named author has substantially contributed to conducting the underlying research and drafting this manuscript. Individual contributions are illustrated in the following statements: Conceptualization, D.A.G., Z.T., A.S. and S.D.B.; methodology, D.A.G., Z.T. and E.D.E.; investigation, D.A.G., Z.T. and E.D.E.; interpretation of data, D.A.G. and Z.T.; writing—Original draft preparation, D.A.G. and Z.T.; writing—Review and editing, D.A.G., Z.T., E.D.E., A.S. and S.D.B.; supervision, A.S. and S.D.B.; funding acquisition, E.D.E., A.S. and S.D.B. All authors have read and agreed to the published version of the manuscript.

References

1. Watanabe, J.H.; McInnis, T.; Hirsch, J.D. Cost of Prescription Drug–Related Morbidity and Mortality. *Ann. Pharmacother.* **2018**, *52*, 829–837. [CrossRef] [PubMed]
2. Fuhr, U.; Hsin, C.-H.; Li, X.; Jabrane, W.; Sörgel, F. Assessment of Pharmacokinetic Drug–Drug Interactions in Humans: In Vivo Probe Substrates for Drug Metabolism and Drug Transport Revisited. *Annu. Rev. Pharmacol. Toxicol.* **2019**, *59*, 507–536. [CrossRef]
3. Magro, L.; Moretti, U.; Leone, R. Epidemiology and characteristics of adverse drug reactions caused by drug–drug interactions. *Expert Opin. Drug Saf.* **2011**, *11*, 83–94. [CrossRef]
4. Subramanian, A.; Adhimoolam, M.; Kannan, S. Study of drug–Drug interactions among the hypertensive patients in a tertiary care teaching hospital. *Perspect. Clin. Res.* **2018**, *9*, 9–14. [CrossRef] [PubMed]
5. Backman, J.T.; Kivistö, K.T.; Olkkola, K.T.; Neuvonen, P.J. The area under the plasma concentration-time curve for oral midazolam is 400-fold larger during treatment with itraconazole than with rifampicin. *Eur. J. Clin. Pharmacol.* **1998**, *54*, 53–58. [CrossRef] [PubMed]
6. de Jong, J.; Skee, D.; Murphy, J.; Sukbuntherng, J.; Hellemans, P.; Smit, J.; de Vries, R.; Jiao, J.J.; Snoeys, J.; Mannaert, E. Effect of CYP3A perpetrators on ibrutinib exposure in healthy participants. *Pharmacol. Res. Perspect.* **2015**, *3*, e00156. [CrossRef]
7. Gessner, A.; König, J.; Fromm, M.F. Clinical Aspects of Transporter-Mediated Drug–Drug Interactions. *Clin. Pharmacol. Ther.* **2019**, *105*, 1386–1394. [CrossRef]
8. Riechelmann, R.P.; del Giglio, A. Drug interactions in oncology: How common are they? *Ann. Oncol.* **2009**, *20*, 1907–1912. [CrossRef]
9. Riechelmann, R.; Girardi, D. Drug interactions in cancer patients: A hidden risk? *J. Res. Pharm. Pr.* **2016**, *5*, 77–78. [CrossRef]
10. Solomon, J.M.; Ajewole, V.B.; Schneider, A.M.; Sharma, M.; Bernicker, E.H. Evaluation of the prescribing patterns, adverse effects, and drug interactions of oral chemotherapy agents in an outpatient cancer center. *J. Oncol. Pharm. Pract.* **2019**, *25*, 1564–1569. [CrossRef]
11. Howlader, N.; Mariotto, A.B.; Besson, C.; Suneja, G.; Robien, K.; Younes, N.; Engels, E.A. Cancer-specific mortality, cure fraction, and noncancer causes of death among diffuse large B-cell lymphoma patients in the immunochemotherapy era. *Cancer* **2017**, *123*, 3326–3334. [CrossRef] [PubMed]
12. Riechelmann, R.P.; Zimmermann, C.; Chin, S.N.; Wang, L.; O'Carroll, A.; Zarinehbaf, S.; Krzyzanowska, M.K. Potential Drug Interactions in Cancer Patients Receiving Supportive Care Exclusively. *J. Pain Symptom Manag.* **2008**, *35*, 535–543. [CrossRef] [PubMed]
13. van Leeuwen, R.; Brundel, D.H.S.; Neef, C.; van Gelder, T.; Mathijssen, R.H.J.; Burger, D.M.; Jansman, F.G.A. Prevalence of potential drug–drug interactions in cancer patients treated with oral anticancer drugs. *Br. J. Cancer* **2013**, *108*, 1071–1078. [CrossRef] [PubMed]
14. Bartel, S. Safe practices and financial considerations in using oral chemotherapeutic agents. *Am. J. Health Pharm.* **2007**, *64*, S8–S14. [CrossRef]
15. Dagher, R.; Cohen, M.; Williams, G.; Rothmann, M.; Gobburu, J.; Robbie, G.; Rahman, A.; Chen, G.; Staten, A.; Griebel, D.; et al. Approval summary: Imatinib mesylate in the treatment of metastatic and/or unresectable malignant gastrointestinal stromal tumors. *Clin. Cancer Res.* **2002**, *8*, 3034–3038. [PubMed]
16. Roskoski, R. Properties of FDA-approved small molecule protein kinase inhibitors. *Pharmacol. Res.* **2019**, *144*, 19–50. [CrossRef]
17. Lemmon, M.A.; Schlessinger, J. Cell Signaling by Receptor Tyrosine Kinases. *Cell* **2010**, *141*, 1117–1134. [CrossRef]
18. Hubbard, S.R.; Till, J.H. Protein Tyrosine Kinase Structure and Function. *Annu. Rev. Biochem.* **2000**, *69*, 373–398. [CrossRef]
19. Robinson, D.R.; Wu, Y.-M.; Lin, S.-F. The protein tyrosine kinase family of the human genome. *Oncogene* **2000**, *19*, 5548–5557. [CrossRef]

20. Arora, A.; Scholar, E.M. Role of Tyrosine Kinase Inhibitors in Cancer Therapy. *J. Pharmacol. Exp. Ther.* **2005**, *315*, 971–979. [CrossRef]
21. Shawver, L.K.; Slamon, D.; Ullrich, A. Smart drugs: Tyrosine kinase inhibitors in cancer therapy. *Cancer Cell* **2002**, *1*, 117–123. [CrossRef]
22. Jeong, W.; Doroshow, J.H.; Kummar, S. United States Food and Drug Administration approved oral kinase inhibitors for the treatment of malignancies. *Curr. Probl. Cancer* **2013**, *37*, 110–144. [CrossRef] [PubMed]
23. Herviou, P.; Thivat, E.; Richard, D.; Roche, L.; Dohou, J.; Pouget, M.; Eschalier, A.; Durando, X.; Authier, N. Therapeutic drug monitoring and tyrosine kinase inhibitors. *Oncol. Lett.* **2016**, *12*, 1223–1232. [CrossRef] [PubMed]
24. Haouala, A.; Widmer, N.; Duchosal, M.A.; Montemurro, M.; Buclin, T.; Decosterd, L.A. Drug interactions with the tyrosine kinase inhibitors imatinib, dasatinib, and nilotinib. *Blood* **2011**, *117*, e75–e87. [CrossRef] [PubMed]
25. Iurlo, A.; Nobili, A.; Latagliata, R.; Bucelli, C.; Castagnetti, F.; Breccia, M.; Abruzzese, E.; Cattaneo, D.; Fava, C.; Ferrero, D.; et al. Imatinib and polypharmacy in very old patients with chronic myeloid leukemia: Effects on response rate, toxicity and outcome. *Oncotarget* **2016**, *7*, 80083–80090. [CrossRef]
26. Hussaarts, K.; Veerman, G.D.M.; Jansman, F.G.A.; van Gelder, T.; Mathijssen, R.H.J.; van Leeuwen, R.W.F. Clinically relevant drug interactions with multikinase inhibitors: A review. *Ther. Adv. Med Oncol.* **2019**, *11*, 1758835918818347. [CrossRef]
27. Fowler, H.; Belot, A.; Ellis, L.; Maringe, C.; Luque-Fernandez, M.A.; Njagi, E.N.; Navani, N.; Sarfati, D.; Rachet, B. Comorbidity prevalence among cancer patients: A population-based cohort study of four cancers. *BMC Cancer* **2020**, *20*, 2–15. [CrossRef]
28. Ergun, Y.; Ozdemir, N.Y.; Toptas, S.; Kurtipek, A.; Eren, T.; Yazici, O.; Sendur, M.A.N.; Akinci, B.; Ucar, G.; Oksuzoglu, B.; et al. Drug-drug interactions in patients using tyrosine kinase inhibitors: A multicenter retrospective study. *J. Buon* **2019**, *24*, 1719–1726.
29. Keller, K.L.; Franquiz, M.J.; Duffy, A.P.; Trovato, J.A. Drug–drug interactions in patients receiving tyrosine kinase inhibitors. *J. Oncol. Pharm. Pract.* **2016**, *24*, 110–115. [CrossRef]
30. da Silva, C.; Honeywell, R.J.; Dekker, H.; Peters, G.J. Physicochemical properties of novel protein kinase inhibitors in relation to their substrate specificity for drug transporters. *Expert Opin. Drug Metab. Toxicol.* **2015**, *11*, 703–717. [CrossRef]
31. Herbrink, M.; Nuijen, B.; Schellens, J.H.; Beijnen, J.H. Variability in bioavailability of small molecular tyrosine kinase inhibitors. *Cancer Treat. Rev.* **2015**, *41*, 412–422. [CrossRef] [PubMed]
32. van Leeuwen, R.; van Gelder, T.; Mathijssen, R.; Jansman, F.G.A. Drug–drug interactions with tyrosine-kinase inhibitors: A clinical perspective. *Lancet Oncol.* **2014**, *15*, e315–e326. [CrossRef]
33. Schulte, R.R.; Ho, R.H. Organic Anion Transporting Polypeptides: Emerging Roles in Cancer Pharmacology. *Mol. Pharmacol.* **2019**, *95*, 490–506. [CrossRef]
34. Ho, R.H.; Kim, R.B. Transporters and drug therapy: Implications for drug disposition and disease. *Clin. Pharmacol. Ther.* **2005**, *78*, 260–277. [CrossRef] [PubMed]
35. Kalliokoski, A.; Niemi, M. Impact of OATP transporters on pharmacokinetics. *Br. J. Pharmacol.* **2009**, *158*, 693–705. [CrossRef]
36. Shitara, Y. Clinical Importance of OATP1B1 and OATP1B3 in DrugDrug Interactions. *Drug Metab. Pharmacokinet.* **2011**, *26*, 220–227. [CrossRef]
37. Zimmerman, E.I.; Hu, S.; Roberts, J.L.; Gibson, A.A.; Orwick, S.J.; Li, L.; Sparreboom, A.; Baker, S. Contribution of OATP1B1 and OATP1B3 to the disposition of sorafenib and sorafenib-glucuronide. *Clin. Cancer Res.* **2013**, *19*, 1458–1466. [CrossRef]
38. Teo, Y.L.; Ho, H.K.; Chan, A. Risk of tyrosine kinase inhibitors-induced hepatotoxicity in cancer patients: A meta-analysis. *Cancer Treat. Rev.* **2013**, *39*, 199–206. [CrossRef]
39. Kellick, K. Organic Ion Transporters and Statin Drug Interactions. *Curr. Atheroscler. Rep.* **2017**, *19*, 65. [CrossRef]
40. Alam, K.; Crowe, A.; Wang, X.; Zhang, P.; Ding, K.; Li, L.; Yue, W. Regulation of Organic Anion Transporting Polypeptides (OATP) 1B1- and OATP1B3-Mediated Transport: An Updated Review in the Context of OATP-Mediated Drug-Drug Interactions. *Int. J. Mol. Sci.* **2018**, *19*, 855. [CrossRef]

41. Lancaster, C.S.; Sprowl, J.A.; Walker, A.L.; Hu, S.; Gibson, A.A.; Sparreboom, A. Modulation of OATP1B-type transporter function alters cellular uptake and disposition of platinum chemotherapeutics. *Mol. Cancer Ther.* **2013**, *12*, 1537–1544. [CrossRef] [PubMed]
42. Chen, M.; Hu, S.; Li, Y.; Gibson, A.A.; Fu, Q.; Baker, S.D.; Sparreboom, A. Role of Oatp2b1 in Drug Absorption and Drug-Drug Interactions. *Drug Metab. Dispos.* **2020**, *48*, 420–426. [CrossRef] [PubMed]
43. Podoll, T.; Pearson, P.G.; Evarts, J.; Ingallinera, T.; Sun, H.; Byard, S.; Fretland, A.J.; Slatter, J.G. Abstract 13: Structure elucidation, metabolism, and drug interaction potential of ACP-5862, an active, major, circulating metabolite of acalabrutinib. *Cancer Res.* **2019**, *79*. [CrossRef]
44. Ellens, H.; Johnson, M.; Lawrence, S.K.; Chen, L.; Richards-Peterson, L.E.; Watson, C. Prediction of the Transporter-Mediated Drug-Drug Interaction Potential of Dabrafenib and Its Major Circulating Metabolites. *Drug Metab. Dispos.* **2017**, *45*, 646–656. [CrossRef] [PubMed]
45. Pahwa, S.; Alam, K.; Crowe, A.; Farasyn, T.; Neuhoff, S.; Hatley, O.; Ding, K.; Yue, W. Pretreatment With Rifampicin and Tyrosine Kinase Inhibitor Dasatinib Potentiates the Inhibitory Effects Toward OATP1B1- and OATP1B3-Mediated Transport. *J. Pharm. Sci.* **2017**, *106*, 2123–2135. [CrossRef] [PubMed]
46. Elsby, R.; Martin, P.; Surry, D.; Sharma, P.; Fenner, K. Solitary Inhibition of the Breast Cancer Resistance Protein Efflux Transporter Results in a Clinically Significant Drug-Drug Interaction with Rosuvastatin by Causing up to a 2-Fold Increase in Statin Exposure. *Drug Metab. Dispos.* **2015**, *44*, 398–408. [CrossRef]
47. Patik, I.; Kovacsics, D.; Német, O.; Gera, M.; Várady, G.; Stieger, B.; Hagenbuch, B.; Szakács, G.; Özvegy-Laczka, C. Functional expression of the 11 human Organic Anion Transporting Polypeptides in insect cells reveals that sodium fluorescein is a general OATP substrate. *Biochem. Pharmacol.* **2015**, *98*, 649–658. [CrossRef]
48. Bergman, E.; Hedeland, M.; Bondesson, U.; Lennernäs, H. The effect of acute administration of rifampicin and imatinib on the enterohepatic transport of rosuvastatinin vivo. *Xenobiotica* **2010**, *40*, 558–568. [CrossRef]
49. Nakamura, Y.; Hirokawa, Y.; Kitamura, S.; Yamasaki, W.; Arihiro, K.; Tatsugami, F.; Iida, M.; Kakizawa, H.; Date, S.; Awai, K. Effect of lapatinib on hepatic parenchymal enhancement on gadoxetate disodium (EOB)-enhanced MRI scans of the rat liver. *Jpn. J. Radiol.* **2013**, *31*, 386–392. [CrossRef]
50. Martin, P.D.; Gillen, M.; Ritter, J.; Mathews, D.; Brealey, C.; Surry, D.; Oliver, S.; Holmes, V.; Severin, P.; Elsby, R. Effects of Fostamatinib on the Pharmacokinetics of Oral Contraceptive, Warfarin, and the Statins Rosuvastatin and Simvastatin: Results From Phase I Clinical Studies. *Drugs R&D* **2016**, *16*, 93–107. [CrossRef]
51. Harvey, R.D.; Aransay, N.R.; Isambert, N.; Lee, J.-S.; Arkenau, T.; Vansteenkiste, J.; Dickinson, P.A.; Bui, K.; Weilert, D.; So, K.; et al. Effect of multiple-dose osimertinib on the pharmacokinetics of simvastatin and rosuvastatin. *Br. J. Clin. Pharmacol.* **2018**, *84*, 2877–2888. [CrossRef]
52. Vishwanathan, K.; Cantarini, M.; So, K.; Masson, E.; Fetterolf, J.; Ramalingam, S.S.; Harvey, R.D. Impact of Disease and Treatment Response in Drug–Drug Interaction Studies: Osimertinib and Simvastatin in Advanced Non-Small Cell Lung Cancer. *Clin. Transl. Sci.* **2019**, *13*, 41–46. [CrossRef] [PubMed]
53. Calvo, E.; Lee, J.-S.; Kim, S.-W.; Moreno, V.; Carpeno, J.D.; Weilert, D.; Laus, G.; Mann, H.; Vishwanathan, K. Modulation of Fexofenadine Pharmacokinetics by Osimertinib in Patients With Advanced EGFR-Mutated Non–Small Cell Lung Cancer. *J. Clin. Pharmacol.* **2019**, *59*, 1099–1109. [CrossRef] [PubMed]
54. Reddy, V.P.; Walker, M.; Sharma, P.; Ballard, P.; Vishwanathan, K. Development, Verification, and Prediction of Osimertinib Drug-Drug Interactions Using PBPK Modeling Approach to Inform Drug Label. *CPT Pharmacomet. Syst. Pharmacol.* **2018**, *7*, 321–330. [CrossRef] [PubMed]
55. Komatsu, H.; Enomoto, M.; Shiraishi, H.; Morita, Y.; Hashimoto, D.; Nakayama, S.; Funakoshi, S.; Hirano, S.; Terada, Y.; Miyamura, M.; et al. Severe hypoglycemia caused by a small dose of repaglinide and concurrent use of nilotinib and febuxostat in a patient with type 2 diabetes. *Diabetol. Int.* **2020**, 1–5. [CrossRef]
56. Kendra, K.; Plummer, R.; Salgia, R.; O'Brien, M.E.R.; Paul, E.M.; Suttle, A.B.; Compton, N.; Xu, C.-F.; Ottesen, L.H.; Villalona-Calero, M.A. A Multicenter Phase I Study of Pazopanib in Combination with Paclitaxel in First-Line Treatment of Patients with Advanced Solid Tumors. *Mol. Cancer Ther.* **2014**, *14*, 461–469. [CrossRef]
57. Poje, D.K.; Božina, N.; Šimičević, L.; Žabić, I. Severe hyperglycaemia following pazopanib treatment: The role of drug-drug-gene interactions in a patient with metastatic renal cell carcinoma—A case report. *J. Clin. Pharm. Ther.* **2020**, *45*, 628–631. [CrossRef]

58. Hamberg, P.; Mathijssen, R.H.J.; de Bruijn, P.; Leonowens, C.; van der Biessen, D.; Eskens, F.A.L.M.; Sleijfer, S. Verweij, J.; de Jonge, M.J.A. Impact of pazopanib on docetaxel exposure: Results of a phase I combination study with two different docetaxel schedules. *Cancer Chemother. Pharmacol.* **2014**, *75*, 365–371. [CrossRef]
59. Xu, C.-F.; Xue, Z.; Bing, N.; King, K.S.; McCann, L.A.; de Souza, P.L.; Goodman, V.L.; Spraggs, C.F. Mooser, V.E.; Pandite, L.N. Concomitant use of pazopanib and simvastatin increases the risk of transaminase elevations in patients with cancer. *Ann. Oncol.* **2012**, *23*, 2470–2471. [CrossRef]
60. Mandery, K.; Glaeser, H.; Fromm, M.F. Interaction of innovative small molecule drugs used for cancer therapy with drug transporters. *Br. J. Pharmacol.* **2011**, *165*, 345–362. [CrossRef]
61. Lawrence, S.K.; Nguyen, D.; Bowen, C.; Richards-Peterson, L.; Skordos, K.W. The Metabolic Drug-Drug Interaction Profile of Dabrafenib: In Vitro Investigations and Quantitative Extrapolation of the P450-Mediated DDI Risk. *Drug Metab. Dispos.* **2014**, *42*, 1180–1190. [CrossRef] [PubMed]
62. Filppula, A.; Neuvonen, P.J.; Backman, J.T. In Vitro Assessment of Time-Dependent Inhibitory Effects on CYP2C8 and CYP3A Activity by Fourteen Protein Kinase Inhibitors. *Drug Metab. Dispos.* **2014**, *42*, 1202–1209 [CrossRef]
63. Grenader, T.; Gipps, M.; Shavit, L.; Gabizon, A. Significant drug interaction: Phenytoin toxicity due to erlotinib. *Lung Cancer* **2007**, *57*, 404–406. [CrossRef] [PubMed]
64. Kuhn, E.L.; Lévêque, D.; Lioure, B.; Gourieux, B.; Bilbault, P. Adverse event potentially due to an interaction between ibrutinib and verapamil: A case report. *J. Clin. Pharm. Ther.* **2016**, *41*, 104–105. [CrossRef]
65. Vaidyanathan, J.; Yoshida, K.; Arya, V.; Zhang, L. Comparing Various In Vitro Prediction Criteria to Assess the Potential of a New Molecular Entity to Inhibit Organic Anion Transporting Polypeptide 1B1. *J. Clin Pharmacol.* **2016**, *56*, S59–S72. [CrossRef] [PubMed]
66. Koide, H.; Tsujimoto, M.; Takeuchi, A.; Tanaka, M.; Ikegami, Y.; Tagami, M.; Abe, S.; Hashimoto, M. Minegaki, T.; Nishiguchi, K. Substrate-dependent effects of molecular-targeted anticancer agents on activity of organic anion transporting polypeptide 1B1. *Xenobiotica* **2017**, *48*, 1059–1071. [CrossRef]
67. Sato, T.; Ito, H.; Hirata, A.; Abe, T.; Mano, N.; Yamaguchi, H. Interactions of crizotinib and gefitinib with organic anion-transporting polypeptides (OATP)1B1, OATP1B3 and OATP2B1: Gefitinib shows contradictory interaction with OATP1B3. *Xenobiotica* **2017**, *48*, 73–78. [CrossRef]
68. Leblanc, A.F.; Sprowl, J.A.; Alberti, P.; Chiorazzi, A.; Arnold, W.D.; Gibson, A.A.; Hong, K.W.; Pioso, M.S. Chen, M.; Huang, K.M.; et al. OATP1B2 deficiency protects against paclitaxel-induced neurotoxicity. *J. Clin Investig.* **2018**, *128*, 816–825. [CrossRef]
69. Febvre-James, M.; Bruyère, A.; Le Vée, M.; Fardel, O. The JAK1/2 Inhibitor Ruxolitinib Reverses Interleukin-6-Mediated Suppression of Drug-Detoxifying Proteins in Cultured Human Hepatocytes. *Drug Metab. Dispos.* **2018**, *46*, 131–140. [CrossRef]
70. Hu, S.; Mathijssen, R.H.J.; de Bruijn, P.; Baker, S.; Sparreboom, A. Inhibition of OATP1B1 by tyrosine kinase inhibitors: In vitro–in vivo correlations. *Br. J. Cancer* **2014**, *110*, 894–898. [CrossRef]
71. Iwase, M.; Fujita, K.-I.; Nishimura, Y.; Seba, N.; Masuo, Y.; Ishida, H.; Kato, Y.; Kiuchi, Y. Pazopanib interacts with irinotecan by inhibiting UGT1A1-mediated glucuronidation, but not OATP1B1-mediated hepatic uptake of an active metabolite SN-38. *Cancer Chemother. Pharmacol.* **2019**, *83*, 993–998. [CrossRef] [PubMed]
72. Taguchi, T.; Masuo, Y.; Sakai, Y.; Kato, Y. Short-lasting inhibition of hepatic uptake transporter OATP1B1 by tyrosine kinase inhibitor pazopanib. *Drug Metab. Pharmacokinet.* **2019**, *34*, 372–379. [CrossRef] [PubMed]
73. Xu, C.F.; Reck, B.H.; Xue, Z.; Huang, L.; Baker, K.L.; Chen, M.; Chen, E.P.; Ellens, H.E.; Mooser, V.E. Cardon, L.R.; et al. Pazopanib-induced hyperbilirubinemia is associated with Gilbert's syndrome UGT1A1 polymorphism. *Br. J. Cancer* **2010**, *102*, 1371–1377. [CrossRef] [PubMed]
74. Izumi, S.; Nozaki, Y.; Maeda, K.; Komori, T.; Takenaka, O.; Kusuhara, H.; Sugiyama, Y. Investigation of the Impact of Substrate Selection on In Vitro Organic Anion Transporting Polypeptide 1B1 Inhibition Profiles for the Prediction of Drug-Drug Interactions. *Drug Metab. Dispos.* **2014**, *43*, 235–247. [CrossRef]
75. McFeely, S.J.; Ritchie, T.K.; Ragueneau-Majlessi, I. Variability in In Vitro OATP1B1/1B3 Inhibition Data: Impact of Incubation Conditions on Variability and Subsequent Drug Interaction Predictions. *Clin. Transl. Sci.* **2020**, *13*, 47–52 [CrossRef]
76. Tátrai, P.; Schweigler, P.; Poller, B.; Domange, N.; de Wilde, R.; Hanna, I.; Gaborik, Z.; Huth, F. A Systematic In Vitro Investigation of the Inhibitor Preincubation Effect on Multiple Classes of Clinically Relevant Transporters. *Drug Metab. Dispos.* **2019**, *47*, 768–778. [CrossRef]

77. Bentz, J.; O'Connor, M.P.; Bednarczyk, D.; Coleman, J.; Lee, C.; Palm, J.; Pak, Y.A.; Perloff, E.S.; Reyner, E.; Balimane, P.; et al. Variability in P-Glycoprotein Inhibitory Potency (IC50) Using Various in Vitro Experimental Systems: Implications for Universal Digoxin Drug-Drug Interaction Risk Assessment Decision Criteria. *Drug Metab. Dispos.* **2013**, *41*, 1347–1366. [CrossRef]
78. Volpe, D.A.; Hamed, S.S.; Zhang, L.K. Use of Different Parameters and Equations for Calculation of IC50 Values in Efflux Assays: Potential Sources of Variability in IC50 Determination. *AAPS J.* **2013**, *16*, 172–180. [CrossRef]
79. Greenblatt, D.J.; Venkatakrishnan, K.; Harmatz, J.S.; Parent, S.J.; von Moltke, L.L. Sources of variability in ketoconazole inhibition of human cytochrome P450 3Ain vitro. *Xenobiotica* **2010**, *40*, 713–720. [CrossRef]
80. Huang, K.M.; Uddin, M.E.; Digiacomo, D.; Lustberg, M.B.; Hu, S.; Sparreboom, A. Role of SLC transporters in toxicity induced by anticancer drugs. *Expert Opin. Drug Metab. Toxicol.* **2020**, *16*, 493–506. [CrossRef]
81. Johnston, R.A.; Rawling, T.; Chan, T.; Zhou, F.; Murray, M. Selective Inhibition of Human Solute Carrier Transporters by Multikinase Inhibitors. *Drug Metab. Dispos.* **2014**, *42*, 1851–1857. [CrossRef] [PubMed]
82. Lacy, S.; Hsu, B.; Miles, D.; Aftab, D.; Wang, R.; Nguyen, L. Metabolism and Disposition of Cabozantinib in Healthy Male Volunteers and Pharmacologic Characterization of Its Major Metabolites. *Drug Metab. Dispos.* **2015**, *43*, 1190–1207. [CrossRef]
83. Khurana, V.; Minocha, M.; Pal, D.; Mitra, A.K. Inhibition of OATP-1B1 and OATP-1B3 by tyrosine kinase inhibitors. *Drug Metab. Drug Interact.* **2014**, *29*, 249–259. [CrossRef] [PubMed]
84. Kotsampasakou, E.; Brenner, S.; Jaeger, W.; Ecker, G.F. Identification of Novel Inhibitors of Organic Anion Transporting Polypeptides 1B1 and 1B3 (OATP1B1 and OATP1B3) Using a Consensus Vote of Six Classification Models. *Mol. Pharm.* **2015**, *12*, 4395–4404. [CrossRef] [PubMed]
85. Polli, J.W.; Humphreys, J.E.; Harmon, K.A.; Castellino, S.; O'mara, M.J.; Olson, K.L.; John-Williams, L.S.; Koch, K.M.; Serabjit-Singh, C.J. The role of efflux and uptake transporters in [N-{3-chloro-4-[(3-fluorobenzyl)oxy]phenyl}-6-[5-({[2-(methylsulfonyl)ethyl]amino}methyl)-2-furyl]-4-quinazolinamine (GW572016, lapatinib) disposition and drug interactions. *Drug Metab. Dispos.* **2008**, *36*, 695–701. [CrossRef] [PubMed]
86. Hayden, E.R. Phosphorylation and function of OATP1B1 with tyrosine kinase inhibitors. *FASEB J.* **2020**, *34*, 1. [CrossRef]
87. Sprowl, J.A.; Chen, M.; Gibson, A.A.; Pasquariello, K.Z.; Sparreboom, A.; Hu, S. Characterization of OATP1B1 and OATP1B3 inhibition by Nilotinib. *FASEB J.* **2019**, *33*, 506–507.
88. Ohya, H.; Shibayama, Y.; Ogura, J.; Narumi, K.; Kobayashi, M.; Iseki, K. Regorafenib Is Transported by the Organic Anion Transporter 1B1 and the Multidrug Resistance Protein 2. *Biol. Pharm. Bull.* **2015**, *38*, 582–586. [CrossRef]

16

Effect of *Rumex Acetosa* Extract, a Herbal Drug, on the Absorption of Fexofenadine

Jung Hwan Ahn †, Junhyeong Kim †, Naveed Ur Rehman, Hye-Jin Kim, Mi-Jeong Ahn and Hye Jin Chung *

College of Pharmacy and Research Institute of Pharmaceutical Sciences, Gyeongsang National University, Jinju 52828, Korea; anjh5803@naver.com (J.H.A.); jhk6914@naver.com (J.K.); naveed.rehman50@gmail.com (N.U.R.); black200203@gmail.com (H.-J.K.); amj5812@gnu.ac.kr (M.-J.A.)

* Correspondence: hchung@gnu.ac.kr

† These authors contributed equally to this work.

Abstract: Herbal drugs are widely used for the auxiliary treatment of diseases. The pharmacokinetics of a drug may be altered when it is coadministered with herbal drugs that can affect drug absorption. The effects of herbal drugs on absorption must be evaluated. In this study, we investigated the effects of *Rumex acetosa (R. acetosa)* extract on fexofenadine absorption. Fexofenadine was selected as a model drug that is a substrate of *P*-glycoprotein (*P*-gp) and organic anion transporting polypeptide 1A2 (OATP1A2). Emodine—the major component of *R. acetosa* extract—showed *P*-gp inhibition in vitro and in vivo. Uptake of fexofenadine via OATP1A2 was inhibited by *R. acetosa* extract in OATP1A2 transfected cells. A pharmacokinetic study showed that the area under the plasma concentration–time curve (AUC) of fexofenadine was smaller in the *R. acetosa* extract coadministered group than in the control group. *R. acetosa* extract also decreased aqueous solubility of fexofenadine HCl. The results of this study suggest that *R. acetosa* extract could inhibit the absorption of certain drugs via intervention in the aqueous solubility and the drug transporters. Therefore, *R. acetosa* extract may cause drug interactions when coadministered with substrates of drug transporters and poorly water-soluble drugs, although further clinical studies are needed.

Keywords: *P*-glycoprotein (*P*-gp); organic anion transporting polypeptide 1A2 (OATP1A2); *Rumex acetosa*; pharmacokinetics; fexofenadine; drug interaction

1. Introduction

Oral drug administration is a preferred route, offering the advantages of convenience and safety. Many drug interactions with foods and other drugs occur via alteration of drug absorption. There are absorptive transporters, such as organic anion transporting polypeptide (OATP) and secretory transporters, including *P*-glycoprotein (*P*-gp), associated with drug absorption. To improve drug therapy, it is necessary to investigate possible interactions mediated by transporters that could alter systemic exposure of drugs.

P-gp, belonging to the ATP binding cassette superfamily, is an ATP-dependent efflux protein that excretes drugs out of cells [1–3]. P-gp is an important factor limiting the absorption of drugs and plays a key role in drug distribution and resistance [3,4]. For example, P-gp overexpression induced by a hypoxic environment in many cancers decreases the effects of chemotherapy [5,6]. Furthermore, drug–drug interactions may occur when substrates of P-gp (e.g., cimetidine, digoxin, doxorubicin, fexofenadine, and vinblastine) are coadministered with inhibitors of P-gp (e.g., atorvastatin, ketoconazole and quinidine) or inducers of P-gp (e.g., rifampin and clotrimazole) [7,8]. The OATP family is also an important transporter for drug disposition. The OATP members of the solute carrier (SLC) family, contributes to the uptake of substrates, including endogenous compounds and drugs [9,10]. Drug–drug interactions and food–drug interactions mediated by these two active transporters—P-gp and OATP—have been reported. In addition, a study on medication use patterns revealed that 50% of 2590 study participants had taken at least one prescription drug during the week prior to the study, and 16% of them had taken one or more herbals/supplements [11,12]. Given that St. John's wort was found to increase *P*-gp expression [13], it is necessary to evaluate the effects of herbal supplements on these transporters. Despite the widespread use of herbal drugs in combination with drugs, there has been little research on the interactions between drugs and herbal medicines.

This study investigated the effects of *Rumex acetosa (R. acetosa)* extract on *P*-gp and OATP1A2 in vitro and on fexofenadine absorption in vivo. *R. acetosa*, used in folk remedies for skin diseases, has been singled out as a natural herbal medicine for its potential to be used in combination with fexofenadine [14]. *R. acetosa* is widely distributed in eastern Asia and decoction of this plant has been used for the treatment of several health disorders such as fever, gastro-intestinal problems, inflammatory diseases. It is belonging in the Polygonaceae family, known to produce many biologic metabolites [15]. Particularly, *R. acetosa* is rich in anthraquinones and flavonoids that have anti-inflammatory and antiproliferative effects [16,17]. Emodin, a major anthraquinone component of *R. acetosa* extract, is reported that has the potential for *P*-gp mediated drug interaction [18] and has various pharmacological effects, such as antidiabetic [19] and anticancer activities [20].

Fexofenadine, a selective histamine H_1 receptor antagonist, is widely used for seasonal allergic rhinitis and chronic idiopathic urticarial treatment [21]. There is no evidence for cardiotoxicity associated with fexofenadine, the active metabolite of terfenadine, even though terfenadine is not used anymore due to the risk of cardiac arrhythmia. Fexofenadine was selected as a model drug that is a marker substrate of *P*-gp [22] and OATP1A2 [23]. Fexofenadine is considered a good model drug, because only around 5% of its dose is metabolized and most of the dose is excreted into urine (11%) and feces (80%) as the unchanged form [24,25], which means that metabolism can be excluded in interpreting the pharmacokinetics of fexofenadine.

To date, there have been many drug interaction studies involving *P*-gp or OATP. However, there have been few studies concerning drug interactions with herbal medicines involving both *P*-gp and OATP1A2. Furthermore, it has been reported that the emodin acts on *P*-gp as an inducer [26] or an inhibitor [18]. Our results clarify the inhibitory effect of emodin on the *P*-gp through in vitro and in vivo study. In addition, our findings include the fact that *R. acetosa* extract could affect drug absorption via intervention in the OATP-mediated influx and the aqueous solubility. These results indicate that the effects of herbal medicines such as plant extracts, on drug absorption must be considered in terms of not only efflux through *P*-gp, but also OATP-mediated influx and the aqueous solubility.

2. Materials and Methods

2.1. Chemicals and Reagents

Fexofenadine hydrochloride and emodin were purchased from Tokyo Chemical Industry (Tokyo, Japan). Dimethyl sulfoxide (DMSO), terfenadine, verapamil, Dulbecco's modified Eagle's medium (DMEM) with high glucose, MEM non-essential amino acid solution (NEAA) and glutamine were purchased from Sigma-Aldrich (St. Louis, MO, USA). HPLC grade acetonitrile and water were purchased from Fisher Scientific Korea (Seoul, Korea). Emodin, emodin-8-*O*-β-D-glucoside, chrysophanol, chrysophanol-8-*O*-β-D-glucoside, physcion and physcion-8-*O*-β-D-glucoside isolated from *R. acetosa* were obtained from the pharmacognosy laboratory of the College of Pharmacy at Gyeongsang National University (Jinju, Korea) [27]. Fetal bovine serum (FBS), N-2-hydroxyethylpiperazine–N′-2-ethanesulfonic acid (HEPES) and Hanks' balanced salt solution (HBSS) were purchased from Corning (Manassas, VA, USA). Penicillin–streptomycin, Opti-MEM and 0.25% (*w/v*) trypsin–EDTA were purchased from Gibco (Carlsbad, CA, USA). Phosphate buffered saline (PBS) was purchased from Welgene (Gyeongsan, Korea). An MDR assay kit (fluorometric) was purchased from Abcam (Cambridge, UK).

2.2. *R. acetosa* Extract

The *R. acetosa* extract was prepared by previously reported procedure [27]. Briefly, the dried whole part of *R. acetosa* was extracted with 70% ethanol. The extraction was performed by the Soxhlet extractor for 3 h at 80 °C. The extract was filtered and lyophilized.

The total phenol content and total flavonoid content of *R. acetosa* extract were 74.5 mg GAE (gallic acid equivalent)/g of dry weight and 180.3 μg QAE (quercetin equivalent)/g of dry weight, respectively The contents of anthraquinones in *R. acetosa* extract were determined by HPLC. The contents of emodin, emodin-8-*O*-β-D-glucoside, chrysophanol, chrysophanol-8-*O*-β-D-glucoside, physcion and physcion-8-*O*-β-D-glucoside in *R. acetosa* extract were 0.94 ± 0.15%, 1.29 ± 0.06%, 0.68 ± 0.09%, 0.77 ± 0.12%, 0.17 ± 0.02% and 0.41% ± 0.05% (*w/w*), respectively. The values were expressed as mean ± standard deviation.

2.3. Cell Culture

The Caco-2 (HTB-37™) cells were purchased from the American Type Culture Collection (ATCC, Manassas, VA, USA). OATP1A2/SLCO1A2 transfected HEK293 cells were purchased from Corning (New York, NY, USA). The Caco-2 cells were cultured in high glucose added DMEM with 10% FBS, 1% NEAA, 10-mM HEPES, 4-mM glutamine, 100 U/mL of penicillin and 100 μg/mL of streptomycin, and maintained in humidified 5% CO_2 at 37 °C. The medium of the Caco-2 cells was replaced 2–3 times per week.

The transfected HEK293 cells were cultured in high glucose added DMEM with 10% FBS and 1% NEAA, and maintained in 8% CO_2 with low humidity at 37 °C for 4 h. After incubation for 4 h, the medium of the transfected HEK293 cells was replaced with high glucose added DMEM with 10% FBS, 1% NEAA and 2-mM sodium butyrate, and incubated for 24 h.

2.4. Cytotoxicity Assay

The cytotoxicity of *R. acetosa* extract on Caco-2 cells and HEK293 cells was measured using an EZ-Cytox cell viability assay kit (Daeil Lab Service, Seoul, Korea). The cells were cultured in DMEM containing 10% FBS, 1% NEAA, 10-mM HEPES, 100 U/mL of penicillin and 100-μg/mL streptomycin without phenol red. The seeding density was 3×10^4 cells/well for Caco-2 cells and 2.5×10^4 cell/well for HEK293 cells, respectively. The Caco-2 cells were incubated for 7 days and the HEK 293 cells were incubated for 24 h after seeding. The medium was replaced with 50 μL of new medium containing *R. acetosa* extract at the concentrations of 1, 2, 5, 10, 20, 50 and 100 μg/mL achieved the 0.5% of DMSO content. After 15 min of incubation, 5 μL of EZ-Cytox reagent (water-soluble tetrazolium) was added to the cells, and the cells were incubated for 3 h. Cell viability was calculated as a percentage of the absorbance at 450 nm compared to untreated cells.

2.5. P-gp Inhibition Test of Anthraquinones and *R. acetosa* Extract

The *P*-gp inhibition effect of anthraquinones from *R. acetosa* was evaluated via MDR assay kit using Caco-2 cells. It was reported that verapamil has concentration-dependent inhibition effects on absorptive and secretory transporters. Accordingly, 100-μM verapamil was used as a positive control [28]. Caco-2 cells were cultured in 96-well plates at a density of 5×10^5 cells/mL and incubated in humidified 5% CO_2 at 37 °C for 24 h. They were treated with 6 test compounds (10 μM) [18] or *R. acetosa* extract in HBSS and incubated for 15 min. The concentration levels of *R. acetosa* extract were 5, 10, 25 and 50 μg/mL. The MDR dye-loading solution was added at a volume of 100 μL and incubated. Fluorescence intensity was detected with a microplate reader Synerge H1 (Biotek, Winooski, VT, USA) at a wavelength of 490 nm for the excitation and 525 nm for the emission.

2.6. Fexofenadine Uptake Test Using OATP1A2/SLCO1A2 Transfected HEK293 Cells

The seeding density of the OATP1A2 overexpressed HEK293 cells was 10^5 cells/well. Verapamil was used as a positive control with a concentration of 100 μM [28]. The cultured cells were washed twice with warmed HBSS with 5-mM MES after removing the medium, then 15-μM fexofenadine was treated with *R. acetosa* extract of 10, 20 and 50 μg/mL. After 15 min of incubation in 8% CO_2 with low humidity at 37 °C, they were washed twice with cold HBSS. They were gently shaken after adding 120 μL of 50-ng/mL terfenadine in 80% acetonitrile. Terfenadine was used as an internal standard. After centrifugation at 10,000× *g* for 5 min, 50 μL of supernatant was mixed with 50 μL of 5-mM ammonium formate (pH 4). The liquid chromatography-tandem mass spectrometry (LC-MS/MS) was used to quantify the fexofenadine uptake amount [28,29].

2.7. LC-MS/MS Analysis

The chromatographic analysis was performed using an Agilent 1260 series (Agilent, Germany) HPLC system. Chromatographic separation was achieved from the Phoroshell® column (C18, 3.0 × 50 mm, 2.7 μm). The mobile phase consisted of 5-mM ammonium formate (pH 4) in water (A) and acetonitrile (B). A gradient method was applied at a flow rate of 0.3 mL/min and, kept on the column temperature at 25 °C. The injection volume was 2 μL. An Agilent 6460 triple-quadruple mass spectrometer (Agilent Technologies, Singapore) with an electrospray ionization (ESI) source was used to detect the signal. It was operated in positive ion mode on multiple reaction monitoring (MRM). The monitored ions of fexofenadine and internal standard (terfenadine) were *m/z* 502→466 and *m/z* 472→436 [30,31], respectively. The collision energy and fragmentor of the ions were 25 V and 175 V for fexofenadine, and 25 V and 130 V for terfenadine, respectively. The data were acquired and processed using Mass Hunter Workstation B.06.00 software (Agilent Technologies, Singapore).

2.8. Animal Study

2.8.1. Animals

Male Sprague-Dawley rats (9 weeks, weighing 300 ± 50 g) were purchased from Koatech (Pyeongtaek, Korea). The rats were acclimated in the Animal Laboratory (Gyeongsang National University) under controlled condition of temperature (between 20 and 23 °C) and humidity (50% ± 5%) and allowed free access to food and water for 7 days. All rats were allowed to recover for 1 day after cannulation into the carotid artery. The rats were fasted for 12 h with free access to water, before the pharmacokinetic experiments.

2.8.2. Pharmacokinetic Study

The pharmacokinetic study was performed on a rat model. The dose of *R. acetosa* extract evaluated was 2 g/kg, the maximum dose without the toxicity in rats (unpublished data). The selected oral dose of emodin was 11 mg/kg that inhibited *P*-gp mediated efflux in rats from the reported study [32]. All test compounds—including 11 mg/kg of emodin and 2 g/kg of *R. acetosa* extract suspended in 0.5% carboxy methyl cellulose (CMC)—were administered orally to rats. Same volume of 0.5% CMC was administered to the vehicle control group rats. After 30 min, a single dose of 10 mg/kg of fexofenadine in 10% ethanol was orally administered to each group of rats [33]. Blood samples of 120 μL were collected from the carotid artery at each time point (0, 0.25, 0.5, 0.75, 1, 1.5, 2, 4, 6, 8, 12 and 24 h) after oral administration of fexofenadine. The samples were then immediately centrifuged at 10,000× *g* and 4 °C for 10 min. All plasma samples were stored at −20 °C. The plasma concentrations of fexofenadine were determined by LC-MS/MS. All experimental procedures of the animal study were approved (GNU-170705-R0030, 5 July 2017) by the Animal Care and Use Committee of Gyeongsang National University, Korea.

2.8.3. Sample Preparation

The method of sample preparation was a modified method of Isleyen et al. [34] for determination of fexofenadine plasma concentration. In summary, 50 µL of 50-ng/mL terfenadine in acetonitrile solution was added to a 50-µL aliquot of plasma, then 20 µL of aqueous 13-µM formic acid solution was added. After vortexing, 50 µL of extraction solvent (a mixture of dichloromethane, ethyl acetate, diethyl ether at the ratio of 30:40:30, *v/v/v*) was added. The sample was then vortexed for 40 s. The protein precipitation was performed via centrifugation at 10,000× *g* and 4 °C for 5 min. The supernatant was cooled at −80 °C for 10 min. The upper fraction of the supernatant was transferred to a polypropylene tube and evaporated with N_2 gas. After being reconstituted with 200 µL of the mobile phase initial composition [5-mM ammonium formate (at a pH of 4): acetonitrile = 60:40], an aliquot of 2 µL was injected into LC-MS/MS.

2.9. Physicochemical Interaction Study

To investigate the possible physicochemical interactions between drug and *R. acetosa* extract, Fourier transform infrared (FT-IR) spectrum measurement and solubility test were carried out.

FT-IR spectra of fexofenadine HCl, *R. acetosa* extract and mixture of fexofenadine-extract (1:1) were measured by Nicolet iS 50 FT-IR spectrometer (Thermo Scientific, Waltham, MA, USA) with attenuated total reflectance (ATR) mode.

The change on the solubility of fexofenadine after mixing with *R. acetosa* extract was tested. The method was modified previously reported method [35,36]. Briefly, 200 µg of fexofenadine and *R. acetosa* extract were placed in the tube after centrifugal vacuum evaporation of solvent. The control group has fexofenadine only, and the mixed group has both fexofenadine and the extract. A 200-µL aliquot of the simulated intestinal fluid (SIF, pH 6.8) without enzyme [37] was added to each tube. The tubes were then incubated in a shaking water bath at 37 °C for 12 h. The concentration of fexofenadine was 1 mg/mL, corresponding to the orally administered concentration to the rats (10 mg/5 mL/kg-fexofenadine with 5-mL/kg extract, total 10 mL). After the incubation, the tubes were centrifuged at 10,000× *g* for 10 min. The supernatant was filtered, diluted with mobile phase, and analyzed by LC-MS/MS.

2.10. Statistical Analysis

The statistical analysis was performed using one-way analysis of variance (ANOVA) followed by a Dunnett's multiple comparison test. A *p*-value of less than 0.05 was considered statistically significant.

3. Results

3.1. Cytotoxicity Assay

Cell viability was expressed as a percentage of the absorbance value obtained from the media only treated control group (Figure 1). Even though there were statistically significant differences in Caco-2 cell viability between control and *R. acetosa* treated groups at concentrations of 20, 10, 2 and 1 µg/mL, the cell viability values were high enough to study (96.4% ± 1.3%, 95.0% ± 2.1%, 95.0% ± 1.2% and 95.5% ± 2.1% at concentrations of 20, 10, 2 and 1 µg/mL, respectively). It is suggested that there is a negligible cytotoxic effect of *R. acetosa* on the Caco-2 cells at the concentration range of 1 to 100 µg/mL.

There was no significant difference on the cell viability on HEK293 cells at the concentration ranges of 1 to 50 µg/mL. The cytotoxic effect of *R. acetosa* was only detected on HEK293 cells at a concentration of 100 µg/mL with the value of 80.9% ± 11.7%. This result suggests a dose window of *R. acetosa* extract for the experiment using HEK293 cells. It also indicates that the inhibitory effect of *R. acetosa* on fexofenadine uptake discussed in Section 3.2 was not due to the cytotoxic effects of *R. acetosa* on HEK293 cells at the concentration range tested.

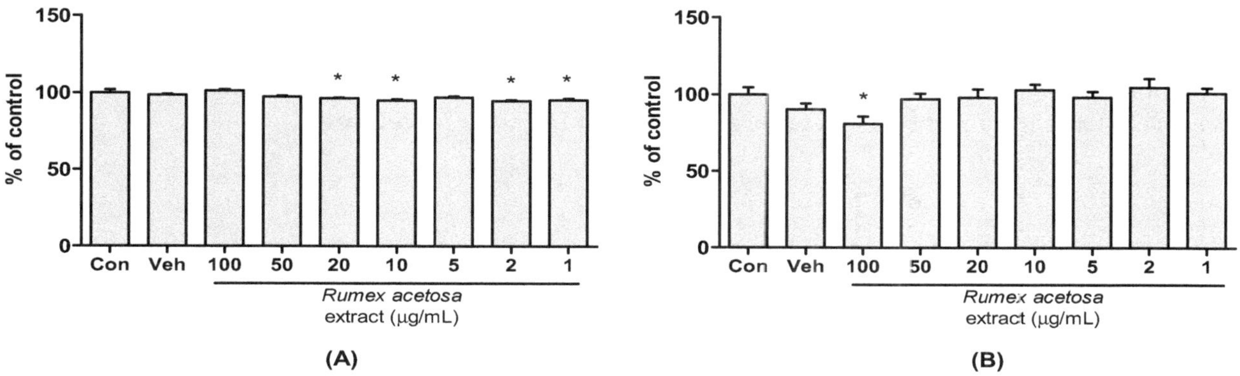

Figure 1. Cytotoxicity of *R. acetosa* extract in (**A**) Caco-2 cells and (**B**) HEK293 cells ($n = 6$). Con—media only treated control; Veh—vehicle treated group; *—$p < 0.05$ compared to media only treated control group.

3.2. *P*-gp Inhibition Test of Anthraquinones and *R. acetosa* Extract

To determine inhibitory effect of anthraquinones on *P*-gp, an MDR kit was used. The accumulated amount of fluorescent dye in the cells represented the *P*-gp inhibition activity. The measured fluorescence intensity is expressed as a percentage of the fluorescence intensity in the control group and is shown in Figure 2. The verapamil, chrysophanol-8-*O*-β-D-glucoside and emodin treated groups displayed significantly different fluorescence intensities in comparison to those of the control group. However, the chrysophanol-8-*O*-β-D-glucoside and emodin treated groups showed significantly higher fluorescence intensities than the control group, with average values of 121.4% ± 2.3% and 147.2% ± 12.4%, respectively (mean ± standard deviation). This result suggests that chrysophanol-8-*O*-β-D-glucoside and emodin affect the efflux of fluorescent dye from Caco-2 cells through *P*-gp inhibition. This is consistent with previous findings that emodin inhibits *P*-gp [18]. It is thus reasonable to suggest that herbal drug containing chrysophanol-8-*O*-β-D-glucoside and emodin may also inhibit *P*-gp.

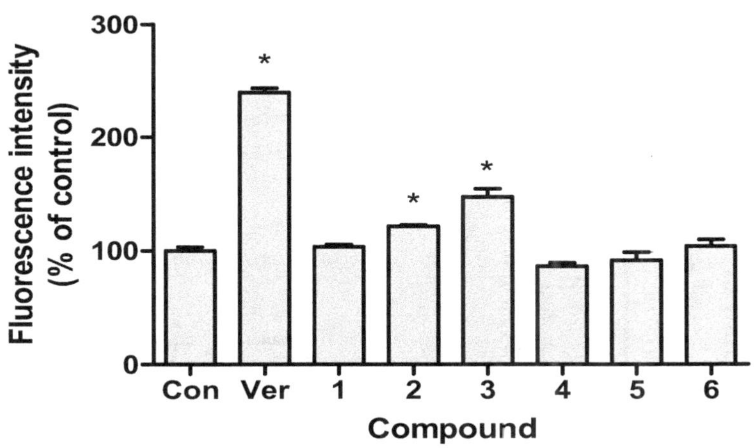

Figure 2. P-gp inhibitory effect of anthraquinones in Caco-2 cells. Cells were treated with 10-μM anthraquinones or 100-μM verapamil ($n = 3$). Con—vehicle treated control; Ver—verapamil; 1—chrysophanol; 2—chrysophanol-8-*O*-β-D-glucoside; 3—emodin; 4—emodin-8-*O*-β-D-glucoside; 5—physcion; 6—physcion-8-*O*-β-D-glucoside; *—$p < 0.05$ compared to control group.

The effects of *R. acetosa* extract on the *P*-gp were also assessed using an MDR kit. The measured fluorescence intensity is expressed as a percentage of the fluorescence intensity in the control group and is shown in Figure 3. There was no significant difference in fluorescence intensity between the control and the *R. acetosa* extract treated group. The significant inhibitory effect at the 95% confidence interval was only detected in the verapamil group used as a positive control. Although *R. acetosa* extract contains chrysophanol-8-*O*-β-D-glucoside and emodin at concentrations of 0.77% ± 0.12% and 0.94% ± 0.15% (*w/w*), respectively [27], inhibitory effects on *P*-gp could not be detected from *R. acetosa* extract at the concentrations tested in this assay. The concentrations of emodin and chrysophanol-8-*O*-β-D-glucoside in *R. acetosa* extract may not be high enough to inhibit *P*-gp in Caco-2 cells.

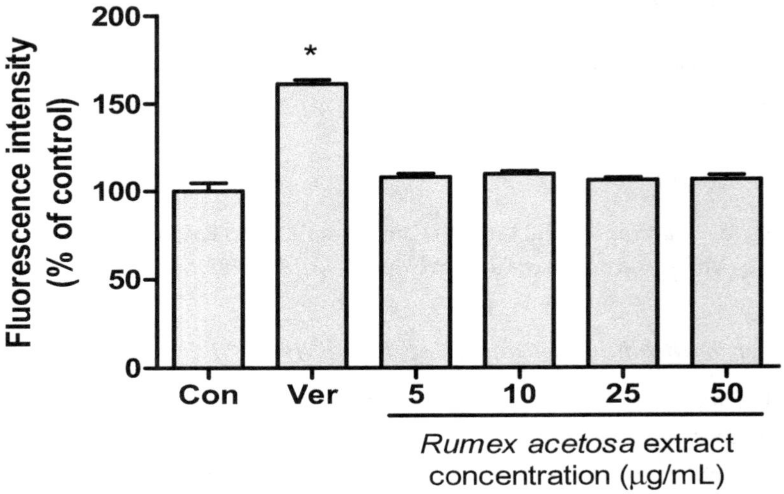

Figure 3. P-gp inhibition test of *R. acetosa* extract using an MDR kit in Caco-2 cells ($n = 6$). Con—vehicle treated control; Ver—100-μM verapamil; *—$p < 0.05$ compared to control group.

3.3. Fexofenadine Uptake Test with OATP1A2/SLCO1A2 Transfected HEK293 Cells

The decreased fexofenadine uptake in the OATP1A2/SLCO1A2 transfected HEK293 cells represented the inhibitory effects on OATP1A2. The accumulated amount of fexofenadine in the OATP/SLCO1A2 transfected cells (the control group) was higher than that of untransfected cells (untransfected control group), which means that the OATP1A2 gene was transfected and expressed sufficiently in the control group. In addition, the fexofenadine uptake was lower in the verapamil cotreated group than in the transfected control group. In the *R. acetosa* extract co-treated group, the uptake amounts of fexofenadine in the OATP1A2 transfected HEK293 cells were significantly lower than that in the control group (Figure 4). This result suggests that *R. acetosa* extract could affect the absorption of fexofenadine through the inhibition of OATP1A2.

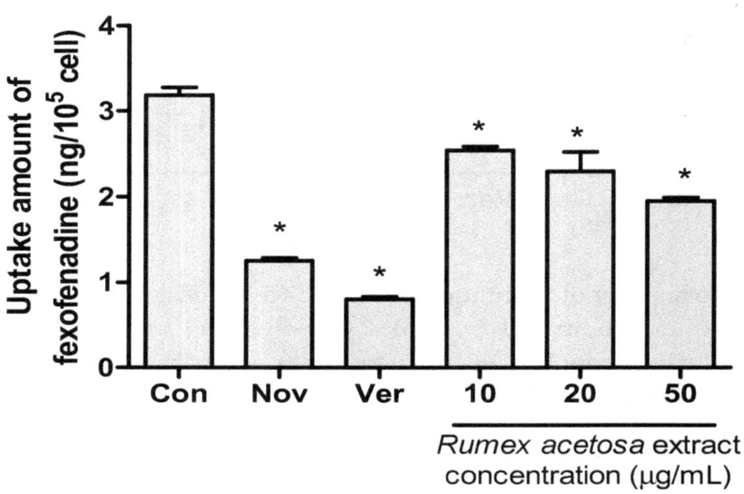

Figure 4. Inhibitory effect of *R. acetosa* extract on fexofenadine uptake in OATP1A2/SLCO1A2 transfected HEK293 cells ($n = 6$). Con—OATP1A2/SLCO1A2 transfected control; Nov—untransfected control; Ver—100-μM verapamil; *—$p < 0.05$ compared to control group.

3.4. *Pharmacokinetic Study*

The mean arterial plasma concentration–time profiles of fexofenadine after the pharmacokinetic study of fexofenadine in a rat drug interaction model, are shown in Figure 5. The pharmacokinetic parameters of fexofenadine after oral coadministration of vehicle, emodin and *R. acetosa* extract are shown in Table 1. The area under the plasma concentration–time curve (AUC) values of fexofenadine were 222.0 ± 85.5 ng·h/mL in the control group and 411.9 ± 189.1 ng·h/mL in the emodin coadministered group. In the emodin group, the absorption of fexofenadine was significantly higher, with a larger fexofenadine AUC and no difference in T_{max}. However, the fexofenadine AUC was lower, with a value of 132.0 ± 50.5 ng·h/mL, in the 2 g/kg *R. acetosa* extract coadministered group. Because fexofenadine is characterized by limited metabolism, it is probable that the lower fexofenadine AUC is due to the inhibitory effect of *R. acetosa* extract on absorption. Consequently, *R. acetosa* extract could inhibit the absorption of fexofenadine. Together with the results of the in vitro assay, this suggests that *R. acetosa* extract inhibits the intracellular uptake of fexofenadine via an intervention in OATP1A2.

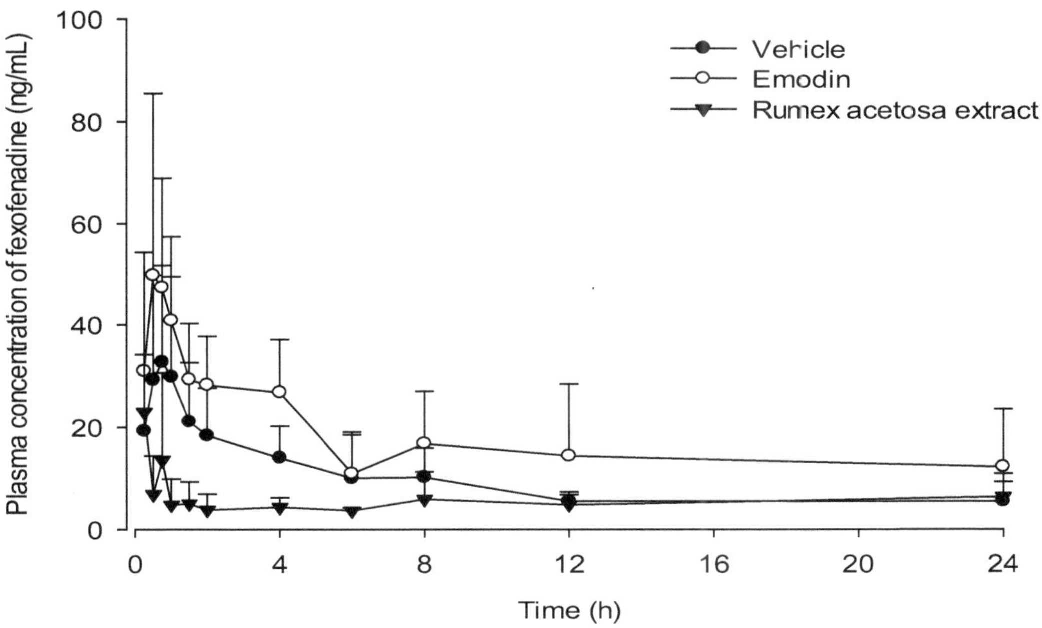

Figure 5. Mean plasma concentration–time profiles of fexofenadine (ng/mL) after oral coadministration of fexofenadine (10 mg/kg) with vehicle (•; $n = 6$), emodin (11 mg/ kg, ○; $n = 6$) and *R. acetosa* extract (2 g/kg, ▼; $n = 6$) to rats. Bars represent standard deviations.

Table 1. Pharmacokinetic parameters of fexofenadine after oral coadministration of fexofenadine (10 mg/kg) with vehicle (control), emodin and *R. acetosa* extract to rats. Values represent means ± standard deviations for $AUC_{0\text{-}24\,h}$ and C_{max} (ng/mL), median (range) for T_{max}.

Parameters	Control ($n = 6$)	Emodin 11 mg/kg ($n = 6$)	*R. acetosa* Extract 2 g/kg ($n = 6$)
$AUC_{0\text{-}24\,h}$ (ng·h/mL)	222.0 ± 85.5	411.9 ± 189.1 *	132.0 ± 50.5
C_{max} (ng/mL)	36.4 ± 22.8	53.4 ± 33.9	32.9 ± 28.5
T_{max} (h)	0.75 (0.5–1)	0.75 (0.5–1)	0.75 (0.25–8)

$AUC_{0\text{-}24\,h}$, total area under the plasma concentration–time curve from time zero to 24 h; C_{max}—maximum plasma concentration; T_{max}—time to reach C_{max}; *—$p < 0.05$ compared to vehicle only control group.

3.5. Physicochemical Interaction Study

To evaluate the possible physicochemical interactions between *R. acetosa* extract and fexofenadine, FT-IR spectra of extract, fexofenadine and mixture were measured and are shown in Figure 6. The FT-IR spectrum of fexofenadine HCl showed the characteristic absorption bands at 3291.03 (OH stretching), 2936.14 (CH stretching), 2639.82 (OH of carboxylate), 1698.68 (CO stretching), 1448.00, 1403.11 (C=C stretching of aromatic ring), 1167.57 (CO stretching of tertiary alcohol) and 1067.94 (CO stretching of secondary alcohol) [38,39]. According to Figure 6, the mixture of *R. acetosa* extract and fexofenadine HCl showed the same bands compared to the pure fexofenadine HCl. It suggests that there is no significant physical interaction between fexofenadine molecule and *R. acetosa* extract component on fexofenadine functional groups.

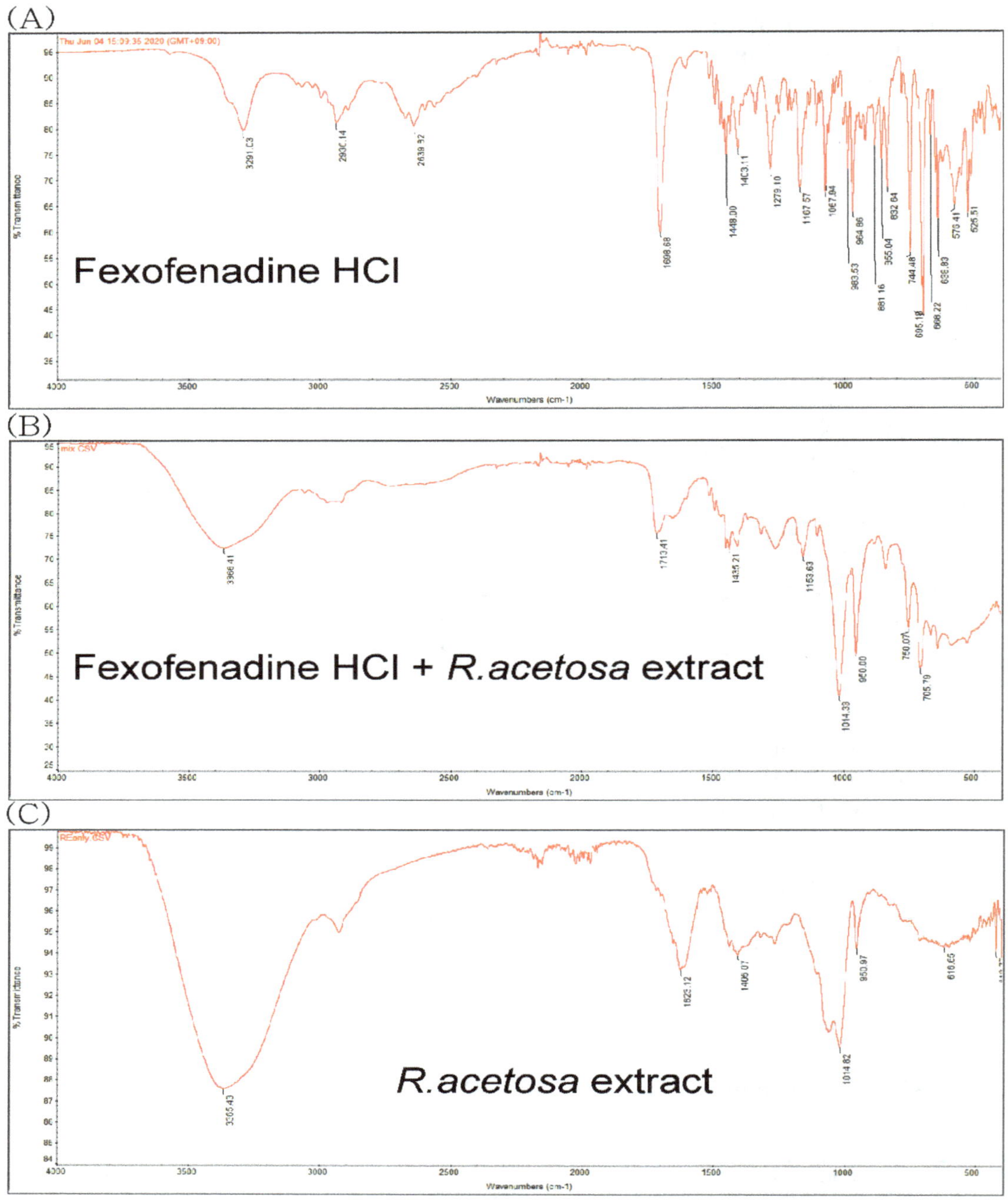

Figure 6. FT-IR spectra of (**A**) fexofenadine, (**B**) a mixture of fexofenadine and *R. acetosa* extract and (**C**) *R. acetosa* extract.

However, there was significant difference on the solubility of fexofenadine after incubation with the extract (Table 2). The average solubilities of fexofenadine in SIF were 1.03 ± 0.04 mg/mL and 0.83 ± 0.10 mg/mL without and with *R. acetosa* extract, respectively. This result indicates that *R. acetosa* extract could alter the solubility of fexofenadine and lead to precipitation in gastro-intestinal tract.

Table 2. The solubility of fexofenadine HCl in simulated intestinal fluid (SIF) with and without *R. acetosa* extract.

Solubility	Without *R. acetosa* Extract($n = 3$)	With *R. acetosa* Extract($n = 3$)
Fexofenadine HCl concentration (mg/mL)	1.03 ± 0.04	0.83 ± 0.10 *

*—$p < 0.05$ compared to without *R. acetosa* extract.

4. Discussion

Pharmacokinetic drug interactions involving drug absorption should be considered for optimum drug therapy, apart from the drug interactions attributed to the oxidative metabolism via the CYP-450 system of different isozymes [40]. Ostensibly harmless natural products—such as juices, fruits, vegetables and herbal products in the form of ayurvedic medicine—have been reported in several studies to potentially cause many drug interactions affecting drug absorption mediated by transporters [41,42]. For example, emodin—a potential antineoplastic drug and a major component of the *Rhamnus, Rumex, Aloe, Rheum* and *Cassia* species—has been reported to be a possible *P*-gp inducer [26] or an inhibitor [18].

This study evaluated the effects of *R. acetosa* extract on the drug transporters discussed above, as well as its potential for drug interactions, while presenting a clear view of the interactions of emodin with the transporter *P*-gp. The major six anthraquinones present in *R. acetosa* were shown in our previous study [27]. A prior cytotoxicity assay was performed to establish the working range for the extract suitable for optimal viability of the cells during the experiment. Afterwards, the effects of these six anthraquinones on *P*-gp were demonstrated individually with an MDR assay kit using Caco-2 cells. Verapamil, being an inhibitor of *P*-gp, served as a positive control. Only groups treated with chrysophanol-8-*O*-β-D-glucoside and emodin showed higher fluorescence intensity than the control group, with average values of 121.4% ± 2.3% and 147.2% ± 12.4%, respectively, suggesting *P*-gp inhibition. This result is consistent with those obtained in a study by Min et al. [18], in which emodin was shown to inhibit *P*-gp. On the other hand, the results from the *P*-gp inhibition test of *R. acetosa* extract suggest no significant inhibition of the efflux transporter, as opposed to the emodin and chrysophanol-8-*O*-β-D-glucoside, which in contrast showed significant inhibition of the *P*-gp transporter when treated individually. A possible explanation is that the emodin content may not be high enough to exert its inhibitory effect in the extract. Chemical contents of herbal plant extracts can vary depending on various factors such as climate, harvesting seasons and extraction solvent. The probability of inhibition of *P*-gp by *R. acetosa* extract cannot be ruled out.

OATP1A2—the uptake transporter used in our in vitro test—is widely expressed in the intestines and serves as a major uptake mechanism for fexofenadine [43,44]. Sometimes, a substrate of *P*-gp—such as this study's selected model drug, fexofenadine—can also be a substrate for the OATP uptake transporter [43,44], making it necessary to differentiate between the contributions of *P*-gp and OATP to potential drug interactions and those of other simultaneously administered drugs that could affect these transporters. Therefore, our in vitro studies were also performed with HEK293 cells transfected with the polypeptide transporter OATP1A2. *R. acetosa* extract was found to inhibit the uptake of fexofenadine through in vitro studies. In other words, the uptake of fexofenadine by OATP1A2 into cells declined when *R. acetosa* extract was used as a co-treatment. This result suggests that *R. acetosa* extract can affect the absorption of fexofenadine through the inhibition of OATP1A2.

A pharmacokinetic study was designed to verify the results of our in vitro study in view of the observed herbal extract's drug interactions at the uptake transporter for fexofenadine in rats. Rat model is considered unsuitable to predict metabolic drug interaction in human [45]. However, there is a correlation in drug intestinal permeability with both carrier-mediated absorption and passive diffusion mechanisms between rat and human [46]. Because the property of our selected model drug, fexofenadine, has little metabolism, it is reasonable to use the rat model for predicting the intervention of extract on absorption. All rats were divided into 3 groups: an emodin administration group, an *R. acetosa* administration group and a control group. Eleven milligrams per kilogram of emodin, 2 g/kg of *R. acetosa* extract and 0.5% CMC as a control was administered orally to each group Fexofenadine at the dose of 10 mg/kg was given orally to each group after 30 min. The results showed a smaller AUC of fexofenadine (132.1 ± 50.3 ng·h/mL) in the *R. acetosa* group in comparison to that of the control group, in which the AUC was 222.0 ± 92.1 ng·h/mL. These results suggest decreased absorption of fexofenadine in the rats treated with *R. acetosa* extract. In other words, the gut uptake transporter OATP1A2, which is responsible for fexofenadine absorption, was inhibited, as predicted by the in vitro results. Moreover, the alteration on the solubility of fexofenadine was also observed by *R. acetosa* extract through the physicochemical interaction study. The FT-IR spectra results suggest that there is no functional group interaction between fexofenadine and the component of *R. acetosa* extract The fexofenadine solubility in SIF changed from 1.03 ± 0.04 mg/mL to 0.83 ± 0.10 mg/mL after mixing with the extract. It means that the solubility alteration could also be the reason for the decreased fexofenadine AUC by *R. acetosa* extract because fexofenadine HCl is Biopharmaceutics Classification System (BCS) class 3 drug with high solubility and low permeability. Drug interactions due to changes in solubility can be avoided by adjusting the administration time. *R. acetosa* extract contains many kinds of compounds, not only anthraquinones, but also flavonoids and polysaccharides [15]. They have also the possibility of interference with the drug absorption through the intervention to the transporters [47,48]. Particularly, one of the flavonoids of *R. acetosa* extract, epicatechin-3-*O*-gallate [49], also has an inhibitory effect on the OATP1A2 [50]. Moreover, there was the possibility that *R. acetosa* extract may change the gastric emptying time [51,52] and the pH in the gastro-intestinal tract when coadministered with the fexofenadine. The effects of anthraquinones on OATP have been rarely reported. Further studies are needed to elucidate the components in *R. acetosa* extract responsible for inhibition of fexofenadine absorption. Meanwhile, emodin increased the AUC for fexofenadine, possibly via the inhibitory effect on an efflux transporter of fexofenadine, *P*-gp [32], the effect of which on the uptake transporter of fexofenadine has yet to be fully understood.

Given the evidence from both in vitro and in vivo studies, *R. acetosa* extract should be used with caution when substrates of the drug transporters or poorly water-soluble drugs are prescribed.

5. Conclusions

The present study evaluated the effects of *R. acetosa* extract on 2 active transporters, P-gp and OATP1A2 and the resulting effects on fexofenadine absorption through in vitro and in vivo studies. The findings suggest that emodin can enhance fexofenadine absorption via an inhibitory effect on *P*-gp. In addition, *R. acetosa* extract could decrease the absorption of fexofenadine via intervention in the aqueous solubility and the drug transporters.

Author Contributions: Conceptualization, H.J.C.; methodology, H.J.C.; validation, J.K. and N.U.R.; formal analysis, J.K.; investigation, J.H.A., J.K. and H.-J.K.; resources, M.-J.A. and H.J.C.; data curation, J.H.A., J.K. and H.J.C.; writing—original draft preparation, J.K. and N.U.R.; writing—review and editing, H.J.C.; visualization, J.K.; supervision, H.J.C. and M.-J.A.; project administration, H.J.C.; funding acquisition, H.J.C. All authors have read and agreed to the published version of the manuscript.

References

1. Dean, M.; Hamon, Y.; Chimini, G. The human ATP-binding cassette (ABC) transporter superfamily. *J. Lipid Res.* **2001**, *42*, 1007–1017. [CrossRef] [PubMed]
2. Anderle, P.; Niederer, E.; Rubas, W.; Hilgendorf, C.; Spahn-Langguth, H.; Wunderli-Allenspach, H.; Merkle, H.P.; Langguth, P. P-Glycoprotein (P-gp) mediated efflux in Caco-2 cell monolayers: The influence of culturing conditions and drug exposure on P-gp expression levels. *J. Pharm. Sci.* **1998**, *87*, 757–762. [CrossRef] [PubMed]

3. Fardel, O.; Lecureur, V.; Guillouzo, A. The P-glycoprotein multidrug transporter. *Gen. Pharm.* **1996**, *27*, 1283–1291. [CrossRef]
4. Chan, L.M.; Lowes, S.; Hirst, B.H. The ABCs of drug transport in intestine and liver: Efflux proteins limiting drug absorption and bioavailability. *Eur. J. Pharm. Sci.* **2004**, *21*, 25–51. [CrossRef]
5. Talks, K.L.; Turley, H.; Gatter, K.C.; Maxwell, P.H.; Pugh, C.W.; Ratcliffe, P.J.; Harris, A.L. The expression and distribution of the hypoxia-inducible factors HIF-1alpha and HIF-2alpha in normal human tissues, cancers, and tumor-associated macrophages. *Am. J. Pathol* **2000**, *157*, 411–421. [CrossRef]
6. Comerford, K.M.; Wallace, T.J.; Karhausen, J.; Louis, N.A.; Montalto, M.C.; Colgan, S.P. Hypoxia-inducible factor-1-dependent regulation of the multidrug resistance (MDR1) gene. *Cancer Res.* **2002**, *62*, 3387–3394.
7. Kim, R.B. Drugs as P-glycoprotein substrates, inhibitors, and inducers. *Drug Metab. Rev.* **2002**, *34*, 47–54. [CrossRef]
8. Palmeira, A.; Sousa, E.; Vasconcelos, M.H.; Pinto, M.M. Three decades of P-gp: Skimming through several generations and scaffolds. *Curr. Med. Che* **2012**, *19*, 1946–2025. [CrossRef]
9. Shitara, Y.; Maeda, K.; Ikejiri, K.; Yoshida, K.; Horie, T.; Sugiyama, Y. Clinical significance of organic anion transporting polypeptides (OATPs) in drug disposition: Their roles in hepatic clearance and intestinal absorption. *Biopharm. Drug Dispos.* **2013**, *34*, 45–78. [CrossRef]
10. Yu, J.; Zhou, Z.; Tay-Sontheimer, J.; Levy, R.H.; Ragueneau-Majlessi, I. Intestinal drug interactions mediated by OATPs: A systematic review of preclinical and clinical findings. *J. Pharm. Sci.* **2017**, *106*, 2312–2325. [CrossRef]
11. Agbabiaka, T.B.; Spencer, N.H.; Khanom, S.; Goodman, C. Prevalence of drug-herb and drug-supplement interactions in older adults: A cross-sectional survey. *Br. J. Gen. Pr.* **2018**, *68*, e711–e717. [CrossRef] [PubMed]
12. Kaufman, D.W.; Kelly, J.P.; Rosenberg, L.; Anderson, T.E.; Mitchell, A.A. Recent patterns of medication use in the ambulatory adult population of the United States: The Slone survey. *JAMA* **2002**, *287*, 337–344. [CrossRef] [PubMed]
13. Durr, D.; Stieger, B.; Kullak-Ublick, G.A.; Rentsch, K.M.; Steinert, H.C.; Meier, P.J.; Fattinger, K. St John's Wort induces intestinal P-glycoprotein/MDR1 and intestinal and hepatic CYP3A4. *Clin. Pharm.* **2000**, *68*, 598–604. [CrossRef] [PubMed]
14. Gescher, K.; Hensel, A.; Hafezi, W.; Derksen, A.; Kuhn, J. Oligomeric proanthocyanidins from Rumex acetosa L. inhibit the attachment of herpes simplex virus type-1. *Antivir. Res.* **2011**, *89*, 9–18. [CrossRef] [PubMed]
15. Vasas, A.; Orban-Gyapai, O.; Hohmann, J. The genus Rumex: Review of traditional uses, phytochemistry and pharmacology. *J. Ethnopharmacol.* **2015**, *175*, 198–228. [CrossRef] [PubMed]
16. Kucekova, Z.; Mlcek, J.; Humpolicek, P.; Rop, O.; Valasek, P.; Saha, P. Phenolic compounds from Allium schoenoprasum, Tragopogon pratensis and Rumex acetosa and their antiproliferative effects. *Molecules* **2011**, *16*, 9207–9217. [CrossRef]
17. Bae, J.Y.; Lee, Y.S.; Han, S.Y.; Jeong, E.J.; Lee, M.K.; Kong, J.Y.; Lee, D.H.; Cho, K.J.; Lee, H.S.; Ahn, M.J. A comparison between water and ethanol extracts of Rumex acetosa for protective effects on gastric ulcers in mice. *Biomol. Ther. (Seoul)* **2012**, *20*, 425–430. [CrossRef] [PubMed]
18. Min, H.; Niu, M.; Zhang, W.; Yan, J.; Li, J.; Tan, X.; Li, B.; Su, M.; Di, B.; Yan, F. Emodin reverses leukemia multidrug resistance by competitive inhibition and downregulation of P-glycoprotein. *PLoS ONE* **2017**, *12*, e0187971. [CrossRef]
19. Feng, Y.; Huang, S.L.; Dou, W.; Zhang, S.; Chen, J.H.; Shen, Y.; Shen, J.H.; Leng, Y. Emodin, a natural product, selectively inhibits 11beta-hydroxysteroid dehydrogenase type 1 and ameliorates metabolic disorder in diet-induced obese mice. *Br. J. Pharm.* **2010**, *161*, 113–126. [CrossRef]
20. Hsu, S.C.; Chung, J.G. Anticancer potential of emodin. *BioMedicine (Taipei)* **2012**, *2*, 108–116. [CrossRef]
21. Simpson, K.; Jarvis, B. Fexofenadine: A review of its use in the management of seasonal allergic rhinitis and chronic idiopathic urticaria. *Drugs* **2000**, *59*, 301–321. [CrossRef] [PubMed]
22. Tahara, H.; Kusuhara, H.; Fuse, E.; Sugiyama, Y. P-glycoprotein plays a major role in the efflux of fexofenadine in the small intestine and blood-brain barrier, but only a limited role in its biliary excretion. *Drug Metab. Dispos.* **2005**, *33*, 963–968. [CrossRef] [PubMed]

23. Shimizu, M.; Fuse, K.; Okudaira, K.; Nishigaki, R.; Maeda, K.; Kusuhara, H.; Sugiyama, Y. Contribution of OATP (organic anion-transporting polypeptide) family transporters to the hepatic uptake of fexofenadine in humans. *Drug Metab. Dispos.* **2005**, *33*, 1477–1481. [CrossRef] [PubMed]
24. Molimard, M.; Diquet, B.; Benedetti, M.S. Comparison of pharmacokinetics and metabolism of desloratadine, fexofenadine, levocetirizine and mizolastine in humans. *Fundam. Clin. Pharm.* **2004**, *18*, 399–411. [CrossRef] [PubMed]
25. Prescribing Information for Allegra®(fexofenadine hydrochloride). Available online: https://www.accessdata.fda.gov/drugsatfda_docs/label/2003/20872se8-003,20625se8-010_allegra_lbl.pdf (accessed on 16 March 2020).
26. Huang, J.; Guo, L.; Tan, R.; Wei, M.; Zhang, J.; Zhao, Y.; Gong, L.; Huang, Z.; Qiu, X. Interactions between emodin and efflux transporters on rat enterocyte by a validated ussing chamber technique. *Front. Pharm.* **2018**, *9*, 646. [CrossRef]
27. Ullah, H.M.A.; Kim, J.; Rehman, N.U.; Kim, H.J.; Ahn, M.J.; Chung, H.J. A simple and sensitive liquid chromatography with tandem mass spectrometric method for the simultaneous determination of anthraquinone glycosides and their aglycones in rat plasma: Application to a pharmacokinetic study of Rumex acetosa extract. *Pharmaceutics* **2018**, *10*, 100. [CrossRef]
28. Petri, N.; Tannergren, C.; Rungstad, D.; Lennernas, H. Transport characteristics of fexofenadine in the Caco-2 cell model. *Pharm. Res.* **2004**, *21*, 1398–1404. [CrossRef]
29. Rebello, S.; Zhao, S.; Hariry, S.; Dahlke, M.; Alexander, N.; Vapurcuyan, A.; Hanna, I.; Jarugula, V. Intestinal OATP1A2 inhibition as a potential mechanism for the effect of grapefruit juice on aliskiren pharmacokinetics in healthy subjects. *Eur. J. Clin. Pharm.* **2012**, *68*, 697–708. [CrossRef]
30. Yamane, N.; Tozuka, Z.; Sugiyama, Y.; Tanimoto, T.; Yamazaki, A.; Kumagai, Y. Microdose clinical trial: Quantitative determination of fexofenadine in human plasma using liquid chromatography/electrospray ionization tandem mass spectrometry. *J. Chromatogr B Anal. Technol Biomed. Life Sci* **2007**, *858*, 118–128. [CrossRef]
31. Bharathi, V.D.; Radharani, K.; Jagadeesh, B.; Ramulu, G.; Bhushan, I.; Naidu, A.; Mullangi, R. LC–MS–MS assay for simultaneous quantification of fexofenadine and pseudoephedrine in human plasma. *Chromatographia* **2008**, *67*, 461–466. [CrossRef]
32. Li, X.; Hu, J.; Wang, B.; Sheng, L.; Liu, Z.; Yang, S.; Li, Y. Inhibitory effects of herbal constituents on P-glycoprotein in vitro and in vivo: Herb-drug interactions mediated via P-gp. *Toxicol. Appl. Pharm.* **2014**, *275*, 163–175. [CrossRef] [PubMed]
33. Kamath, A.V.; Yao, M.; Zhang, Y.; Chong, S. Effect of fruit juices on the oral bioavailability of fexofenadine in rats. *J. Pharm. Sci.* **2005**, *94*, 233–239. [CrossRef] [PubMed]
34. İşleyen, E.A.Ö.; Özden, T.; Özilhan, S.; Toptan, S. Quantitative determination of fexofenadine in human plasma by HPLC-MS. *Chromatographia* **2007**, *66*, 109–113. [CrossRef]
35. Dai, W.G. In vitro methods to assess drug precipitation. *Int. J. Pharm.* **2010**, *393*, 1–16. [CrossRef] [PubMed]
36. Saito, Y.; Usami, T.; Katoh, M.; Nadai, M. Effects of thylakoid-rich spinach extract on the pharmacokinetics of drugs in rats. *Biol. Pharm. Bull.* **2019**, *42*, 103–109. [CrossRef] [PubMed]
37. Stippler, E.; Kopp, S.; Dressman, J.B. Comparison of US pharmacopeia simulated intestinal fluid TS (without pancreatin) and phosphate standard buffer pH 6.8, TS of the international pharmacopoeia with respect to their use in in vitro dissolution testing. *Dissolution Technol.* **2004**, *11*, 6–10. [CrossRef]
38. Singh, B.; Saini, G.; Vyas, M.; Verma, S.; Thakur, S. Optimized chronomodulated dual release bilayer tablets of fexofenadine and montelukast: Quality by design, development, and in vitro evaluation. *Future J. Pharm. Sci.* **2019**, *5*, 5. [CrossRef]
39. Arefin, P.; Hasan, I.; Reza, M.S. Design, characterization and in vitro evaluation of HPMC K100 M CR loaded fexofenadine HCl microspheres. *Springerplus* **2016**, *5*, 691. [CrossRef]
40. Hansten, P.D.; Levy, R.H. Role of P-glycoprotein and organic anion transporting polypeptides in drug absorption and distribution. *Clin. Drug Investig.* **2001**, *21*, 587–596. [CrossRef]
41. Mallhi, T.H.; Sarriff, A.; Adnan, A.S.; Khan, Y.H.; Qadir, M.I.; Hamzah, A.A.; Khan, A.H. Effect of fruit/vegetable-drug interactions on CYP450, OATP and p-glycoprotein: A systematic review. *Trop. J. Pharm. Res.* **2015**, *14*, 1927–1935. [CrossRef]
42. Bailey, D.G. Fruit juice inhibition of uptake transport: A new type of food-drug interaction. *Br. J. Clin. Pharm.* **2010**, *70*, 645–655. [CrossRef] [PubMed]

43. Cvetkovic, M.; Leake, B.; Fromm, M.F.; Wilkinson, G.R.; Kim, R.B. OATP and P-glycoprotein transporters mediate the cellular uptake and excretion of fexofenadine. *Drug Metab. Dispos.* **1999**, *27*, 866–871. [PubMed]
44. Niemi, M.; Kivisto, K.T.; Hofmann, U.; Schwab, M.; Eichelbaum, M.; Fromm, M.F. Fexofenadine pharmacokinetics are associated with a polymorphism of the SLCO1B1 gene (encoding OATP1B1). *Br. J. Clin. Pharm.* **2005**, *59*, 602–604. [CrossRef] [PubMed]
45. Jaiswal, S.; Sharma, A.; Shukla, M.; Vaghasiya, K.; Rangaraj, N.; Lal, J. Novel pre-clinical methodologies for pharmacokinetic drug-drug interaction studies: Spotlight on "humanized" animal models. *Drug Metab. Rev.* **2014**, *46*, 475–493. [CrossRef] [PubMed]
46. Cao, X.; Gibbs, S.T.; Fang, L.; Miller, H.A.; Landowski, C.P.; Shin, H.C.; Lennernas, H.; Zhong, Y.; Amidon, G.L.; Yu, L.X.; et al. Why is it challenging to predict intestinal drug absorption and oral bioavailability in human using rat model. *Pharm. Res.* **2006**, *23*, 1675–1686. [CrossRef]
47. Mandery, K.; Bujok, K.; Schmidt, I.; Keiser, M.; Siegmund, W.; Balk, B.; Konig, J.; Fromm, M.F.; Glaeser, H. Influence of the flavonoids apigenin, kaempferol, and quercetin on the function of organic anion transporting polypeptides 1A2 and 2B1. *Biochem. Pharm.* **2010**, *80*, 1746–1753. [CrossRef]
48. Masumoto, K.; Quan, Z.; Ishiuchi, K.i.; Matsumoto, T.; Watanabe, J.; Makino, T. Drug interaction between shoseiryuto extract or catechins and fexofenadine through organic-anion-transporting polypeptide 1A2 in vitro. *Pharmacogn. Mag.* **2019**, *15*, 304–308. [CrossRef]
49. Bicker, J.; Petereit, F.; Hensel, A. Proanthocyanidins and a phloroglucinol derivative from *Rumex acetosa* L. *Fitoterapia* **2009**, *80*, 483–495. [CrossRef]
50. Roth, M.; Timmermann, B.N.; Hagenbuch, B. Interactions of green tea catechins with organic anion-transporting polypeptides. *Drug Metab. Dispos.* **2011**, *39*, 920–926. [CrossRef]
51. Bajad, S.; Bedi, K.L.; Singla, A.K.; Johri, R.K. Piperine inhibits gastric emptying and gastrointestinal transit in rats and mice. *Planta Med.* **2001**, *67*, 176–179. [CrossRef]
52. Hu, M.L.; Rayner, C.K.; Wu, K.L.; Chuah, S.K.; Tai, W.C.; Chou, Y.P.; Chiu, Y.C.; Chiu, K.W.; Hu, T.H. Effect of ginger on gastric motility and symptoms of functional dyspepsia. *World J. Gastroenter.* **2011**, *17*, 105–110. [CrossRef] [PubMed]

Permissions

All chapters in this book were first published by MDPI; hereby published with permission under the Creative Commons Attribution License or equivalent. Every chapter published in this book has been scrutinized by our experts. Their significance has been extensively debated. The topics covered herein carry significant findings which will fuel the growth of the discipline. They may even be implemented as practical applications or may be referred to as a beginning point for another development.

The contributors of this book come from diverse backgrounds, making this book a truly international effort. This book will bring forth new frontiers with its revolutionizing research information and detailed analysis of the nascent developments around the world.

We would like to thank all the contributing authors for lending their expertise to make the book truly unique. They have played a crucial role in the development of this book. Without their invaluable contributions this book wouldn't have been possible. They have made vital efforts to compile up to date information on the varied aspects of this subject to make this book a valuable addition to the collection of many professionals and students.

This book was conceptualized with the vision of imparting up-to-date information and advanced data in this field. To ensure the same, a matchless editorial board was set up. Every individual on the board went through rigorous rounds of assessment to prove their worth. After which they invested a large part of their time researching and compiling the most relevant data for our readers.

The editorial board has been involved in producing this book since its inception. They have spent rigorous hours researching and exploring the diverse topics which have resulted in the successful publishing of this book. They have passed on their knowledge of decades through this book. To expedite this challenging task, the publisher supported the team at every step. A small team of assistant editors was also appointed to further simplify the editing procedure and attain best results for the readers.

Apart from the editorial board, the designing team has also invested a significant amount of their time in understanding the subject and creating the most relevant covers. They scrutinized every image to scout for the most suitable representation of the subject and create an appropriate cover for the book.

The publishing team has been an ardent support to the editorial, designing and production team. Their endless efforts to recruit the best for this project, has resulted in the accomplishment of this book. They are a veteran in the field of academics and their pool of knowledge is as vast as their experience in printing. Their expertise and guidance has proved useful at every step. Their uncompromising quality standards have made this book an exceptional effort. Their encouragement from time to time has been an inspiration for everyone.

The publisher and the editorial board hope that this book will prove to be a valuable piece of knowledge for researchers, students, practitioners and scholars across the globe.

List of Contributors

Bo Tang
School of Pharmacy, Nantong University, 19 Qixiu Road, Nantong 226001, China
Yabang Medical Research Institute, 66 Changhong Road, Changzhou 213145, China

Yu Qian and Guihua Fang
School of Pharmacy, Nantong University, 19 Qixiu Road, Nantong 226001, China
School of Pharmacy, Shenyang Pharmaceutical University, 103 Wenhua Road, Shenyang 110016, China

Noriaki Nagai, Ryotaro Seiriki, Saori Deguchi and Hiroko Otake
Faculty of Pharmacy, Kindai University, 3-4-1 Kowakae, Higashi-Osaka, Osaka 577-8502, Japan

Noriko Hiramatsu
Laboratory of Molecularbiology and Histochemistry, Fujita Health University Institute of Joint Research, 1-98 Dengakugakubo, Kutsukake, Toyoake, Aichi 470-1192, Japan

Hiroshi Sasaki and Naoki Yamamoto
Department of Ophthalmology, Kanazawa Medical University, 1-1 Daigaku, Uchinada, Kahoku, Ishikawa 920-0293, Japan

Sanjita Paudel, Piljoung Cho, Riya Shrestha, Younah Kim, Taeho Lee and Sangkyu Lee
BK21 Plus KNU Multi-Omics based Creative Drug Research Team, College of Pharmacy, Research Institute of Pharmaceutical Sciences, Kyungpook National University, Daegu 41566, Korea

Aarajana Shrestha, Ju-Hyun Kim, Tae Cheon Jeong and Eung-Seok Lee
College of Pharmacy, Yeungnam University, Gyeongsan 38541, Korea

Marta Kus-Slowinska
Department of Toxicology, Poznan University of Medical Sciences, 30 Dojazd St., 60-631 Poznan, Poland
Research and Development Department of Ethifarm, Ethifarm Manufacturing Plant, 9 Stefana Zeromskiego St., 60-544 Poznan, Poland

Monika Wrzaskowska, Izabela Ibragimow and Piotr Igor Czaklosz
Research and Development Department of Ethifarm, Ethifarm Manufacturing Plant, 9 Stefana Zeromskiego St., 60-544 Poznan, Poland

Anna Olejnik
Department of Biotechnology and Food Microbiology, Poznan University of Life Sciences, 48 Wojska Polskiego St., 60-627 Poznan, Poland

Hanna Piotrowska-Kempisty
Department of Toxicology, Poznan University of Medical Sciences, 30 Dojazd St., 60-631 Poznan, Poland
Department of Basic and Preclinical Sciences, Institute of Veterinary Medicine, Nicolaus Copernicus University in Toruń, 7 Gagarina St., 87-100 Torun, Poland

So-Young Park, Su-Nyeong Jang, Ga-Hyun Lee and Kwang-Hyeon Liu
BK21 Plus KNU Multi-Omics based Creative Drug Research Team, College of Pharmacy and Research Institute of Pharmaceutical Sciences, Kyungpook National University, Daegu 41566, Korea
College of Pharmacy and Research Institute of Pharmaceutical Sciences, Kyungpook National University, Daegu 41566, Korea

Phi-Hung Nguyen
Institute of Natural Products Chemistry, Vietnam Academy of Science and Technology, 18-Hoang Quoc Viet, Cau Giay, Hanoi 100000, Vietnam

Gahyun Kim and Zhexue Wu
College of Pharmacy and Research Institute of Pharmaceutical Sciences, Kyungpook National University, Daegu 41566, Korea

Nguyen Minh Phuc
College of Pharmacy and Research Institute of Pharmaceutical Sciences, Kyungpook National University, Daegu 41566, Korea
Vietnam Hightech of Medicinal and Pharmaceutical JSC, Group 11 Quang Minh town, Hanoi 100000, Vietnam

Hyeon-Cheol Jeong, Yoojeong Jang and Kwang-Hee Shin
College of Pharmacy, Research Institute of Pharmaceutical Sciences, Kyungpook National University, Daegu 41566, Korea

Soo Hyeon Bae
Korea Institute of Radiological & Medical Sciences, Seoul 01812, Korea
Q-fitter, Inc., Seoul 06578, Korea
College of Pharmacy and Integrated Research Institute of Pharmaceutical Sciences, The Catholic University, Korea, Bucheon 14662, Korea

Jung-Woo Bae and Sooyeun Lee
College of Pharmacy, Keimyung University, Daegu 42601, Korea

Anhye Kim
Department of Clinical Pharmacology and Therapeutics, CHA Bundang Medical Center, CHA University, Seongnam 13496, Korea

Yoshihiro Noguchi and Tomoya Tachi
Laboratory of Clinical Pharmacy, Gifu Pharmaceutical University, 1-25-4, Daigakunishi, Gifu-shi, Gifu 501-1196, Japan

Hitomi Teramachi
Laboratory of Clinical Pharmacy, Gifu Pharmaceutical University, 1-25-4, Daigakunishi, Gifu-shi, Gifu 501-1196, Japan
Laboratory of Community Healthcare Pharmacy, Gifu Pharmaceutical University, Daigakunishi, Gifu-shi, Gifu 501-1196, Japan

Malavika Deodhar, Sweilem B Al Rihani, Meghan J. Arwood, Lucy Darakjian and Pamela Dow
Tabula Rasa HealthCare Precision Pharmacotherapy Research and Development Institute, Orlando, FL 32827, USA

Jacques Turgeon and Veronique Michaud
Tabula Rasa HealthCare Precision Pharmacotherapy Research and Development Institute, Orlando, FL 32827, USA
Faculty of Pharmacy, Université de Montréal, Montreal, QC H3C 3J7, Canada

Young Hee Choi
College of Pharmacy and Integrated Research Institute for Drug Development, Dongguk University Seoul, 32 Dongguk-lo, Ilsandong-gu, Goyang-si 10326, Gyeonggi-do, Korea

Yu Fen Zheng
School of Basic Medicine and Clinical Pharmacy, China Pharmaceutical University, 639 Longmian Road, Jiangning District, Nanjing 211198, China

Zhouchi Huang, Soon Uk Chae, Seong Jun Jo, Hyung Joon Shim, Chae Bin Lee and Soo Kyung Bae
College of Pharmacy and Integrated Research Institute of Pharmaceutical Sciences, The Catholic University, Korea, Bucheon 14662, Korea

Doyun Kim
College of Pharmacy and Integrated Research Institute of Pharmaceutical Sciences, The Catholic University, Korea, Bucheon 14662, Korea
Life Science R&D Center, SK Chemicals, 310 Pangyoro, Sungnam 13494, Korea

Hunseung Yoo
Life Science R&D Center, SK Chemicals, 310 Pangyoro, Sungnam 13494, Korea

Young-Guk Na, Jin-Ju Byeon, Hyun Wook Huh, Min-Ki Kim, Young G. Shin, Hong-Ki Lee and Cheong-Weon Cho
College of Pharmacy and Institute of Drug Research and Development, Chungnam National University, 99, Daehak-ro, Yuseong-gu, Daejeon 34134, Korea

Milica Markovic, Moran Zur, Inna Ragatsky and Arik Dahan
Department of Clinical Pharmacology, School of Pharmacy, Faculty of Health Sciences, Ben-Gurion University of the Negev, Beer-Sheva 8410501, Israel

Sandra Cvijić
Department of Pharmaceutical Technology and Cosmetology, Faculty of Pharmacy, University of Belgrade, Vojvode Stepe 450, 11221 Belgrade, Serbia

Florian Klomp and Stefan Oswald
Institute of Pharmacology and Toxicology, Rostock University Medical Center, 18057 Rostock, Germany

Christoph Wenzel
Department of Pharmacology, Center of Drug Absorption and Transport, University Medicine Greifswald, 17487 Greifswald, Germany

Marek Drozdzik
Department of Experimental and Clinical Pharmacology, Pomeranian Medical University, 70-111 Szczecin, Poland

Gracia Santos-Díaz and Pedro Dorado
Biosanitary Research Institute of Extremadura (INUBE), University of Extremadura, 06006 Badajoz, Spain

Ana María Pérez-Pico
Department of Nursing, University of Extremadura, 10600 Plasencia, Spain

Miguel Ángel Suárez-Santisteban
Biosanitary Research Institute of Extremadura (INUBE), University of Extremadura, 06006 Badajoz, Spain
Nephrology Department, Virgen del Puerto Hospital, Servicio Extremeño de Salud, 10600 Plasencia, Spain

Vanesa García-Bernalt
Nephrology Department, Virgen del Puerto Hospital, Servicio Extremeño de Salud, 10600 Plasencia, Spain

Raquel Mayordomo
Department of Anatomy, Cellular Biology and Zoology, University of Extremadura, 10600 Plasencia, Spain

Dominique A. Garrison, Zahra Talebi, Eric D. Eisenmann, Alex Sparreboom and Sharyn D. Baker
Division of Pharmaceutics and Pharmacology, College of Pharmacy, The Ohio State University, Columbus, OH 43210, USA

Jung Hwan Ahn, Junhyeong Kim, Naveed Ur Rehman, Hye-Jin Kim, Mi-Jeong Ahn and Hye Jin Chung
College of Pharmacy and Research Institute of Pharmaceutical Sciences, Gyeongsang National University, Jinju 52828, Korea

Index